Vascular Emergencies

Expert Management for the Emergency Physician

Vascular Emergencies

Expert Management for the Emergency Physician

Editor-in-Chief

Robert L. Rogers, MD, FACEP

Associate Professor of Emergency Medicine and Medicine, and Director of the
Medical Education Fellowship, Department of Emergency Medicine,
The University of Maryland School of Medicine, Baltimore, MD, USA

Editor

Thomas Scalea, MD, FACS, FCCM

Francis X. Kelly Professor of Trauma Surgery, Director of Program in Trauma,
Physician-in-Chief, R. Adams Cowley Shock Trauma Center,
The University of Maryland School of Medicine, Baltimore, MD, USA

Associate Editors

Lee Wallis

Professor of Emergency Medicine, University of Cape Town,
Cape Town, South Africa

Heike Geduld

Clinical Head of Education and Training for Emergency Medicine,
Department of Emergency Medicine, University of Cape Town,
Cape Town, South Africa

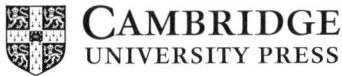
CAMBRIDGE
UNIVERSITY PRESS

CAMBRIDGE UNIVERSITY PRESS
Cambridge, New York, Melbourne, Madrid, Cape Town,
Singapore, São Paulo, Delhi, Mexico City

Cambridge University Press
The Edinburgh Building, Cambridge CB2 8RU, UK

Published in the United States of America by Cambridge
University Press, New York

www.cambridge.org
Information on this title: www.cambridge.org/9781107035027

© Cambridge University Press 2013

First published 2013

Printed and bound in the United Kingdom by the MPG Books
Group

*A catalogue record for this publication is available from the British
Library*

Library of Congress Cataloguing in Publication data
Vascular emergencies: expert management for the emergency
physician / editor-in-chief, Robert L. Rogers ; editor, Thomas
Scalea ; associate editors, Lee Wallis, Heike Geduld.
    p.   ;   cm.
Includes bibliographical references and index.
ISBN 978-1-107-03502-7 (hardback)
I. Rogers, Robert L., 1970–
[DNLM: 1. Vascular Diseases – therapy.   2. Emergencies.
3. Vascular Diseases – diagnosis. WG 500]
616.8′1025 – dc23   2012035055

ISBN 978-1-107-03502-7 Hardback

Contents

Contributors

Majid Afshar, MD, MCR
Division of Pulmonary and Critical Care Medicine, Department of Internal Medicine, The University of Maryland School of Medicine, Baltimore, MD, USA

Leah Bright, DO
Johns Hopkins Medical Institute, Baltimore, MD, USA

Karan Chopra, BS
The University of Maryland School of Medicine, Baltimore, MD, USA

Daan den Hollander, Artsexamen (Amsterdam); M Phil (UKZN); FCS (SA); Trauma Surgery (HPCSA)
Head of Burn Unit and Paediatric Trauma Consultant, Inkosi Albert Luthuli Central Hospital, Honorary Lecturer in Surgery, University of KwaZulu-Natal, Durban, South Africa

James T. DeVries, MD, FACC, FSCAI
Dartmouth Medical School, Hanover, NH, USA

Sharon Dowell
Department of Medicine, Division of Rheumatology, The University of Maryland School of Medicine, Baltimore, MD, USA

Jonathan A. Edlow, MD, FACEP
Vice-chair and Director of Quality, Department of Medicine, Beth Israel Deaconess Medical Center (BIOMC), Professor of Medicine, Harvard Medical School, Boston, MA, USA

John A. Elefteriades, MD
Yale University School of Medicine, New Haven, CT, USA

Brian Euerle, MD, RDMS
Associate Professor, Director of Emergency Ultrasound, Department of Emergency Medicine, The University of Maryland School of Medicine, Baltimore, MD, USA

Christopher M. Fischer, MD
Department of Emergency Medicine, Beth Israel Deaconess Medical Center (BIMOC), Boston, MA, USA

Raymond Flores, MD
Associate Professor, The University of Maryland School of Medicine, Baltimore, MD, USA

Matthew K. Folstein, MD
Resident, Department of Surgery, The University of Maryland School of Medicine, Baltimore, MD, USA

Alisa Gibson, MD, DMD
Department of Emergency Medicine, The University of Maryland School of Medicine, Baltimore, MD, USA

Joshua N. Goldstein, MD, PhD
Assistant Professor, Harvard Medical School, Massachusetts General Hospital, Department of Emergency Medicine, Boston, MA, USA

Kapil Gopal, MD, MBA
Assistant Professor of Surgery, Division of Vascular Surgery, The University of Maryland School of Medicine, Baltimore, MD, USA

Timothy Craig Hardcastle, MB, ChB (Stell); M Med (Chir) (Stell); FCS (SA); Trauma Surgery (HPCSA)
Trauma Surgeon, Deputy Director, Trauma Unit, Inkosi Albert Luthuli Central Hospital, Honorary Senior Lecturer in Surgery and Director of Trauma Sub-specialty Training Program, University of KwaZulu-Natal, Durban, South Africa

Beatrice Hoffmann, MD, PhD
Johns Hopkins Medical Institute, Baltimore, MD, USA

Sam Hsu, MD, RDMS
Assistant Professor, The University of Maryland School of Medicine, Baltimore, MD, USA

Jeffrey Indes, MD
Yale University School of Medicine, New Haven, CT, USA

Akhilesh Jain, MD
Yale University School of Medicine, New Haven, CT, USA

Jonathan Kittredge, MD
Fellow, Division of Vascular Surgery, The University of Maryland School of Medicine, Baltimore, MD, USA

Sa'ad Lahri, MBChB (UCT), FCEM (SA)
Division of Emergency Medicine, UCT and Stellenbosch University, Cape Town, South Africa

Bo E. Madsen, MD, MPH
Beth Israel Deaconess Medical Center (BIDMC), Boston, MA, USA

Selim H. Magdy, MD, PhD
Beth Israel Deaconess Medical Center (BIDMC), Boston, MA, USA

Haney A. Mallemat, MD
Assistant Professor in Emergency Medicine, The University of Maryland School of Medicine, Baltimore, MD, USA

Joseph P. Martinez, MD
Assistant Professor of Emergency Medicine, Assistant Dean for Student Affairs, The University of Maryland School of Medicine, Baltimore, MD, USA

Michael T. McCurdy, MD
Director, Critical Care Consult Service, Program Director, Critical Care Medicine Fellowship, Assistant Professor, Pulmonary and Critical Care Medicine, Assistant Professor, Emergency Medicine, The University of Maryland School of Medicine, Baltimore, MD, USA

Jay Menaker, MD
Associate Professor, Department of Surgery, Department of Emergency Medicine (Secondary), The University of Maryland School of Medicine, Baltimore, MD, USA

Thomas S. Monahan, MD
Assistant Professor of Surgery, The University of Maryland School of Medicine, Division of Vascular Surgery, Department of Surgery, Baltimore, MD, USA

Bart E. Muhs, MD, PhD
Associate Professor of Surgery and Radiology, Yale University School of Medicine, New Haven, CT, USA

Lauren M. Nentwich, MD
Attending, Department of Emergency Medicine, Instructor, Boston University School of Medicine, Boston Medical Center, Boston, MA, USA

Niels K. Rathlev, MD
Professor and Chair, Department of Emergency Medicine, Baystate Medical Center and Tufts University School of Medicine, Springfield, MA, USA

Robert M. Reed, MD
Division of Pulmonary and Critical Care Medicine, The University of Maryland School of Medicine, Baltimore, MD, USA

Jonathan C. Roberts, MD
Department of Emergency Medicine, Beth Israel Deaconess Medical Center, Boston (BIOMC), MA, USA

Joseph C. Schmidt, MD
Department of Emergency Medicine, Baystate Medical Center and Tufts University School of Medicine Springfield, MA, USA

Eugene J. Schweitzer, MD
Professor, Department of Surgery, The University of Maryland School of Medicine, Baltimore, MD, USA

Phillip A. Scott, MD
Department of Emergency Medicine, University of Michigan, Ann Arbor, MI, USA

Nirav G. Shah, MD
Assistant Professor of Medicine, Division of Pulmonary and Critical Care Medicine, Department of Internal Medicine, The University of Maryland School of Medicine, Baltimore, MD, USA

Leann L. Silhan, MD
Division of Pulmonary and Critical Care Medicine, The University of Maryland School of Medicine, Baltimore, MD, USA

David J. Skarupa, MD
Recent Fellow, Surgical Critical Care, R Adams Cowley Shock Trauma Center, Baltimore, MD, USA, Current Assistant Professor of Surgery, Department of Surgery, Division of Trauma and Surgical Critical Care, East Carolina University, Brody School of Medicine, Greenville, NC, USA

Sarah K. Sommerkamp, MD, RDMS
Department of Emergency Medicine, The University of Maryland School of Medicine, Baltimore, MD, USA

Cemal B. Sozener, MD, MEng
Department of Emergency Medicine, University of Michigan, Ann Arbor, MI, USA

Ronald Tesoriero, MD
Assistant Professor, Department of Surgery, The University of Maryland School of Medicine, Baltimore, MD, USA

Kristian A. Ulloa, MD, FACS
Vascular Surgery Associates, Baltimore, MD, USA

Kamil Vallabh, MBBCh(Wits), FCEM(SA)
Specialist Emergency Physician, GF Jooste Hospital, Cape Town, South Africa

Christopher Venter, N Dip (EMC&R) (DUT)
Advanced Life Support Paramedic, VEMA Voluntary Emergency Medical Assistance, Hillcrest, KwaZulu-Natal, Durban, South Africa

George C. Willis, MD
Assistant Professor, Department of Emergency Medicine, The University of Maryland School of Medicine, Baltimore, MD, USA

Samantha L. Wood, MD
Department of Emergency Medicine, The University of Maryland School of Medicine, Baltimore, MD, USA

Samuel Youssef, MD
Yale University School of Medicine, New Haven, CT, USA

Preface

Vascular emergencies are common in the practice of emergency medicine, and emergency care providers will no doubt encounter these entities on a day-to-day basis in the emergency department. Of all of the clinical entities in the house of medicine, vascular emergencies typically are the most time sensitive, and the patients with these conditions tend to be the sickest. Vascular emergencies by their very nature are limb and life threatening, and emergency physicians and other acute care providers should be expert in the care and disposition of this group of patients in order to ensure an optimal outcome. This book, developed by emergency physicians, vascular surgeons, and trauma surgeons who know what it is like to see patients day in and day out, focuses on the acute presentation of vascular emergencies in the emergency department. The overall aim of the book is to provide practical, useful information that will allow for the delivery of excellent medical care.

Most books covering the topic of vascular emergencies are usually aimed at surgeons and tend to focus on in-depth surgical management and other inpatient issues. This book has been written for you – the practicing emergency physician. What you do on a day-to-day basis truly does matter, and it is our hope that this book helps you better care for your patients.

Acknowledgments

I would like to thank my wife, Tricia, and my wonderful children, Harrison and Gabriella, for tolerating me while I put this very important book together. They are my sole inspiration.

To Linda Kesselring, who helped me to organize my cluttered brain and develop a truly wonderful book that is aimed at helping emergency physicians throughout the world.

To our patients, who teach us every day that we still have so much to learn.

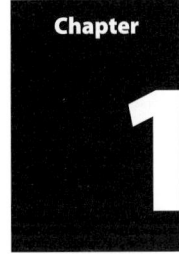

Cerebral venous sinus thrombosis

Jonathan C. Roberts and Christopher M. Fischer

Cerebral venous sinus thrombosis (CVST) is an uncommon cause of stroke. Arterial strokes are much more common. CVST more commonly affects younger adults and children and can be associated with significant rates of morbidity and mortality.

Diagnosing CVST requires a high index of suspicion, as the presenting symptoms can be highly variable and their onset can be subacute. Few large clinical investigations of CVST have been performed; therefore, much controversy and misunderstanding persist surrounding its clinical presentation, diagnosis, and management.

Anatomy

The cerebral venous sinus network, a series of vascular channels suspended within the dura mater, drains cerebrospinal fluid (CSF) and venous blood from the brain into the systemic venous circulation. CSF bathes the central nervous system (CNS) and provides the brain and spinal column with a protective cushion. CSF is produced by the choroid plexus and modified ependymal cells found within the lateral third and fourth ventricles. It flows through a ventricular system into the subarachnoid space, where it eventually passes through arachnoid villi into cerebral venous sinuses. Venous blood also drains from deeper cortical veins into this same sinus system.

The major cerebral venous sinuses are the superior and inferior sagittal sinuses, the straight sinus, the transverse sinuses, the sigmoid sinuses, the cavernous sinuses, and the superior and inferior petrosal sinuses. Disruption of this vascular sinus network can impair venous and CSF outflow, causing hydrocephalus and catastrophic changes in cerebral perfusion pressure, along with possible infarction and hemorrhage.

Pathophysiology

CVST is a rare form of stroke, caused by a blockage of this drainage system. Thrombosis may be confined to the large cerebral venous sinuses or may involve the deeper cortical veins. Isolated thrombosis of a large cerebral venous sinus impairs venous drainage and CSF absorption, which results in an elevation of intracranial pressures. This can cause abrupt alterations in consciousness and impaired vital functions by affecting perfusion of the brainstem. Thrombosis of draining cortical veins results in cytotoxic and vasogenic edema with possible subsequent capillary rupture, hemorrhage, and infarction from impaired perfusion.

If collateral circulation remains intact, patients may present with extremely subtle symptoms and physical examination findings. Thrombus progression to multiple venous sinuses and cortical veins with impaired collateral circulation may cause more focal neurologic signs, seizures, and altered mental status.[1,2]

Epidemiology and risk factors

CVST has an annual incidence of two to four per million[3] and an overall mortality rate approximating 8%.[4] Although the exact incidence is unknown, CVST is thought to account for 1 to 2% of all strokes. While arterial stroke tends to affect older patients, with a slight male predominance,[5] CVST affects predominantly younger patients, with peaks in childhood and in the fourth and fifth decades of life, and with a 3 : 1 female predominance.[4]

There are numerous risk factors for the development of CVST (Table 1.1). Genetic or acquired prothrombotic states are found in more than 85%

Vascular Emergencies, ed. Robert L. Rogers, Thomas Scalea, Lee Wallis, and Heike Geduld. Published by Cambridge University Press. © Cambridge University Press 2013.

Table 1.1 Causes of and risk factors for development of cerebral venous sinus thrombosis

Medications

Oral contraceptives

Genetic prothrombotic tendencies

Factor V Leiden mutation

Protein C and protein S deficiency

Antithrombin deficiency

Prothrombin mutation

Acquired prothrombotic states

Pregnancy and peripartum period

Nephrotic syndrome

Dehydration

Hematologic conditions

Polycythemia

Thrombocytosis

Leukemia

Mechanical causes

Head trauma

Neurosurgical procedures

Lumbar puncture

Infection

Mastoiditis, otitis, sinusitis

Meningitis

Inflammatory disease

Inflammatory bowel disease

Systemic lupus erythematosus

Sarcoidosis

Adapted from Stam.[1]

of patients with CVST.[1,6] Oral contraceptive use is the most commonly identified risk factor for CVST; several case-control studies demonstrated a greater than 10-fold increase in risk among women using those medications.[7,8] Infections, including otitis media and mastoiditis, may also predispose individuals to CVST. Trauma can disrupt the normal vascular channel anatomy and lead to thrombosis. The risk of CVST increases during pregnancy and the immediate postpartum period.[1] Other risk factors include disease processes that induce a prothrombotic state. These include factor V Leiden mutation, protein S and C deficiency, antithrombin III deficiencies, inflammatory bowel disease, and malignancy. Despite extensive evaluation, no clear cause is identified in

approximately 20% of cases. Case reports have described rare associations between CVST and paroxysmal nocturnal hemoglobinuria,[9] heparin-induced thrombocytopenia,[10] and even lumbar puncture.[11]

Clinical presentation

CVST is a very rare form of stroke with variable presentations. The variable nature of the symptoms and the subtle presentation can often delay diagnosis. In one study, investigators found the median delay between symptom onset and diagnosis of CVST was seven days.

History

Headache is the most common presenting symptom of CVST, present in more than 75% of patients. The nature of the headache can be highly variable and is not helpful in distinguishing CVST from other causes of headache. Up to 15% of patients may report sudden onset of a thunderclap headache more typical of subarachnoid hemorrhage.[12] Other neurologic symptoms may be associated with increased intracranial pressure and include dizziness, nausea, and visual disturbances. Focal or generalized seizures may be part of the initial presentation and occur in as many as half of patients.[13] Seizures may be even more common in peripartum women with CVST.[14] Other possible focal neurologic symptoms include focal weakness, sensory deficits, aphasia, and visual field deficits. Coma and stupor may result from dramatic increases in intracranial pressure and are a poor prognostic sign.

CVST can mimic other conditions. The combination of headache, visual disturbances, and papilledema can also be found in idiopathic intracranial hypertension (pseudotumor cerebri). In one study, 10% of 106 patients diagnosed with presumed idiopathic intracranial hypertension were ultimately found to have CVST.[15]

Physical examination

Careful neurologic examination is important to elicit the sometimes subtle findings that can be associated with CVST. Cranial nerve examinations may demonstrate papilledema, nerve palsies, or visual field deficits. Focused neurologic examination may elicit focal weakness or signs that accompany increased intracranial pressure, including gait instability and abnormal reflexes.

Diagnosis

Diagnosing CVST depends on a high index of suspicion and appropriate imaging studies. Imaging may also provide prognostic information for patients with CVST. The extent of venous sinus involvement and the presence of intraparenchymal hemorrhage may correlate with functional outcome.[2]

Non-invasive imaging

Unenhanced brain computed tomography (CT) is useful in identifying secondary signs of CVST, including hemorrhagic infarction, brain edema, mass effect, hydrocephalus, subdural effusion, and subarachnoid hemorrhage. It may also infrequently identify primary signs of CVST, including the dense triangle sign and the cord sign. The dense triangle sign or delta sign represents a hyperintense thrombus within the superior sagittal sinus and may be visible on axial images through the superior sagittal sinus. The cord sign represents a hyperintense thrombus within a deeper cortical vein.[16] However, only 25% of patients with CVST demonstrate these signs on unenhanced brain CT.[17] The most common finding on an unenhanced CT scan is a non-arterial distribution of areas of hemorrhage – this finding represents the venous congestion resulting from venous thrombosis.

Enhanced brain CT has emerged as a possible alternative to magnetic resonance imaging/magnetic resonance venography (MRI/MRV) for non-invasive diagnosis of CVST. Computed tomography venography (CTV) imaging protocols use intravenous contrast to highlight draining cortical and dural venous sinuses and can thus readily identify filling defects. The empty delta sign represents an occlusive thrombus within the venous sinus, which prevents contrast-mediated enhancement, and is found in 30% of patients with known CVST.[17] Disadvantages of CTV include exposure to ionizing radiation, exposure to iodinated contrast, and hyperdense bony artifact requiring digital subtraction techniques for optimal image quality. Many authors suggest that CTV's sensitivity and specificity for identifying CVST are equivalent to those for the more time-consuming magnetic resonance (MR) techniques.

Unenhanced brain MRI is more sensitive than unenhanced brain CT in identifying CVST. Using intravenous contrast and time-of-flight techniques, enhanced brain MRV is able to reliably detect alterations in cerebral venous flow, identifying CVST with an overall sensitivity and specificity similar to those for CTV. In addition, MR techniques may be able to identify deeper cortical vein thrombus more readily than CT.[18]

A proposed CVST management algorithm published by the American Heart Association and the American Stroke Association in 2011 recommends T2-MRI + MRV as the initial diagnostic modality of choice. CT + CTV is the preferred alternative if MR is not readily available or is contraindicated.[18]

Invasive imaging

Cerebral angiography provides detailed images of the deep cortical veins and cerebral venous sinus network. It can serve as an alternative imaging modality when CT and MR prove inconclusive or are unavailable.

Additional diagnostics

Many patients with the symptoms of CVST undergo lumbar puncture during their initial evaluation. The most common finding on lumbar puncture is an elevated opening pressure (>20 cm H_2O), which is found in more than 80% of cases. In addition, the diagnosis of CVST should be entertained if an elevated opening pressure is encountered during the workup of the headache patient. This may very well be the one clue that leads to the diagnosis.

Treatment

Treatment of CVST can involve multiple approaches, including systemic anticoagulation, chemical or mechanical endovascular thrombectomy, and surgical decompression or open clot retrieval.[19]

Few studies have investigated the safety and efficacy of systemic anticoagulation for CVST. Concern that this procedure can precipitate hemorrhage or exacerbate pre-existing hemorrhage in CVST creates barriers to aggressive and effective treatment. This unproven risk of progressive hemorrhage must be weighed against the real risk of withholding anticoagulation and thus promoting venous infarction with hemorrhagic conversion.[20]

Two randomized trials have evaluated systemic anticoagulation in CVST. They were combined in a Cochrane Review meta-analysis,[3] which found a non-significant trend toward reduced death and disability (relative risk [RR] 0.33 and 0.46, respectively) in patients treated with systemic anticoagulation. No cases of spontaneous or progressive hemorrhage were documented.

The best available evidence supporting the safety and efficacy of systemic anticoagulation for CVST is based on observational cohorts of undifferentiated CVST patients (including those with intracerebral hemorrhage).[3] The International Study on Cerebral Vein and Dural Sinus Thrombosis (ISCVT) CVST cohort (624 patients known to have CVST and treated with systemic anticoagulation) demonstrated a non-significant reduction in death and disability (12.7% and 18.3%, respectively). The rates of spontaneous and progressive hemorrhage did not increase.

Additional studies support systemic anticoagulation as a safe and effective therapeutic approach for patients with CVST in the emergency department (ED). However, given the rarity of this condition, all clinical trials conducted thus far are underpowered to establish statistical significance.[19]

Not all patients respond to systemic anticoagulation, so alternative methods to re-establish normal outflow have been explored. Systemic or localized fibrinolysis has been evaluated in small trials and has yielded mixed results. At best, thrombolytics provide a safe and effective alternative for CVST that is resistant to systemic anticoagulation. At worst, they might increase the risk of spontaneous or progressive hemorrhage. A handful of small studies have investigated mechanical thrombectomy as an alternative to systemic or localized chemical thrombolysis. Balloon angioplasty, stenting, clot maceration, and rheolytic thrombectomy are promising alternatives for CVST resistant to systemic anticoagulation and might be associated with reduced rates of hemorrhage compared with chemical thrombolysis. Surgical intervention via intracerebral pressure monitor placement or hemicraniectomy for hematoma evacuation may be indicated for management of elevated intracranial pressure.[19]

Multiple studies have evaluated risk factors for and prognostic implications of early seizures in CVST. A prospective observational study of 194 patients found a threefold increase in the mortality rate among patients with CVST who experienced early seizure.[21] A second prospective observational study found that supratentorial hemorrhage, seizures at the time of presentation, and motor deficits were predictive of subsequent seizure activity and clinical deterioration.[22] The use of antiepileptic drugs may be indicated in this subgroup of CVST patients; however, no studies have demonstrated that their use reduces the morbidity or mortality rate.

Clinical approach when resources are limited

In most cases, CVST can be diagnosed definitively only with the use of advanced imaging modalities, including unenhanced CT, contrast CT, MRI, and magnetic resonance angiography (MRA). When these advanced modalities are not available, the diagnosis might be suspected but cannot be confirmed easily. The diagnosis should be considered in patients with focal neurologic deficits and risk factors for CVST, especially those who are using oral contraceptives or have a genetic predisposition for thrombosis. Close coordination with consulting neurologists, when available, should be part of the management of these patients.

Pearls and pitfalls

- Consider CVST in patients with headache, neurologic findings, and risk factors.
- Consider CVST in patients with a history suggestive of pseudotumor cerebri (idiopathic intracranial hypertension).
- Anticoagulation should be considered in patients with CVST even if there is concurrent hemorrhagic infarction.

Critical actions

- CVST can be associated with subtle symptoms and a subacute onset. Knowledge of the epidemiology and risk factors for CVST can help raise suspicion for this often-overlooked diagnosis.
- Prompt attention to airway, breathing, circulation (ABCs) in patients who present with stupor or coma is essential.
- A thorough neurologic examination is important to elicit findings that indicate CVST (focal weakness, sensory deficits, aphasia, papilledema, visual field deficits).
- Recognition of a non-arterial distribution of hemorrhage, caused by venous congestion, on a brain CT scan suggests the diagnosis and should prompt further investigation and consultation.

- Anticoagulation should be initiated promptly in appropriate patients.
- If a patient does not respond to systemic anticoagulation, more invasive options should be considered.

References

1. Stam J. Thrombosis of the cerebral veins and sinuses. *N Engl J Med* 2005; 352: 1791–8.

2. Zubkov AY, McBane RD, Brown RD, Rabinstein AA. Brain lesions in cerebral venous sinus thrombosis. *Stroke* 2009; 40: 1509–11.

3. Stam J, De Bruijn SF, DeVeber G. Anticoagulation for cerebral sinus thrombosis. *Cochrane Database Syst Rev* 2002; (4): CD002005.

4. Ferro JM, Canhão P, Stam J, *et al.* Prognosis of cerebral vein and dural sinus thrombosis: results of the International Study on Cerebral Vein and Dural Sinus Thrombosis (ISCVT). *Stroke* 2004; 35: 664–70.

5. Rosamond W, Flegal K, Friday G, *et al.* Heart disease and stroke statistics–2007 update: a report from the American Heart Association Statistics Committee and Stroke Statistics Subcommittee. *Circulation* 2007; 115: e69–171.

6. Otrock ZK, Taher AT, Shamseddeen WA, Mahfouz RA. Thrombophilic risk factors among 16 Lebanese patients with cerebral venous and sinus thrombosis. *J Thromb Thrombolysis* 2008; 26: 41–3.

7. De Bruijn SF, Stam J, Koopman MM, Vandenbroucke JP. Case-control study of risk of cerebral sinus thrombosis in oral contraceptive users who are carriers of hereditary prothrombotic conditions. The Cerebral Venous Sinus Thrombosis Study Group. *BMJ* 1998; 316: 589–92.

8. Martinelli I, Bucciarelli P, Passamonti SM, *et al.* Long-term evaluation of the risk of recurrence after cerebral sinus-venous thrombosis. *Circulation* 2010; 121: 2740–6.

9. Misra UK, Kalita J, Bansal V, *et al.* Paroxysmal nocturnal haemoglobinuria presenting as cerebral venous sinus thrombosis. *Transfus Med* 2008; 18: 308–11.

10. Fesler MJ, Creer MH, Richart JM, *et al.* Heparin-induced thrombocytopenia and cerebral venous sinus thrombosis: case report and literature review. *Neurocrit Care* 2011; 15: 161–5.

11. Todorov L, Laurito CE, Schwartz DE. Postural headache in the presence of cerebral venous sinus thrombosis. *Anesth Analg* 2005; 101: 1499–500.

12. Cortez O, Schaeffer CJ, Hatem SF, *et al.* Cases from the Cleveland Clinic: cerebral venous sinus thrombosis presenting to the emergency department with worst headache of life. *Emerg Radiol* 2009; 16: 79–82.

13. Masuhr F, Mehraein S, Einhäupl K. Cerebral venous and sinus thrombosis. *J Neurol* 2004; 251: 11–23.

14. Cantú C, Barinagarrementeria F. Cerebral venous thrombosis associated with pregnancy and puerperium: review of 67 cases. *Stroke* 1993; 24: 1880–4.

15. Lin A, Foroozan R, Danesh-Meyer HV, *et al.* Occurrence of cerebral venous sinus thrombosis in patients with presumed idiopathic intracranial hypertension. *Ophthalmology* 2006; 113: 2281–4.

16. Roland T, Jacobs J, Rappaport A, *et al.* Unenhanced brain CT is useful to decide on further imaging in suspected venous sinus thrombosis. *Clin Radiol* 2010; 65: 34–9.

17. Leach JL, Fortuna RB, Jones BV, *et al.* Imaging of cerebral venous thrombosis: current techniques, spectrum of findings, and diagnostic pitfalls. *Radiographics* 2006; 26(suppl 1): S19–43.

18. Saposnik G, Barinagarrementeria F, Brown RD, *et al.* Diagnosis and management of cerebral venous thrombosis: a statement for healthcare professionals from the American Heart Association/American Stroke Association. *Stroke* 2011; 42: 1158–92.

19. Medel R, Monteith SJ, Crowley RW, *et al.* A review of therapeutic strategies for the management of cerebral venous sinus thrombosis. *Neurosurg Focus* 2009; 27: E6.

20. Stam J, Majoie CBLM, van Delden OM, *et al.* Endovascular thrombectomy and thrombolysis for severe cerebral sinus thrombosis: a prospective study. *Stroke* 2008; 39: 1487–90.

21. Masuhr F, Busch M, Amberger N, *et al.* Risk and predictors of early epileptic seizures in acute cerebral venous and sinus thrombosis. *Eur J Neurol* 2006; 13: 852–6.

22. Ferro JM, Canhão P. Acute treatment of cerebral venous and dural sinus thrombosis. *Curr Treat Options Neurol* 2008; 10: 126–37.

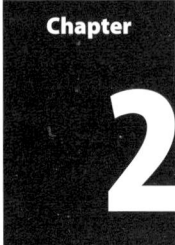

Chapter 2

Acute ischemic stroke

Cemal B. Sozener and Phillip A. Scott

Stroke is the third leading cause of death and the leading cause of disability in the United States. In addition, it is an extremely common condition around the world and has become a global health threat, along with diabetes and heart disease. Ischemic stroke afflicts more than 795,000 Americans each year, 610,000 of whom have a first attack. Stroke accounts for 1 in every 18 deaths in the United States, or just over 130,000 deaths, per year.[1] An additional 200,000 to 500,000 Americans experience transient ischemic attack (TIA). *Stroke* refers to any disease process that alters blood flow to a focal region of the brain. This chapter focuses on ischemic causes, which account for 87% of strokes. Timely diagnosis and appropriate management of acute ischemic stroke (AIS) and TIA can reduce morbidity and mortality rates.

Pathophysiology

Ischemic strokes are generally divided into three major categories: thrombotic, embolic, and hypoperfusion associated (watershed strokes). A substantial portion of strokes (30–40%) defy etiologic categorization and are considered cryptogenic. Vasculitic causes of stroke include Takayasu's arteritis, systemic lupus erythematosus, and polyarteritis nodosa. Hypercoagulable states and arterial dissection may also result in cerebral infarction.

Thrombotic strokes, the most common subtype, are characterized by a narrowing of the vascular lumen, typically as a result of atherosclerotic disease, with subsequent platelet adhesion and local clot formation. Thrombosis occurs most commonly in the internal carotid and the middle cerebral and basilar arteries. Clinically, thrombotic stroke symptoms may wax and wane in severity depending on direct flow as well as collateral circulation to the affected tissue.

Embolic strokes, the second most common subtype, account for approximately 20% of ischemic strokes. They result from the release of material into the vascular lumen, which travels distally to occlude a cerebral vessel. The majority of these emboli are cardiac in origin, either from mural thrombi (arising from untreated cardiac dysrhythmias or myocardial infarction) or valvular abnormalities. Other causes include paradoxic emboli (related to right-to-left shunting in patients with a patent foramen ovale or other septal defect), artery-to-artery embolization (resulting from the migration of proximal clots from atherosclerotic disease in larger vessels), or emboli from fat (fractures) or air (injection, diving). Embolic strokes are typically abrupt in onset and manifest maximal deficits early.

Hypoperfusion-related strokes, the least common type of ischemic stroke, are typically the result of systemic disease from cardiac failure, causing diminished blood flow to watershed regions of the cerebral vasculature. The neurologic symptoms of this type of infarct are more diffuse than those associated with strokes of other cause and correlate with the magnitude of reduction in blood pressure.

Epidemiology

In 2006, more than 6.4 million American adults had a stroke.[1] At younger ages, the incidence of stroke is higher among men than women; this trend is reversed in older age groups. Blacks have a higher incidence than whites, particularly in younger populations. The stroke-related mortality rates in the two racial groups are similar. Mexican Americans have a higher incidence of stroke than non-Hispanic whites.[2] Among patients ≥65 years of age, stroke has a 30-day mortality of 8.1%.[3]

Vascular Emergencies, ed. Robert L. Rogers, Thomas Scalea, Lee Wallis, and Heike Geduld. Published by Cambridge University Press. © Cambridge University Press 2013.

Risk factors for stroke parallel those for cardiovascular disease. The degree and duration of hypertension strongly correlate with stroke risk.[1] Atrial fibrillation leads to a fivefold increase in lifetime stroke risk throughout all age groups.[4,5] Cigarette smoking doubles the lifetime risk. Diabetes increases incidence at all age groups; however, the risk is magnified in blacks younger than 55 and whites younger than 65.[6] Female sex, advancing age, prior TIA, obesity, high cholesterol, pregnancy (particularly the peripartum to six weeks postpartum period), physical inactivity, and sickle cell disease are also independent risk factors.

Recovery following stroke is variable. Approximately 50 to 70% of stroke survivors regain functional independence, but 15 to 30% are permanently disabled. Approximately 20% of survivors require institutional care 90 days after a stroke.[1] In the Framingham Study, residual disabilities included hemiparesis in 50% of patients, aphasia in 18%, difficulty with activities of daily living in 26%, and inability to ambulate without assistance in 30%.[7] Disability is associated with substantial economic costs. In 2010, total direct and indirect costs attributed to ischemic stroke in the United States were estimated at $73.3 billion.[1] The majority of direct medical costs are attributed to rehabilitation and nursing home expenditures.[8]

Worldwide, 15 million people experience stroke annually, and 5.5 million of them die, making stroke the second leading cause of death among people over the age of 60. Although the incidence of stroke is declining in some developed countries secondary to better blood pressure control and decreased rates of smoking, the absolute number of strokes continues to increase because of the aging of the population.[9]

Diagnosis

History

Patients with stroke symptoms require immediate evaluation because diagnosis and treatment are time sensitive. The paramount initial historical element to obtain from either the patient or bystander is the time of the onset of symptoms. This is defined as the time the patient was last at his or her neurologic baseline. Care should be taken in determining this time in patients who wake up with symptoms ("wake-up strokes").

Establishing stroke risk factors may aid in identifying the subtype of ischemic stroke. The presence of comorbid conditions such as hypertension, diabetes mellitus, atherosclerotic disease, sickle cell disease, pregnancy, drug abuse, migraine headache, seizure disorder, trauma, and infection should be determined. Inclusion and exclusion criteria for thrombolytic eligibility are reviewed below.

Stroke syndromes

Common stroke presentations are described here based on the vascular structures that are involved.[10]

Anterior cerebral artery (ACA) syndrome. Patients with this syndrome present with contralateral weakness in the leg greater than the arm, with mild deficits in sensation. They may exhibit slowness of speech or motor actions. Proximal lesions are less symptomatic, owing to collateral flow from the paired anterior communicating artery. Distal lesions tend to produce more severe presentations.

Middle cerebral artery (MCA) syndrome. The MCA is the most common site of ischemic stroke. Occlusion leads to contralateral hemiplegia and hemianesthesia. Symptoms generally affect the face and arm more than the leg. If the dominant hemisphere is involved, aphasia may be encountered. The left hemisphere is dominant in right-handed patients and in approximately 80% of those who are left handed. Proximal lesions create substantial clinical deficits and can result in significant cerebral edema.

Posterior cerebral artery (PCA) syndrome. The PCA supplies blood to the occipital lobe, parts of the temporal lobe, thalamus, upper brainstem, and midbrain. Proximal occlusions lead to minor deficits, as the posterior communicating artery often provides collateral circulation. Distal occlusions lead to complications such as homonymous hemianopsia. Occipital cortex lesions resulting in visual deficits can be difficult to determine unless visual fields are formally tested. Light touch and pinprick sensation may also be reduced.

Vertebrobasilar syndrome. The vertebrobasilar circulation provides blood to the brainstem and cerebellum. Crossed neurologic deficits (e.g., ipsilateral facial weakness with contralateral weakness of the body) are the hallmark of posterior fossa involvement. Physical findings may be subtle and easily attributed to other conditions. Commonly encountered symptoms include vertigo, ataxia, diplopia, dysarthria, and dysphagia.

Cerebellar stroke syndrome. This is a subset of posterior circulation stroke and presents as sudden onset of vertigo and inability to stand. Patients may also complain of associated headache, nausea, vomiting, and cervical pain. Early identification and neurosurgical consultation is critical in order to monitor for potential herniation or brainstem compression due to posterior fossa edema.

Lacunar stroke syndrome. This syndrome results from occlusion of small penetrating arteries, typically due to chronic hypertension. There are five classic lacunar syndromes: hemiparesis (pure motor, most common), ataxic hemiparesis (combines motor and cerebellar symptoms), clumsy hand dysarthria (manifests as hand weakness and clumsiness with dysarthria), pure sensory (persistent or transient unilateral numbness, tingling, pain, or burning), and mixed sensorimotor (hemiparesis or hemiplegia with ipsilateral sensory impairment).

Physical examination

The clinical examination begins with assessment of the airway, breathing, and circulation. The general inspection should evaluate for signs of trauma, particularly of the head and neck. Examination of the oropharyngeal space should include inspection of the tongue for lacerations, which would suggest an alternate cause (seizure). The neck should be examined for the presence of carotid bruit or jugular venous distension. The cardiac examination should screen for tachycardia, irregular rhythm, and murmur. The skin should be examined to identify petechiae suggestive of coagulopathies or platelet dysfunction.

Neurologic examination

The goal of the neurologic examination is to localize the lesion and exclude other disease processes. Review of the entire examination is beyond the scope of this text, but we advocate the use of a formal stroke scale, such as the National Institutes of Health (NIH) Stroke Scale (NIHSS) (Table 2.1), as a component of it. Determining a patient's score can enhance the emergency practitioner's assessment, enhance

Table 2.1 National Institutes of Health Stroke Scale

Tested item	Title	Responses and scores
1A	Level of consciousness	0 – Alert 1 – Drowsy 2 – Obtunded 3 – Coma/unresponsive
1B	Orientation questions (2)	0 – Answers both correctly 1 – Answers one correctly 2 – Answers neither correctly
1C	Response to commands (2)	0 – Performs both tasks correctly 1 – Performs one task correctly 2 – Performs neither
2	Gaze	0 – Normal horizontal movements 1 – Partial gaze palsy 2 – Complete gaze palsy
3	Visual fields	0 – No visual field deficit 1 – Partial hemianopia 2 – Complete hemianopia 3 – Bilateral hemianopia
4	Facial movement	0 – Normal 1 – Minor facial weakness 2 – Partial facial weakness 3 – Complete unilateral palsy
5	Motor function (arm) a. Left b. Right	0 – No drift 1 – Drift before 5 seconds 2 – Falls before 10 seconds 3 – No effort against gravity 4 – No movement
6	Motor function (leg) a. Left b. Right	0 – No drift 1 – Drift before 5 seconds 2 – Falls before 5 seconds 3 – No effort against gravity 4 – No movement
7	Limb ataxia	0 – No ataxia 1 – Ataxia in one limb 2 – Ataxia in two limbs
8	Sensory	0 – No sensory loss 1 – Mild sensory loss 2 – Severe sensory loss
9	Language	0 – Normal 1 – Mild aphasia 2 – Severe aphasia 3 – Mute or global aphasia
10	Articulation	0 – Normal 1 – Mild dysarthria 2 – Severe dysarthria
11	Extinction or inattention	0 – Absent 1 – Mild (loss of one sensory modality) 2 – Severe (loss of two modalities)

communication with consultants, and allow quantifications of changes in the patient's condition. In addition to its good reproducibility over serial examinations, the NIHSS has been shown to correlate with subsequent infarct volume. Caution is warranted because the NIHSS favors evaluation of the anterior circulation and can miss subtle posterior circulation stroke syndromes.

The station and gait portion of the neurologic examination is frequently not obtained or documented in the emergency department, but it can greatly assist in the difficult stroke diagnosis. Because station and gait are a culmination of motor, sensory, and central integration, subtle asymmetries and signs of stroke can be magnified with this part of the physical examination.

Laboratory tests to obtain in the emergency department

The following blood tests should be obtained rapidly upon the patient's arrival: blood glucose level (preferably a rapid, point-of-care test), complete blood count with platelets (CBCP), electrolytes, renal function, prothrombin time (PT), activated partial thromboplastin time (aPTT), international normalized ratio (INR), and type and screen.[11] Measuring cardiac ischemia markers can be useful, because cardiac disease is prevalent in these patients. Depending on the context, consider hepatic function tests (if coagulopathy related to liver disease is suspected), toxicology screening (for possible sympathomimetic abuse), measurement of the blood alcohol level, a pregnancy test, and arterial blood gas measurement (if altered mental status is suspected as a result of hypoxia or hypercarbia). Having a predetermined panel of tests speeds the process.

Imaging in the emergency department

A non-contrast computed tomography (CT) scan of the brain should be performed early during the evaluation. The CT scan assists in differentiating hemorrhagic and ischemic stroke. Typically, in patients with ischemic stroke less than six hours old, no acute changes are identified on CT imaging. For stroke patients who might be eligible for reperfusion therapies, the goals are to obtain CT imaging within 25 minutes after arrival in the emergency department (ED) and to interpret the study within 45 minutes.[12] Some hospitals have the capability to perform advanced neuroimaging using magnetic resonance imaging (MRI) sequences, CT perfusion, and CT angiography (CTA). These studies, however, should not be obtained at the expense of early initiation of thrombolytic therapy in eligible patients unless they are required because of diagnostic uncertainty or other clinical indications. MRI is superior to CT in the assessment of stroke patients; if it can be performed and interpreted as rapidly as CT, it is preferred.

Pearls and pitfalls related to specific presentations

Young adults (age < 50) with stroke

In young adults, consider the possibility of arterial dissection, sympathomimetic or injection drug use, a cardioembolic event (or paradoxic embolism via a patent foramen ovale), and air emboli as potential causes of the stroke.

Uncooperative patients

In uncooperative patients, particularly in the elderly, consider the possibility of a non-dominant hemisphere stroke or other stroke syndrome as the cause of the behavior, especially if the change is abrupt. A thorough history and physical examination will aid in the diagnosis of a stroke.

Patients with vertigo and vomiting

Consider posterior circulation infarcts in patients presenting with vertigo and nausea or vomiting. Early identification of a cerebellar stroke and neurosurgical consultation for possible decompressive surgery may be life-saving.

Emergency department management

Prehospital care/triage

Between 29% and 65% of patients with signs or symptoms of acute stroke access the medical system via emergency medical services (EMS) systems.[11] When prehospital care personnel notify the receiving facility that a potential stroke patient is en route, the time from symptom onset to physician evaluation can be reduced, as is the time to diagnostic imaging; therefore, evaluation of the patient for eligibility for thrombolytic treatment is facilitated.[13–21] Successful hospital systems use a multidisciplinary approach for the identification and treatment of patients with AIS.

First 15 minutes

Patients with acute stroke symptoms should be evaluated similarly to those with other time-sensitive conditions, such as myocardial infarction or trauma. Critical pathways for stroke patients should be in place and utilized for urgent evaluation of these patients.

Initial assessment

The emergency physician should obtain a quick, but thorough, history and physical examination. Critical pathway order sets should be initiated for intravenous (IV) line placement, with blood being sent for testing as previously described, a 12-lead electrocardiogram (ECG), and an emergent non-contrast head CT scan. If CT imaging is unavailable, arrangements should be made to transfer the patient immediately to a facility with that capability. If a stroke team is available, it should be contacted at the earliest possible opportunity.

The last time the patient was known to be normal must be established rapidly in order to identify patients who are eligible for reperfusion therapy. This information might be available from family members, caregivers, or EMS personnel. Context clues such as what television show was playing at the time of symptom onset can be particularly helpful in establishing onset time. Thrombolytic therapy is not indicated if a reliable time of symptom onset cannot be determined.

Critical actions

- Rapid evaluation of the suspected stroke patient.
- Initiation of an acute stroke care pathway.
- Quick, but thorough, history and physical examination, with special attention to time of onset of stroke symptoms (last time the patient was known to be normal).
    - Application of a formal stroke scale such as the NIHSS.
    - Stroke team activation, if available.
- Placement of IV line, with blood drawn and sent to the lab.

Table 2.2 Differential diagnosis of stroke

Condition	Specific causes
Metabolic	Hyperglycemia/hypoglycemia Hyponatremia Hepatic encephalopathy
Toxicologic	Lithium, phenytoin, alcohol intoxication, Wernicke's encephalopathy
Vascular	Polyarteritis nodosa, systemic lupus erythematosus, Takayasu's arteritis, hypertensive encephalopathy, arterial dissection, cerebral venous sinus thrombosis
Idiopathic	Meniere's disease
Central nervous system	Trauma (subdural/epidural hematoma) Seizure with post-ictal (Todd's) paralysis Migraine Mass lesion Multiple sclerosis Bell's palsy
Psychiatric	Factitious disorders Conversion disorder Functional hemiparesis
Miscellaneous	Positional vertigo, syncope

- Glucose determination.
- CBCP, basic metabolic panel.
- Coagulation profile (PT, INR, aPTT).
- Type and screen.
- Twelve-lead ECG.
- Initiation of an emergent head CT scan, with notification to radiologist that images will need to be rapidly interpreted.

Differential diagnosis

Specific causes of stroke are presented in Table 2.2.

Treatment

General management

Patients with low oxygen saturation levels should receive oxygen by nasal cannula unless airway protection becomes an issue necessitating emergent treatment. If appropriate, the head of the patient's bed should be elevated to 30°. Intravenous fluids should be used judiciously. Fever leads to a worse neurologic outcome, so it should be treated and the source identified.[22–27] The patient should be maintained on a cardiorespiratory monitor.

Table 2.3 Management of hypertension in AIS patients potentially eligible for recombinant tissue-type plasminogen activator (rtPA)

Patients otherwise eligible for acute reperfusion therapy except that blood pressure (BP) is > 185/110 mmHg:

- labetalol, 10–20 mg IV, over 1–2 minutes, may repeat ×1, or
- nicardipine IV, 5 mg/h, titrate up by 2.5 mg/h every 5–15 minutes, maximum 15 mg/h; when desired BP is reached, lower to 3 mg/h, or
- consider other agents (e.g., hydralazine, enalaprilat) when appropriate.

If BP is not maintained at or below 185/110 mmHg, do not administer rtPA.

Management of BP during and after rtPA or other acute reperfusion therapy:

- monitor BP every 15 minutes for 2 hours from the start of rtPA therapy, then every 30 minutes for 6 hours, and then every hour for 16 hours.

If systolic BP is 180–230 mmHg or diastolic BP is 105–120 mmHg:

- labetalol, 10 mg IV, followed by continuous IV infusion, 2–8 mg/min, or
- nicardipine IV, 5 mg/h, titrate to desired effect by 2.5 mg/h every 5–15 minutes; maximum, 15 mg/h.

If BP is not controlled or diastolic BP is > 140 mmHg, consider sodium nitroprusside.

Blood pressure

During the first few hours after stroke, blood pressure is elevated (systolic > 160 mmHg) in 60% of patients.[11] In AIS, it is appropriate to allow permissive hypertension unless the blood pressure elevation is severe (systolic > 220 mmHg or diastolic > 120 mmHg). Abruptly lowering the blood pressure may reduce blood flow to the ischemic penumbra, causing neurologic worsening. If antihypertensive agents are indicated, careful management is warranted, with a goal of no more than a 15 to 25% drop in blood pressure during the first day of treatment. Easily titratable parenteral agents such as labetalol and nicardipine are preferred. Sublingual calcium channel blockers are contraindicated because they can induce rapid and prolonged drops in blood pressure.[28]

Patients eligible for thrombolytic therapy must have a systolic blood pressure < 185 mmHg and a diastolic pressure < 110 mmHg. Antihypertensives are indicated to decrease blood pressure prior to thrombolytic use (Table 2.3). If the blood pressure remains > 185 / 110 mmHg despite treatment, thrombolytic treatment is contraindicated.

Persistent hypotension in AIS, though rare, is associated with poor outcome.[29] The cause of hypotension should be determined and corrected. Volume should be replaced and arrhythmias corrected if applicable; the patient should be flat in the bed. Vasopressor agents may be required for persistent hypotension (< 110 / 70 mmHg).

Glycemic monitoring

Hypoglycemia should be corrected, because it could be the cause of the patient's neurologic deficits. Data suggest that persistent hyperglycemia during the first 24 hours after ischemic stroke independently predicts expansion of stroke volume and leads to worse neurologic outcome.[30] Although there currently is no evidence to indicate a benefit of tight glycemic control in the ED, the level should be monitored in the inpatient setting.

Reperfusion therapies

Intravenous rtPA (Activase® [alteplase])

Intravenous thrombolytic therapy using recombinant tissue-type plasminogen activator (rtPA) for the treatment of AIS was approved by the US Food and Drug Administration (FDA) in 1996 and subsequently by similar regulatory bodies in Canada (1999) and the European Union (2002). These approvals were based on data from the National Institutes of Neurological Disorders and Stroke rtPA Stroke Study, in which 624 patients with AIS were treated with placebo or rtPA within three hours after symptom onset. The trial assessed four neurologic scales, 90 days post-stroke. All of them favored treatment. The primary outcome (a global statistic combining all scales) found treated patients were at least 30% more likely to have a favorable outcome compared with those who received placebo.[31] A similar benefit was identified one year post-stroke as well.[32] Benefit was found regardless of stroke subtype or severity.

The major risk of treatment was symptomatic intracerebral hemorrhage (ICH), which occurred in 6.4% of rtPA-treated patients versus 0.6% in the placebo group. Even with the increased hemorrhage rate, the mortality rates between the two groups were similar at both three-month (17% rtPA group, 21% placebo group) and one-year (24% rtPA group, 28% placebo group) follow-up.[31,32]

Data indicate greater likelihood of benefit if treatment is initiated earlier after the onset of symptoms. A 2008 randomized, placebo-controlled

Table 2.4 Inclusion and exclusion criteria for use of rtPA in AIS within three hours after onset

Inclusion criteria:

- diagnosis of ischemic stroke causing measurable neurologic deficit;
- onset of symptoms less than 3 hours before beginning treatment;
- age $\geq$ 18 years.

Exclusion criteria:

- head trauma or stroke in the previous 3 months;
- symptoms suggest subarachnoid hemorrhage;
- arterial puncture at non-compressible site in the previous 7 days;
- history of intracranial hemorrhage;
- elevated blood pressure (systolic > 185 mmHg or diastolic > 110 mmHg);
- evidence of active bleeding on examination;
- acute bleeding diathesis, including but not limited to:
  - platelet count < 100,000 / mm^3;
  - heparin received within 48 hours, resulting in aPTT > upper limit of normal;
  - current use of anticoagulant, with INR > 1.7 or PT > 15 seconds;
- blood glucose concentration < 50 mg/dL (2.7 mmol/L);
- CT demonstrates multilobar infarction (hypodensity or more than one-third of the cerebral hemisphere).

Relative exclusion criteria

Experience suggests that under some circumstances – with careful consideration and weighing of risk to benefit – patients may receive fibrinolytic therapy despite one or more relative contraindications. Consider risk to benefit of rtPA administration carefully if any of these relative contraindications is present:

- only minor or rapidly improving stroke symptoms (clearing spontaneously);
- seizure at onset with post-ictal residual neurologic impairments;
- major surgery or serious trauma within the previous 14 days;
- recent gastrointestinal or urinary tract hemorrhage (within the previous 21 days);
- recent acute myocardial infarction (within the previous 3 months).

Table 2.5 Additional inclusion and exclusion criteria for use of rtPA in AIS within 3 to 4.5 hours after onset

Inclusion criteria:

- diagnosis of ischemic stroke causing measurable neurologic deficit;
- onset of symptoms 3 to 4.5 hours before beginning treatment.

Exclusion criteria:

- age > 80 years;
- severe stroke (NIHSS > 25);
- taking an oral anticoagulant regardless of INR;
- history of both diabetes and prior ischemic stroke.

Notes

- The checklist includes some FDA-approved indications and contraindications for administration of rtPA for AIS. Recent guideline revisions modified the original FDA criteria. A physician with expertise in acute stroke care can modify this list.
- Onset time is either witnessed or last known normal.
- In patients without recent use of oral anticoagulants or heparin, treatment with rtPA can be initiated before availability of coagulation study results but should be discontinued if INR is greater than 1.7 or PT is elevated by local laboratory standards.
- In patients without a history of thrombocytopenia, treatment with rtPA can be initiated before the platelet count is known but should be discontinued if the platelet count is less than 100,000/mm^3.

study (European Cooperative Acute Stroke Study [ECASS-3]) demonstrated improved clinical outcome in selected stroke patients treated with the standard National Institute of Neurological Disorders and Stroke (NINDS) dose 3 to 4.5 hours after onset. The benefit, while superior to placebo, was smaller than that achieved with earlier treatment in the NINDS trial.[33,34] This underscores that, within any time window, earlier treatment results in better outcomes. ECASS-3 used similar inclusion and exclusion criteria to the NINDS trial (Table 2.4), with the additional exclusions found in Table 2.5.

Other randomized controlled trials testing different intravenous thrombolytic drugs (streptokinase), dosing regimens (cardiac dosing), time windows (six hours), and patient populations (inclusion of

hypertensive patients) have failed to identify additional clinical scenarios in which treatment was successful beyond those presented above. A full discussion of the individual merits and limitations of these studies is beyond the scope of this chapter, so the reader is referred to the source documents.[33,35–39]

In summary, broad regulatory approval for the use of intravenous rtPA in AIS exists for patients treated within three hours of symptom onset. Furthermore, its use as long as 4.5 hours after stroke in select patients is supported by data from ECASS-3 and a science advisory statement from the American Stroke Association.[34]

Intravenous rtPA (Activase® [alteplase]) administration

The total dose of rtPA for the treatment of AIS is 0.9 mg/kg IV, with a maximum dose of 90 mg. Ten percent of the dose is given as a bolus, and the remainder is infused intravenously over 60 minutes. Care should be taken not to administer cardiac doses of rtPA. Tables 2.4 and 2.5 contain the inclusion and exclusion criteria for selection of appropriate patients for treatment.

Patients should be monitored closely for alterations in neurologic status and blood pressure after administration. Blood pressure should be measured and neurologic checks performed every 15 minutes for the first two hours after rtPA administration.

Intra-arterial thrombolytic therapy

Administration of thrombolytic drugs through an intra-arterial (IA) approach delivers higher drug concentrations directly to the thrombus surface, theoretically improving clot dissolution. Controlled trials investigating this approach have yielded mixed results. Current recommendations describe IA thrombolytic therapy as an option for treatment within six hours after symptom onset.[40] Eligible patients are generally characterized as having a major stroke due to occlusion of the MCA and/or not being eligible for treatment with intravenous (systemic) therapy. Treatment should be performed at an experienced stroke center with readily available cerebral angiography and intervention personnel.

Endovascular interventions

There is active investigation into benefits of many endovascular therapies for the treatment of AIS, including angioplasty and stenting, mechanical clot disruption, and clot extraction. In the Mechanical Embolus Removal in Cerebral Embolism (MERCI) Trial, thrombi were successfully removed from intracranial vessels in 45% of patients within eight hours after symptom onset.[41] The FDA subsequently approved the MERCI device for the re-establishment of cerebral blood flow; however, its clinical efficacy has not been established in randomized controlled trials. Current recommendations state that, while the MERCI device may be useful at extracting intra-arterial thrombi in appropriately selected patients, its utility in improving outcomes after stroke remains unclear.[40] The usefulness of other endovascular devices is not yet established, but they might be beneficial in specific circumstances.[40] Use of these devices should be limited to comprehensive stroke centers with the appropriate personnel and resources.[11] The availability of IA thrombolytic or endovascular treatment should not preclude administration of intravenous rtPA in the otherwise eligible patient.[11,40]

First few hours

Patients with AIS are at risk for neurologic deterioration and require close monitoring while in the ED.

They should be kept NPO (nothing by mouth) to prevent aspiration until a swallowing assessment can be completed. After the assessment, patients who are not eligible for thrombolysis should receive aspirin.[11] Standard precautions to prevent decubitus ulcers are indicated, particularly in hemiplegic patients.

In patients not eligible for thrombolytic therapy, permissive hypertension is recommended unless other comorbidities or acute processes require tight blood pressure control (e.g., acute myocardial infarction, congestive heart failure, aortic dissection).[12]

For patients recently treated with rtPA, any deterioration of neurologic status should prompt an emergent head CT scan to evaluate for ICH. Similarly, any sudden increase in blood pressure should trigger a search for painful stimulus, including urinary retention or ICH. If ICH is suspected or confirmed, both neurosurgical and hematologic consultations should be requested to determine the optimum management approach. Cryoprecipitate and/or fresh frozen plasma and platelets should be requested.

In rtPA-treated patients, hypertension is a significant risk factor for ICH.[42] Blood pressure should be checked every 15 minutes for 2 hours after administration of rtPA, every 30 minutes for the subsequent 6 hours, and hourly afterward for the first 24 hours. Systolic blood pressure (SBP) > 180 mmHg and diastolic blood pressure (DBP) > 105 mmHg should be treated aggressively using labetalol, nicardipine, or nitroprusside (Table 2.3).[12]

Admission/level of care

Ideally, thrombolytic-treated patients and those with cerebellar infarctions or large deficits should be admitted to either a stroke unit or an intensive care unit for close monitoring. Patients with stroke can be admitted to general inpatient beds, but admission to special areas providing stroke care provides long-term benefits comparable to the use of thrombolytics.[12]

Inpatient care

Ideally, admission to the hospital for AIS patients will achieve many goals: (1) observation for changes in clinical condition requiring further medical or surgical interventions, (2) monitoring and providing treatment to reduce the chance of bleeding following rtPA administration, (3) facilitation of medical and surgical measures that can improve outcomes after stroke, (4) prevention of subacute complications, (5) planning for and initiating long-term therapies to prevent recurrent stroke, and (6) beginning efforts to restore neurologic function through rehabilitation and supportive care.[11] Approximately 25% of patients with AIS have deterioration in neurologic status in the first 24 to 48 hours.[11,43] This may result from infarct progression or complications from comorbid conditions or treatment. The most serious neurologic complications are those resulting from mass effect secondary to post-infarct edema or hemorrhage.

Disposition

In a recent large study of patients admitted with stroke, 46% went home at discharge, 21% went to rehabilitation, 20% went to a skilled nursing facility, 4% went to a hospice, and 6% were deceased. This underscores the substantial personal and societal toll of ischemic stroke.[44]

Clinical approach when resources are limited

Treatment of AIS in some emergency centers may be limited secondary to lack of resources, particularly imaging modalities such as CT. In this setting, history and physical examination skills are paramount in the detection of stroke. If a patient is a thrombolytic or intervention candidate, arrangements for transfer to a higher level of care should be made quickly. Clinical distinction between ischemic and hemorrhagic stroke is not accurate; treatment with IV rtPA is contraindicated without neuroimaging to rule out hemorrhage.

In areas of the world where reperfusion treatment of AIS is not possible because of a lack of diagnostic or therapeutic resources, attention should focus on public health strategies of diet, lifestyle, and risk factor modification (hypertension, tobacco use, glucose control in diabetics) in an attempt to prevent AIS. Aspirin is also an effective and inexpensive method to reduce the likelihood of subsequent strokes. Estimates suggest that, with improved treatment of hypertension, stroke risk can be decreased 40% worldwide.[9]

Transient ischemic attacks

Transient ischemic attacks are brief episodes of neurologic dysfunction caused by brief focal cerebral ischemia. In the past, TIAs were defined as neurologic deficits resolving within 24 hours after symptom onset. More recently, this definition has come

Table 2.6 Determining ABCD^2 score and stroke risk

Criteria	Score (points)
Age $\geq$ 60 years	1
Blood pressure $\geq$ 140/90 mmHg on first evaluation	1
Clinical symptoms of focal weakness with the spell	2
Speech impairment without weakness	1
Duration $\geq$ 60 minutes	2
Duration 10–59 minutes	1
Total score (points)	**Two-day stroke risk**
0 or 1	0%
2 or 3	1.3%
4 or 5	4.1%
6 or 7	8.1%

Source: Johnston *et al.*[54]

under scrutiny, as 30 to 50% of patients experiencing TIA were found to have MRI evidence of brain infarction.[45] A revised definition of TIA is "a transient episode of neurologic dysfunction caused by focal brain, spinal cord, or retinal ischemia, without acute infarction."[45] The typical duration of TIAs is less than one to two hours, with occasional prolonged episodes.[45]

The diagnosis of TIA is important because of the high risk of subsequent ischemic stroke. Several studies have shown that the short-term risk of stroke in patients with TIA exceeds 10% within 90 days, with up to 50% of these strokes occurring in the first two days.[46–53] Formal prediction rules have been developed to determine the short-term risk of stroke following TIA. The ABCD^2 scores patients with TIA on multiple risk factors to predict the risk of stroke (Table 2.6).[54]

The evaluation of TIA is similar to that of AIS. Current guidelines recommend neuroimaging within 24 hours after symptom onset. Although MRI is preferred in the evaluation of TIA, CT imaging should be performed if MRI is unavailable. Imaging studies of the cervicocephalic vessels utilizing Doppler ultrasound, magnetic resonance angiography (MRA), or CTA are routinely indicated.[45] Transthoracic or transesophageal echocardiography may be needed in some patients.

There is no current consensus for admission versus "discharge with close outpatient evaluation" for patients diagnosed with TIA. The American Heart

Association's 2009 guidelines state that it is reasonable to hospitalize patients with TIA if they present within 72 hours after their event with an $ABCD^2$ score ≥ 3, have an $ABCD^2$ score of 0 to 2 and uncertainty that the diagnostic workup can be completed as an outpatient within two days, or an $ABCD^2$ score 0 to 2 and other evidence that indicates that the event was caused by focal ischemia.[45] Importantly, validation of the $ABCD^2$ rule had been inconsistent.

Patients with non-cardioembolic TIA should be started on antiplatelet therapy. Aspirin (50–325 mg/day), combination aspirin/extended-release dipyridamole, and clopidogrel are all reasonable first-line therapies. Aspirin combined with clopidogrel increases hemorrhage risk and is not routinely recommended.[55,56] Patients with TIA secondary to a cardioembolic source may require anticoagulation. A specific regimen should be selected with specialty consultation.

Conclusion

Stroke and TIA are medical conditions that, without treatment, carry substantial rates of morbidity and mortality. Efforts should be made to improve care through rapid and accurate diagnosis. Early identification of AIS allows early intervention and thus decreases the likelihood and severity of neurologic consequences. Prehospital, emergency department, and inpatient resources should be mobilized quickly to provide treatment with proven benefit to patients and thus maximize recovery from ischemic stroke.

References

1. Lloyd-Jones D, Adams RJ, Brown TM, et al. Heart disease and stroke statistics–2010 update: a report from the American Heart Association. *Circulation* 2010; 121(7): e46–215.

2. Morgenstern LB, Smith MA, Lisabeth LD, et al. Excess stroke in Mexican Americans compared with non-Hispanic Whites: the Brain Attack Surveillance in Corpus Christi Project. *Am J Epidemiol* 2004; 160(4): 376–83.

3. El-Saed A, Kuller LH, Newman AB, et al. Geographic variations in stroke incidence and mortality among older populations in four US communities. *Stroke* 2006; 37(8): 1975–9.

4. Wolf PA, Abbott RD, Kannel WB. Atrial fibrillation as an independent risk factor for stroke: the Framingham Study. *Stroke* 1991; 22(8): 983–8.

5. Wang TJ, Massaro JM, Levy D, et al. A risk score for predicting stroke or death in individuals with new-onset atrial fibrillation in the community: the Framingham Heart Study. *JAMA* 2003; 290(8): 1049–56.

6. Kissela BM, Khoury J, Kleindorfer D, et al. Epidemiology of ischemic stroke in patients with diabetes: the greater Cincinnati/Northern Kentucky Stroke Study. *Diabetes Care* 2005; 28(2): 355–9.

7. Kelly-Hayes M. The influence of gender and age on disability following ischemic stroke: the Framingham Study. *J Stroke Cerebrovasc Dis* 2003; 12(3): 119–26.

8. Fagan SC, Morgenstern LB, Petitta A, et al. Cost-effectiveness of tissue plasminogen activator for acute ischemic stroke. NINDS rt-PA Stroke Study Group. *Neurology* 1998; 50(4): 883–90.

9. Mackay J, Mensah GA, Mendis S, Greenlund K, World Health Organization. *The Atlas of Heart Disease and Stroke*. Geneva: World Health Organization; 2004.

10. Gavrilescu T, Kase CS. Clinical stroke syndromes: clinical-anatomical correlations. *Cerebrovasc Brain Metab Rev* 1995; 7(3): 218–39.

11. Adams HP Jr, del Zoppo G, Alberts MJ, et al. Guidelines for the early management of adults with ischemic stroke: a guideline from the American Heart Association/American Stroke Association Stroke Council, Clinical Cardiology Council, Cardiovascular Radiology and Intervention Council, and the Atherosclerotic Peripheral Vascular Disease and Quality of Care Outcomes in Research Interdisciplinary Working Groups: The American Academy of Neurology affirms the value of this guideline as an educational tool for neurologists. *Circulation* 2007; 115(20): e478–534.

12. Jauch EC, Cucchiara B, Adeoye O, et al. Part 11: adult stroke: 2010 American Heart Association Guidelines for Cardiopulmonary Resuscitation and Emergency Cardiovascular Care. *Circulation* 2010; 122(18 suppl 3): S818–28.

13. Morris DL, Rosamond WD, Hinn AR, Gorton RA. Time delays in accessing stroke care in the emergency department. *Acad Emerg Med* 1999; 6(3): 218–23.

14. Porteous GH, Corry MD, Smith WS. Emergency medical services dispatcher identification of stroke and transient ischemic attack. *Prehosp Emerg Care* 1999; 3(3): 211–16.

15. Morris DL, Rosamond W, Madden K, Schultz C, Hamilton S. Prehospital and emergency department delays after acute stroke: the Genentech Stroke Presentation Survey. *Stroke* 2000; 31(11): 2585–90.

16. Schroeder EB, Rosamond WD, Morris DL, Evenson KR, Hinn AR. Determinants of use of emergency

medical services in a population with stroke symptoms: the Second Delay in Accessing Stroke Healthcare (DASH II) Study. *Stroke* 2000; 31(11): 2591–6.

17. Wein TH, Staub L, Felberg R, *et al.* Activation of emergency medical services for acute stroke in a nonurban population: the T.L.L. Temple Foundation Stroke Project. *Stroke* 2000; 31(8): 1925–8.

18. Williams JE, Rosamond WD, Morris DL. Stroke symptom attribution and time to emergency department arrival: the Delay in Accessing Stroke Healthcare Study. *Acad Emerg Med* 2000; 7(1): 93–6.

19. Lacy CR, Suh DC, Bueno M, Kostis JB. Delay in presentation and evaluation for acute stroke: Stroke Time Registry for Outcomes Knowledge and Epidemiology (S.T.R.O.K.E.). *Stroke* 2001; 32(1): 63–9.

20. Handschu R, Poppe R, Rauss J, Neundorfer B, Erbguth F. Emergency calls in acute stroke. *Stroke* 2003; 34(4): 1005–9.

21. Rossnagel K, Jungehulsing GJ, Nolte CH, *et al.* Out-of-hospital delays in patients with acute stroke. *Ann Emerg Med* 2004; 44(5): 476–83.

22. Castillo J, Davalos A, Marrugat J, Noya M. Timing for fever-related brain damage in acute ischemic stroke. *Stroke* 1998; 29(12): 2455–60.

23. Ginsberg MD, Busto R. Combating hyperthermia in acute stroke: a significant clinical concern. *Stroke* 1998; 29(2): 529–34.

24. Hajat C, Hajat S, Sharma P. Effects of poststroke pyrexia on stroke outcome: a meta-analysis of studies in patients. *Stroke* 2000; 31(2): 410–14.

25. Wang Y, Lim LL, Levi C, Heller RF, Fisher J. Influence of admission body temperature on stroke mortality. *Stroke* 2000; 31(2): 404–9.

26. Kammersgaard LP, Jorgensen HS, Rungby JA, *et al.* Admission body temperature predicts long-term mortality after acute stroke: the Copenhagen Stroke Study. *Stroke* 2002; 33(7): 1759–62.

27. Zaremba J. Hyperthermia in ischemic stroke. *Med Sci Monit* 2004; 10(6): RA148–53.

28. Grossman E, Messerli FH, Grodzicki T, Kowey P. Should a moratorium be placed on sublingual nifedipine capsules given for hypertensive emergencies and pseudoemergencies? *JAMA* 1996; 276(16): 1328–31.

29. Leonardi-Bee J, Bath PM, Phillips SJ, Sandercock PA. Blood pressure and clinical outcomes in the International Stroke Trial. *Stroke* 2002; 33(5): 1315–20.

30. Baird TA, Parsons MW, Phanh T, *et al.* Persistent poststroke hyperglycemia is independently associated

with infarct expansion and worse clinical outcome. *Stroke* 2003; 34(9): 2208–14.

31. Tissue plasminogen activator for acute ischemic stroke. The National Institute of Neurological Disorders and Stroke rt-PA Stroke Study Group. *N Engl J Med* 1995; 333(24): 1581–7.

32. Kwiatkowski TG, Libman RB, Frankel M, *et al.* Effects of tissue plasminogen activator for acute ischemic stroke at one year. National Institute of Neurological Disorders and Stroke Recombinant Tissue Plasminogen Activator Stroke Study Group. *N Engl J Med* 1999; 340(23): 1781–7.

33. Hacke W, Kaste M, Bluhmki E, *et al.* Thrombolysis with alteplase 3 to 4.5 hours after acute ischemic stroke. *N Engl J Med* 2008; 359(13): 1317–29.

34. Del Zoppo GJ, Saver JL, Jauch EC, Adams HP Jr. Expansion of the time window for treatment of acute ischemic stroke with intravenous tissue plasminogen activator: a science advisory from the American Heart Association/American Stroke Association. *Stroke* 2009; 40(8): 2945–8.

35. Randomised controlled trial of streptokinase, aspirin, and combination of both in treatment of acute ischaemic stroke. Multicentre Acute Stroke Trial–Italy (MAST-I) Group. *Lancet* 1995; 346(8989): 1509–14.

36. Hacke W, Kaste M, Fieschi C, *et al.* Intravenous thrombolysis with recombinant tissue plasminogen activator for acute hemispheric stroke. The European Cooperative Acute Stroke Study (ECASS). *JAMA* 1995; 274(13): 1017–25.

37. Donnan GA, Davis SM, Chambers BR, *et al.* Streptokinase for acute ischemic stroke with relationship to time of administration: Australian Streptokinase (ASK) Trial Study Group. *JAMA* 1996; 276(12): 961–6.

38. Hacke W, Kaste M, Fieschi C, *et al.* Randomised double-blind placebo-controlled trial of thrombolytic therapy with intravenous alteplase in acute ischaemic stroke (ECASS II). Second European-Australasian Acute Stroke Study Investigators. *Lancet* 1998; 352(9136): 1245–51.

39. Jaillard A, Cornu C, Durieux A, *et al.* Hemorrhagic transformation in acute ischemic stroke. The MAST-E Study. MAST-E Group. *Stroke* 1999; 30(7): 1326–32.

40. Meyers PM, Schumacher HC, Higashida RT, *et al.* Indications for the performance of intracranial endovascular neurointerventional procedures: a scientific statement from the American Heart Association Council on Cardiovascular Radiology and Intervention, Stroke Council, Council on Cardiovascular Surgery and Anesthesia, Interdisciplinary Council on Peripheral Vascular

Disease, and Interdisciplinary Council on Quality of Care and Outcomes Research. *Circulation* 2009; 119(16): 2235–49.

41. Gobin YP, Starkman S, Duckwiler GR, *et al.* MERCI 1: a phase 1 study of Mechanical Embolus Removal in Cerebral Ischemia. *Stroke* 2004; 35(12): 2848–54.

42. Gebel JM, Sila CA, Sloan MA, *et al.* Thrombolysis-related intracranial hemorrhage: a radiographic analysis of 244 cases from the GUSTO-1 trial with clinical correlation. Global Utilization of Streptokinase and Tissue Plasminogen Activator for Occluded Coronary Arteries. *Stroke* 1998; 29(3): 563–9.

43. Davalos A, Cendra E, Teruel J, Martinez M, Genis D. Deteriorating ischemic stroke: risk factors and prognosis. *Neurology* 1990; 40(12): 1865–9.

44. Schwamm LH, Fonarow GC, Reeves MJ, *et al.* Get With the Guidelines – Stroke is associated with sustained improvement in care for patients hospitalized with acute stroke or transient ischemic attack. *Circulation* 2009; 119(1): 107–15.

45. Easton JD, Saver JL, Albers GW, *et al.* Definition and evaluation of transient ischemic attack: a scientific statement for healthcare professionals from the American Heart Association/American Stroke Association Stroke Council; Council on Cardiovascular Surgery and Anesthesia; Council on Cardiovascular Radiology and Intervention; Council on Cardiovascular Nursing; and the Interdisciplinary Council on Peripheral Vascular Disease. The American Academy of Neurology affirms the value of this statement as an educational tool for neurologists. *Stroke* 2009; 40(6): 2276–93.

46. Johnston SC, Gress DR, Browner WS, Sidney S. Short-term prognosis after emergency department diagnosis of TIA. *JAMA* 2000; 284(22): 2901–6.

47. Coull AJ, Lovett JK, Rothwell PM. Population based study of early risk of stroke after transient ischaemic attack or minor stroke: implications for public education and organisation of services. *BMJ* 2004; 328(7435): 326.

48. Daffertshofer M, Mielke O, Pullwitt A, Felsenstein M, Hennerici M. Transient ischemic attacks are more than "ministrokes". *Stroke* 2004; 35(11): 2453–8.

49. Eliasziw M, Kennedy J, Hill MD, Buchan AM, Barnett HJ. Early risk of stroke after a transient ischemic attack in patients with internal carotid artery disease. *CMAJ* 2004; 170(7): 1105–9.

50. Gladstone DJ, Kapral MK, Fang J, Laupacis A, Tu JV. Management and outcomes of transient ischemic attacks in Ontario. *CMAJ* 2004; 170(7): 1099–104.

51. Hill MD, Yiannakoulias N, Jeerakathil T, *et al.* The high risk of stroke immediately after transient ischemic attack: a population-based study. *Neurology* 2004; 62(11): 2015–20.

52. Lisabeth LD, Ireland JK, Risser JM, *et al.* Stroke risk after transient ischemic attack in a population-based setting. *Stroke* 2004; 35(8): 1842–6.

53. Kleindorfer D, Panagos P, Pancioli A, *et al.* Incidence and short-term prognosis of transient ischemic attack in a population-based study. *Stroke* 2005; 36(4): 720–3.

54. Johnston SC, Rothwell PM, Nguyen-Huynh MN, *et al.* Validation and refinement of scores to predict very early stroke risk after transient ischaemic attack. *Lancet* 2007; 369(9558): 283–92.

55. Diener HC, Cunha L, Forbes C, *et al.* European Stroke Prevention Study. 2. Dipyridamole and acetylsalicylic acid in the secondary prevention of stroke. *J Neurol Sci* 1996; 143(1-2): 1–13.

56. Sacco RL, Adams R, Albers G, *et al.* Guidelines for prevention of stroke in patients with ischemic stroke or transient ischemic attack: a statement for healthcare professionals from the American Heart Association/American Stroke Association Council on Stroke: co-sponsored by the Council on Cardiovascular Radiology and Intervention: the American Academy of Neurology affirms the value of this guideline. *Circulation* 2006; 113(10): e409–49.

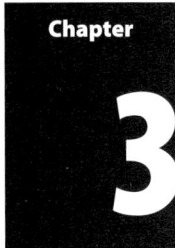

Intracerebral hemorrhage

Lauren M. Nentwich and Joshua N. Goldstein

Intracerebral hemorrhage (ICH) is defined as spontaneous, non-traumatic bleeding into the brain parenchyma.[1] ICH constitutes 10 to 15% of all first-ever strokes,[2] with a worldwide incidence of 10 to 20 cases per 100,000 population.[1] It is a medical emergency with a 30-day mortality rate of 35 to 52% and a high morbidity rate. Only 20% of patients are expected to be functionally independent at six months.[2] ICH also places a large financial burden on the healthcare system. The average per-patient hospitalization cost is estimated to be $15,256, with lifetime costs estimated at more than $123,500.[3]

Risk factors

Intracranial hemorrhage has genetic, demographic, medical, and environmental risk factors. Genetic risk factors include the presence of apolipoprotein E2 or E4 alleles, associated with cerebral amyloid angiopathy (CAA), and a first-degree relative with ICH.[4] Other risk factors include older age, African American ethnicity, hypertension, low levels of low-density lipoprotein cholesterol or triglycerides, high alcohol intake, previous ischemic or hemorrhagic stroke,[4–7] and oral anticoagulation use.[8] The most important modifiable risk factor for ICH is hypertension, and the risk of ICH increases with its worsening severity.[4–7] Oral anticoagulation with warfarin is another important risk factor. Randomized trials in patients with atrial fibrillation show a 0.3 to 1.8% annual rate of ICH for patients anticoagulated with warfarin.[8]

Classification

ICH can be classified as either primary or secondary depending on the underlying cause. Primary ICH originates from the spontaneous rupture of small vessels caused by chronic hypertension or CAA.[1] It is the most common cause of ICH, accounting for 78 to 88% of all cases. Secondary ICH occurs in a minority of patients and can be associated with vascular abnormalities (e.g., arteriovenous malformation, intracranial aneurysm, cavernous angioma, venous angioma), venous sinus thrombosis, intracranial neoplasm, coagulopathy, vasculitis, eclampsia, cerebral endometriosis, cocaine or alcohol use, hemorrhagic transformation of ischemic stroke, or trauma.[1,9] This chapter focuses on primary spontaneous non-traumatic ICH. Intracerebral hemorrhage resulting from secondary causes such as cerebral venous sinus thrombosis, hemorrhagic conversion of ischemic stroke, and intracranial aneurysm are addressed elsewhere in this book.

Pathophysiology

Primary ICH is often classified according to the region of the brain in which it occurs. Lobar ICH occurs at the junction of the cortical gray matter and subcortical white matter. Non-lobar, or deep, ICH occurs in the thalamus, basal ganglia, brainstem, or cerebellum.[10] Chronic hypertension is more often associated with non-lobar ICH, whereas CAA-related ICH is more often seen in lobar bleeds. However, overlap can be seen between the various causes (Figure 3.1).[11]

Longstanding chronic hypertension is thought to cause lipohyalinosis of small, deep-penetrating arteries, resulting in degenerative changes and reduced compliance of the vessel wall[1,11] as well as microaneurysms at the bifurcation of the arterioles, which are prone to rupture.[12] In CAA, amyloid protein infiltrates the media and adventitia of the cerebral microvasculature, causing brittle vessels that can rupture.[13] Either pathology causes acute vessel rupture

Vascular Emergencies, ed. Robert L. Rogers, Thomas Scalea, Lee Wallis, and Heike Geduld. Published by Cambridge University Press. © Cambridge University Press 2013.

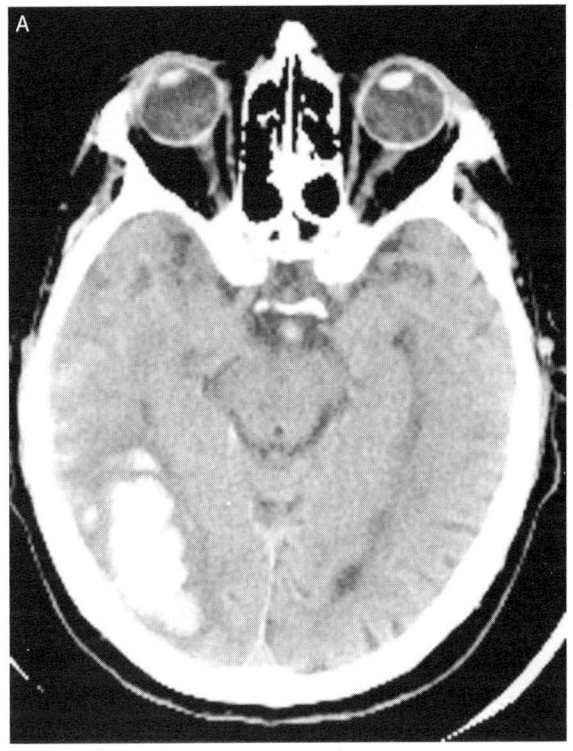
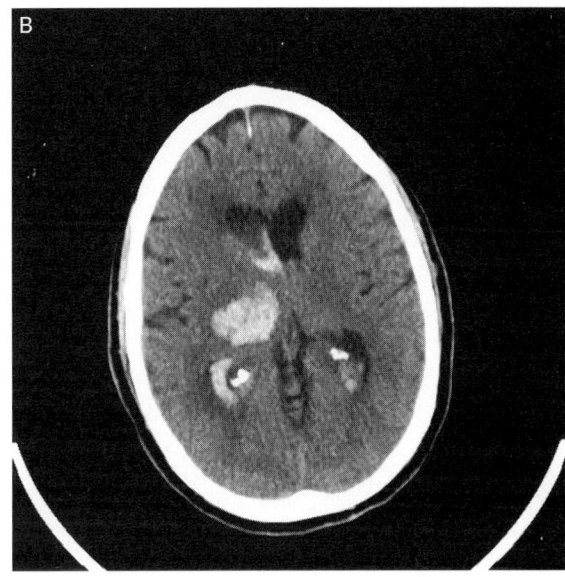

Figure 3.1 Primary intracerebral hemorrhage. (A) Lobar ICH, typically associated with cerebral amyloid angiopathy. (B) Deep ICH, typically associated with chronic hypertension.

and acute hemorrhage, which initiates a cascade of brain injury.

First, the initial injury and the resulting deficit are caused by mass effect of the hematoma on the brain.[11] Second, perihematomal brain edema develops immediately after the onset of hemorrhage and peaks 10 to 20 days after the ictus.[12] Early edema results from the accumulation of osmotically active serum proteins from the clot. Later, vasogenic and cytotoxic edema is caused by disruption of the blood–brain barrier, failure of the sodium pump, death of neurons, erythrocyte lysis, and hemoglobin toxicity.[1] Edema formation after ICH may cause additional mass effect and increase intracranial pressure (ICP), causing midline shift and herniation.[12] Third, blood and plasma products appear to mediate a number of secondary injury processes. Iron from hemoglobin degradation appears to be particularly neurotoxic and causes delayed neuronal injury and edema formation.[1,12,14] An inflammatory response occurs soon after ICH and aggravates hemorrhagic brain injury. Activation of the coagulation cascade, including thrombin production,

occurs immediately after ICH; at high concentrations, thrombin may induce early perihematomal edema and is thought to cause the death of neurons.[12] Finally, continued bleeding occurs in 20 to 38% of patients, and this hematoma growth (or expansion) is associated with an increased risk of neurologic deterioration and ICH-related death.[15–17] Expansion of the hematoma may be multifactorial; contributing factors are thought to include continued bleeding from the primary source, secondary bleeding at the periphery of the hemorrhage due to mechanical disruption of surrounding vessels, acute hypertension, and a local coagulation deficit.[1,11] Most hematoma growth occurs within the first 24 hours after the inciting event.[12]

Diagnosis

Clinical presentation

Much like ischemic stroke, the presentation of ICH depends on its location, size, and speed of development.[9] Both ICH and ischemic stroke cause sudden dysfunction of neural tissue in a specific territory of the

Computed tomography

Magnetic resonance imaging (GRE)

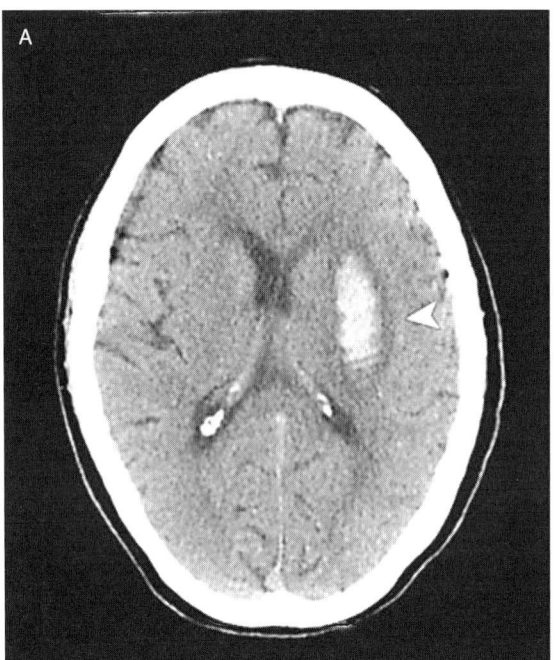
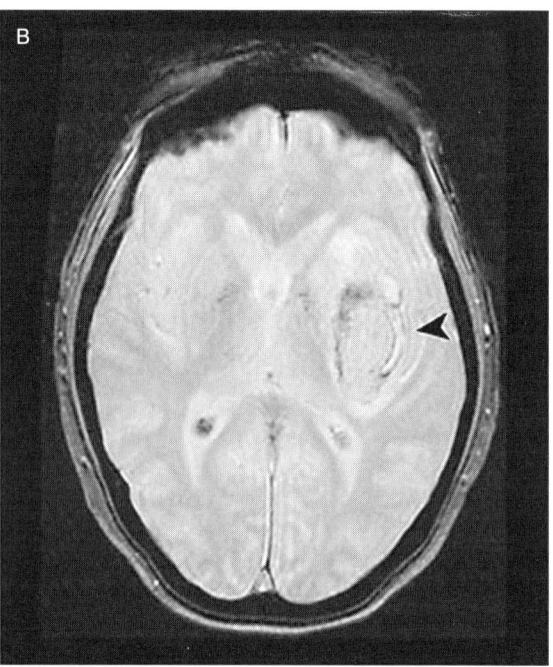

Figure 3.2 Acute intracerebral hemorrhage imaged with computed tomography (A) and magnetic resonance imaging, gradient-recalled echo (B).

brain, which results in focal neurologic deficits, such as gaze palsy, visual field cuts, hemiparesis, hemisensory loss, ataxia, vertigo, or speech disturbances.[18] If the hematoma is large or continues to grow, it may lead to coma and death due to increased ICP and compression on the brainstem.[9]

ICH causes leakage of blood into the brain parenchyma, resulting in mass effect with compression of adjacent tissues, increased ICP, and occasional extension of blood into the ventricles or subarachnoid space. Initial findings more likely to be associated with ICH versus ischemic stroke include loss of consciousness, coma, neck stiffness, seizure accompanying the neurologic deficit, diastolic blood pressure greater than 110 mmHg, vomiting, and headache. Several clinical findings significantly decrease the likelihood of ICH versus ischemic stroke, including the presence of a cervical bruit, history of transient ischemic attack (TIA), peripheral artery disease, and history of atrial fibrillation.[18]

In patients with stroke, findings characteristic of ICH – loss of consciousness, coma, neck stiffness, seizure, vomiting, headache – increase the likelihood of a patient having ICH, but many patients with ICH

lack any of these distinctive findings. The diagnosis of ICH, and its differentiation from ischemic stroke, cannot be made clinically and requires definitive neuroimaging.[18] Both the American Heart Association (AHA) and the European Stroke Initiative (EUSI) recommend rapid neuroimaging to distinguish ischemic stroke from ICH.[9,19]

Neuroimaging

Initial neuroimaging

Computed tomography (CT) and magnetic resonance imaging (MRI) can both be used in the initial evaluation of patients presenting with possible ICH (Figure 3.2). Non-contrast CT is thought to be 100% sensitive for clinically relevant acute hemorrhage and is considered the gold standard for diagnosing ICH.[19] Computed tomography scanners are now rapidly available to almost all emergency department (ED) patients in the United States[20] but may not be available in some developing countries.

Gradient-echo (GRE) and T2* susceptibility-weighted MRI are as sensitive as CT for the detection of acute intracranial hemorrhage. MRI has the added benefit of being more sensitive for acute ischemic stroke and chronic hemorrhage, making it the more accurate imaging modality for definitive diagnosis of patients presenting with acute focal neurologic deficits and possible stroke.[21,22] However, many patient- and hospital-related factors can make MRI impossible or impractical in the acute setting. Availability of MRI, proximity of MRI to the ED, patient contraindications, diminished level of consciousness, vomiting, agitation, and medical instability may preclude emergent MRI in a large proportion of cases. In one prospective study, 73% of patients presenting with acute stroke who were too medically unstable for MRI were diagnosed with ICH.[23]

Additional neuroimaging

Once ICH is diagnosed, additional neuroimaging may be performed to identify patients at risk for hematoma expansion and investigate for secondary causes of ICH that are amenable to intervention.

Computed tomography angiography (CTA) and contrast-enhanced CT may identify patients at risk for hematoma expansion. With these two modalities, contrast extravasation appears as small, enhancing foci within the hematoma (a "spot sign") (Figure 3.3). Patients with a spot sign are at high risk for hematoma expansion.[24,25] The clinical use of this radiologic marker is an area of active research.

Magnetic resonance imaging/angiography/venography (MRI/A/V) and CT angiography/venography (CTA/V) can exclude secondary causes of ICH, such as arteriovenous malformations, fistulas, aneurysms, tumors, and cerebral vein thrombosis.[19] Non-lobar hemorrhages involving the putamen, globus palidum, thalamus, internal capsule, periventricular white matter, pons, and cerebellum in patients with known hypertension are often, but not exclusively, caused by hypertensive vasculopathy. However, patients with hemorrhages in other locations, including isolated intraventricular hemorrhage (IVH); younger patients; and those without a history of hypertension are at higher risk of secondary ICH.[9,26] A practical scoring system using baseline clinical and non-contrast CT characteristics has been developed to predict a vascular cause of a patient's ICH. The Secondary Intracerebral Hemorrhage Score is tallied by combining various characteristics: non-contrast CT imaging that indicates a high probability of a vascular anomaly based on ICH location and other imaging characteristics, younger age, female

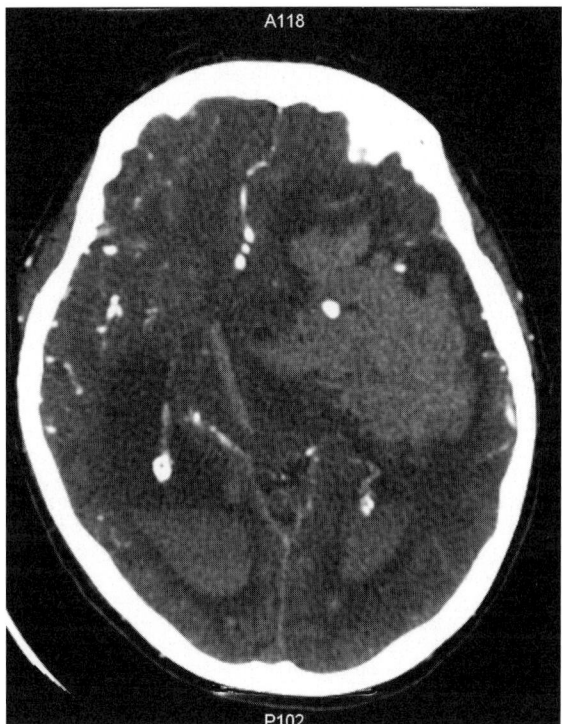

Figure 3.3 Contrast extravasation into the hematoma: the "spot sign."

sex, and either known hypertension or impaired coagulation.[27]

Laboratory data

As part of the workup and as a means of guiding treatment decisions, rapid serum and urine tests should be obtained in all patients presenting with suspected or known ICH. A complete blood count should be obtained, with consideration of a platelet disorder. Chemistry tests should be obtained, as electrolyte disturbances are not uncommon, and hyperglycemia may be a modifiable risk factor for poor outcome. Liver function tests, prothrombin time (or INR), and activated partial thromboplastin time should be considered because patients with coagulopathy have increased risk of hematoma expansion and therefore increased morbidity and mortality rates. A toxicology screen can be considered for detection of abuse of cocaine or other sympathomimetic drugs. A pregnancy test should be performed in all women of child-bearing age.[11,19] The management of hyperglycemia and anticoagulation-related hemorrhages are addressed later in this chapter.

Table 3.1 Critical actions in the emergency management and diagnosis of acute ICH

- On arrival, obtain vital signs and assess and stabilize the ABCs. Intubation may be necessary but should be weighed against the impact of the loss of the neurologic examination.
- Obtain rapid neuroimaging with CT or MRI (GRE) in all patients presenting with acute focal neurologic deficits and suspicion of ICH.
- Consider vascular imaging to evaluate for secondary causes of ICH amenable to intervention in patients who are young, have lobar hemorrhage or isolated IVH, or do not have a history of hypertension.
- Place two large-bore IV lines and obtain full labs, especially complete blood count and coagulation studies.
- Lower significantly elevated blood pressure with IV antihypertensive medications with a short half-life. Current recommendations for blood pressure treatment can be found in the guidelines from the AHA and the EUSI and are listed in Table 3.2.
- Coagulopathy-associated ICH requires rapid correction of the coagulopathy. Warfarin-associated ICH should have the INR corrected using fresh frozen plasma (FFP) or prothrombin complex concentrate (PCC) infusions as well as IV vitamin K. Transfuse platelets in cases of thrombocytopenia.
- Treat clinical seizures with antiepileptics, but do not give antiepileptics prophylactically.
- Obtain urgent specialty consultation (typically neurology and/or neurosurgery) in the ED.
- Admit patients with ICH to an intensive care unit (ICU), preferably a neurologic or neurosurgical ICU, if available.
- New DNR orders or withdrawal of care are not recommended in the first 24 hours. Aggressive full care early after ICH onset is recommended.

Emergency department workup

As discussed previously, patients with ICH present with acute stroke symptoms, so rapid assessment, including neuroimaging, is necessary to differentiate patients with hemorrhage from those with ischemia. Though no individual therapy has yet been demonstrated to improve outcome in patients with ICH, two lines of evidence suggest that aggressive medical care offers substantial benefit.[11] First, admission to a stroke unit appears to improve outcomes, compared with admission to a general medical unit.[28] Second, institutions with a higher rate of DNR (do not resuscitate) order use show higher risk-adjusted mortality rates.[29,30] Critical actions for the emergency diagnosis and treatment of patients with ICH are summarized in Table 3.1.

General principles of treatment

General treatment of patients with ICH does not differ from the stabilization of most acutely ill patients. Particular attention should be paid to close monitoring of neurologic status and vital signs.[9]

On arrival in the ED, patients with suspected acute stroke should receive priority triage. Vital signs should be obtained rapidly, and an initial primary survey should be performed to assess the patient's airway, breathing, and circulation. Any acute abnormalities on the primary survey should be managed and stabilized. Once stabilized, a secondary examination looking for evidence of trauma, bleeding, and other abnormalities should be performed quickly as well as a rapid assessment of the patient's neurologic status. Neurologic status is best monitored using the National Institutes of Health Stroke Scale (NIHSS) and the Glasgow Coma Scale (GCS). Intravenous access should be established, and laboratory testing, including complete blood count, chemistry panel, coagulation tests, and cardiac enzymes, should be obtained. Patients with suspected stroke should undergo rapid neuroimaging, as discussed previously. If ICH is diagnosed on neuroimaging, neurologic consultation should be obtained urgently.

Airway management

Many patients with ICH are unable to protect their airway; as a result, emergency airway management is often needed. Early intubation for airway protection may be necessary but should be weighed against the impact of the loss of the neurologic examination. In a study that evaluated characteristics of patients with stroke and ICH requiring mechanical ventilation, Gujjar *et al.* found that the majority of patients requiring mechanical ventilation were intubated for neurologic deterioration on presentation and that 30% of patients with ICH were intubated sometime during their hospitalization. Signs of brainstem dysfunction as well as older age and early intubation predicted higher rates of mortality in these patients.[31]

If airway management is required in the emergency setting, rapid-sequence endotracheal intubation should be performed. Pretreatment with lidocaine may be considered, as it may blunt the rise in ICP that is associated with intubation. Consider using etomidate as the induction agent, as it may preserve cerebral perfusion pressure. Paralytic agents to consider include succinylcholine, rocuronium, and vecuronium. Given its short duration of clinical effect, propofol is a reasonable choice for sedation, as it provides effective sedation yet allows the patient to retain the ability to participate in the neurologic examination.[11]

Glucose management

Admission hyperglycemia is associated with mortality and morbidity rates; therefore, many clinicians advocate strict glucose control. Of note, one randomized trial found no benefit to intensive insulin therapy over subcutaneous sliding-scale insulin;[32] therefore, while normoglycemia is recommended to minimize neurotoxicity, it is not clear that continuous insulin infusion is necessary. At present, the best management of hyperglycemia and the target glucose in patients with ICH are unknown. The AHA recommends that glucose should be monitored, hypoglycemia should be avoided, and normoglycemia should be maintained.[19]

Temperature management

Fever is common after supratentorial ICH, especially in patients with IVH. The exact cause of fever in ICH is unknown, but hyperthermia augments neuronal damage and worsens clinical outcome after brain injury. The duration of fever during the first 72 hours in patients with ICH has been found to be a prognostic factor and is associated with poor outcome.[33] ICH patients with fever should undergo an infectious workup to rule out alternative and treatable causes of fever. The fever should be treated to maintain normothermia, though there are currently no data linking fever treatment with outcome.[19]

Blood pressure management

Acutely elevated BP is frequently observed in patients with ICH. It may lead to adverse outcomes via hematoma expansion or perihematomal edema formation. However, it is unclear whether reducing the BP can improve the outcome.[19] One clinical trial, Intensive Blood Pressure Reduction in Acute Cerebral Haemorrhage (INTERACT), randomized patients to a target systolic blood pressure (SBP) of 140 versus 180 mmHg. There was a trend toward reduced hematoma growth in the intensive treatment group but no clear difference in clinical outcome.[34] A second study, Antihypertensive Treatment of Acute Cerebral Hemorrhage (ATACH), confirmed the feasibility of rapid BP lowering using intravenous nicardipine.[35] Given the success of these two trials, INTERACT2 (ClinicalTrials.gov #NCT00716079) and ATACH-II (ClinicalTrials.gov #NCT01176565) are currently recruiting patients to investigate whether intensive BP

Table 3.2 AHA Stroke Council and European Stroke Initiative recommendations for the treatment of acute hypertension in ICH

AHA treatment recommendations:[19]

- If SBP > 200 mmHg or MAP > 150 mmHg, consider aggressive reduction of BP with continuous intravenous infusion and frequent BP monitoring every five minutes.
- If SBP > 180 mmHg or MAP > 130 mmHg and there is a possibility of elevated ICP, consider monitoring ICP and reducing BP using intermittent or continuous IV medications while maintaining CPP ≥ 60 mmHg.
- If SBP > 180 mmHg or MAP > 130 mmHg and there is no evidence of elevated ICP, consider a modest reduction of BP using intermittent or continuous IV medications to control BP and then clinically re-examine the patient.

The EUSI recommends treatment if blood pressure remains elevated above the following levels, confirmed by repeated measurements:[9]

- Patients with known history of hypertension or signs of chronic hypertension: SBP > 180 mmHg and/or DBP > 105 mmHg. Target blood pressure is 170 / 100 mmHg (or MAP of 125 mmHg).
- Patients without known hypertension: SBP > 160 mmHg and/or DBP > 95 mmHg. Target blood pressure is 150 / 90 mmHg (or a MAP of 110 mmHg).
- Reduction of MAP by >20% should be avoided.
- These limits and targets should be adapted to higher values in patients undergoing monitoring of increased ICP, to guarantee a sufficient CPP > 70 mmHg.

SBP, systolic blood pressure; MAP, mean arterial pressure; BP, blood pressure; ICP, intracranial pressure; DBP, diastolic blood pressure; CPP, cerebral perfusion pressure.

lowering improves clinical outcomes. Both the AHA and the EUSI provide guidelines for the acute BP management of patients with ICH (Table 3.2).[9,19] Intravenous antihypertensive medications with a short half-life should be used as first-line treatment.[9] The AHA recommends considering IV labetalol, nicardipine, esmolol, enalapril, hydralazine, sodium nitroprusside, or nitroglycerin.[2] The EUSI recommends IV labetalol, urapidil, sodium nitroprusside, nitroglycerin, or captopril.[9]

Management of coagulopathy
Warfarin reversal

Warfarin-associated ICH is a devastating complication of oral anticoagulation treatment. It is associated with a high mortality rate and poor neurologic outcomes in survivors. Many authors believe that early action to rapidly correct the coagulopathy may prevent continued bleeding. A number of therapeutic options are available for warfarin reversal, though an optimal strategy has yet to be defined.

Because warfarin inhibits vitamin-K-dependent carboxylation of factors II, VII, IX, and X, vitamin K is an integral component in the restoration of these factors and reversal of warfarin's effects. Vitamin K given intravenously lowers the INR as early as four hours. Of note, intravenous vitamin K carries a rare risk of anaphylaxis and should be given slowly, with close monitoring of the airway to minimize complications.

Since vitamin K requires hours to take effect, emergency warfarin reversal also requires an infusion of coagulation factors. Coagulation factor replacement may be accomplished by giving fresh frozen plasma (FFP) or prothrombin complex concentrates (PCCs). FFP is readily available and can be effective when adequately dosed, but it can require large volumes of fluid and is associated with long processing delays in time to infusion in standard practice. PCCs correct the INR more quickly than FFP and require smaller volumes of fluid, but their availability is limited in the United States. Activated recombinant factor VII (rFVIIa) given as a supplement to FFP and vitamin K appears to reduce time to INR reversal, but it is not clear that rFVIIa in isolation can restore clinical hemostasis.[36–38]

The AHA and EUSI recommendations for warfarin reversal in patients with ICH and an elevated INR are similar. Clinical recommendations include withholding warfarin, giving intravenous vitamin K, and normalizing the INR with FFP or PCCs.[9,19] The AHA states that further research is required before recommendations can be made regarding the use of rFVIIa.[19]

Dabigatran etexilate reversal

Dabigatran etexilate is an oral, reversible direct thrombin inhibitor that has recently been approved by the FDA for the prevention of stroke in patients with non-valvular atrial fibrillation. The incidence of ICH is 1.0 per 1000 patients treated with dabigatran at the recommended dose. In the event of ICH in a patient on dabigatran, there is no currently known antidote for reversal of the anticoagulant effects. Dabigatran should be stopped immediately and symptomatic treatment should be initiated. Specific reversal agents such as rFVIIa and PCCs may be considered, though data on their use in patients on dabigatran are limited.[39] One recently published study showed that the administration of a PCC (Cofact) did not reverse the anticoagulant effect of dabigatran in healthy subjects. Further clinical studies are necessary regarding PCC use in patients with bleeding events who are anticoagulated with dabigatran.[40]

Platelet disorders

Studies are conflicting on whether antiplatelet therapy worsens outcome in patients with ICH, but a recent meta-analysis suggested a small but statistically significant increase in the mortality rate.[41] However, the utility and safety of platelet transfusion in patients with normal platelet count who are on antiplatelet therapy are unknown and considered investigational by the AHA.[19] Platelet transfusion is not recommended by the EUSI.[9] However, in patients with thrombocytopenia (platelet count <100,000/μL), the AHA recommends platelet transfusion.[19]

Management of elevated intracranial pressure

Elevated ICP in patients with ICH is usually the result of hydrocephalus from IVH or mass effect from the hematoma or surrounding edema. Data regarding the frequency and management of elevated ICP in patients with ICH are limited,[19] but patients with radiologic or clinical evidence of elevated ICP should be considered for therapies aimed at lowering the pressure. Given the paucity of data, the management principles for elevated ICP are borrowed from the traumatic brain injury guidelines. Those guidelines recommend a cerebral perfusion pressure of 50 to 70 mmHg (depending on cerebral autoregulation) and initiating treatment to lower ICP once it rises above an upper threshold of 20 to 25 mmHg. Medical methods for lowering elevated ICP include administration of mannitol or hypertonic saline, induction of paralysis, and hyperventilation. Hyperventilation with a goal PCO_2 of 30 to 35 mmHg is a temporizing method and should be used only in cases of impending herniation while awaiting surgical decompression. Induction of coma with high-dose barbiturate therapy may be considered to control elevated ICP that is refractory to optimal medical and surgical management; it should be managed by critical care providers.[42]

In patients with suspected elevated ICP who receive ICP monitoring, an external ventricular drain (EVD) should be considered and neurosurgery should be consulted (or the patient transferred to a center with neurosurgical capabilities).[42] The EVD allows drainage of cerebrospinal fluid, which can reduce ICP in patients with hydrocephalus. ICP can also be monitored via a parenchymal catheter, which is thought to have a lower risk of infection than EVDs.[19] The AHA recommends that ICP monitoring and treatment be considered in patients with a GCS score ≤ 8, those with clinical evidence of transtentorial herniation, and those with significant IVH or hydrocephalus.[19] The EUSI recommends considering continuous ICP monitoring in patients who need mechanical ventilation and recommends medical treatment of elevated ICP if clinical deterioration is related to increasing edema.[9]

Management of seizure

Clinical seizures occur more often in patients with ICH than in those with ischemic stroke. The majority of seizures occur early, at or near the onset of hemorrhage. Cortical location of the hemorrhage appears to be a risk factor for the development of seizures in patients with ICH.[43] Studies of continuous electroencephalography have reported electrographic seizures in 28 to 31% of ICH patients.[19] However, the development of seizures in patients with ICH has not been associated with worsened disability or mortality.[19,43] In fact, recent studies have shown the use of antiepileptics, particularly phenytoin, following acute ICH to be associated with severe disability and death.[44] As a result, current AHA recommendations state that, although clinical seizures should be treated with antiepileptic drugs, antiepileptics should not be used prophylactically. In patients with depressed mental status out of proportion to the degree of brain injury, continuous electroencephalographic monitoring is indicated, and patients found to have electrographic seizures should be treated with antiepileptics.[19] The EUSI recommends treatment of seizures only if they occur, with the exception that prophylactic treatment may be considered for select patients with lobar ICH.[9]

Admission

Given that they are often medically and neurologically unstable, patients with ICH should be admitted to an intensive care unit (ICU) for frequent monitoring of vital signs and neurologic status and to receive intensive treatments as needed. If possible, admission to a specialty ICU is beneficial, as admission to a neurologic or neurosurgical ICU versus a general ICU is associated with a reduced mortality rate.[28] Patients with ICH should be admitted preferentially to hospitals that have neurology, neuroradiology, and neurosurgical capabilities.

Definitive treatment

Intraventricular hemorrhage and hydrocephalus

Intraventricular hemorrhage occurs in 45% of patients with spontaneous ICH and can be either primary, confined to the ventricles, or secondary, originating as an extension of the ICH. The majority of IVH is secondary, originating from deep hypertensive hemorrhages.[19] The presence of IVH is an independent risk factor for death and poor functional outcome, as prolonged exposure of the ventricles to blood can lead to altered consciousness, tissue inflammation and fibrosis, and hydrocephalus. Small studies suggest that ventricular drainage can improve outcome.[45]

Theoretically, removal of IVH and treatment of hydrocephalus can be accomplished via the placement of an EVD, which drains cerebrospinal fluid (CSF) and blood. However, EVD drainage may be ineffective because of the difficulty in maintaining catheter patency and the slow removal caused by blood clots. Injection of thrombolytic agents may accelerate lysis and evacuation of IVH. The Clot Lysis: Evaluating Accelerated Resolution of IVH (CLEAR-IVH) clinical trial prospectively evaluated the safety of intraventricular injection of low-dose rtPA in patients with IVH. Preliminary analyses found that low-dose rtPA can be administered safely to patients with stable IVH clots and may increase lysis rates,[46] but the efficacy of this treatment requires confirmation. The AHA recommendations state that ventricular drainage as treatment for hydrocephalus is reasonable in patients with a decreased level of consciousness, though intraventricular administration of rtPA to maintain catheter patency remains uncertain and investigational.[19] All patients with IVH and/or hydrocephalus should undergo urgent consultation by a neurosurgeon.

Surgery

Surgery as treatment to remove ICH remains controversial and is typically reserved for select candidates, depending on the location of the hemorrhage, time from ictus, and other clinical factors. Patients with cerebellar hematomas larger than 3 cm, brainstem compression, or hydrocephalus likely bene-fit from surgical evacuation; however, for non-cerebellar hematomas, the potential benefit is less clear.[19] The International Surgical Trial in Intracere-bral Haemorrhage (STICH) was a large, prospective randomized study of 1,033 patients, which showed no overall benefit from early hematoma evacuation in patients with supratentorial ICH. A subgroup analysis suggested a benefit to early surgery for patients with ICH within 1 cm of the cortical surface.[47] A follow-up study, STICH II (ClinicalTrials.gov #NCT01320423), is ongoing. Minimally invasive clot evacuation techniques have been developed util-izing stereotactic or endoscopic aspiration with and without thrombolytics; the effectiveness of these techniques remains investigational.[19]

The AHA recommends surgery for patients with cerebellar hemorrhage who are deteriorating neurologically or who have brainstem compression and/or hydrocephalus from ventricular obstruction. For supratentorial ICH, the AHA states that standard craniotomy may be considered in patients with lobar clots >30 mL within 1 cm of the cortical surface.[19] The EUSI recommends considering craniotomy if there is deterioration in consciousness, if the ICH is superficial and less than 1 cm from the surface, or if the hemorrhage is located in the cerebellum.[9]

Prognosis

ICH is associated with a high early mortality rate and significant morbidity among survivors.[2] Mul-tiple grading scores allow evidence-based risk strati-fication in the acute phase. The ICH score is a clinical grading score used to predict 30-day mortality. Fac-tors associated with higher 30-day mortality include high ICH volume, low initial GCS score, the presence of IVH, older age, and an infratentorial origin of the ICH.[48] Alternatively, the FUNC score is a clinical grading score that predicts functional independence at 90 days. Factors associated with reduced functional independence are similar to those associated with high 30-day mortality and include older age, low GCS score, non-lobar ICH location, and ICH volume. Addition-ally, pre-ICH cognitive impairment is associated with reduced functional independence but not with mor-bidity.[49]

Family members often want to know the patient's likely ultimate outcome when making decisions regarding aggressiveness of care. Prognostic models

are often used by physicians to attempt to provide an answer. There is concern that preconceived notions about futility of care in patients may lead to death due to self-fulfilling prophecies of an initial poor prog-nosis. Studies have shown that the most important prognostic variable in determining outcome after ICH is the level of medical support provided. Patients who are initially predicted to have a poor outcome can achieve reasonable neurologic recovery if they are treated aggressively.[29] Limiting care in response to early DNR orders, withdrawal of care, or deferral of other life-sustaining interventions is independently associated with both short- and long-term mortality after ICH, independent from other predictors of death.[30] As such, new DNR orders or withdrawal of care are generally not recommended in the emergency department. The AHA recommends aggressive full care early after ICH onset and postponement of new DNR orders until at least the second full day of hospitalization.[19]

Clinical approach when resources are limited

The burden of stroke is increasing in low- and middle-income countries where resources are likely to be scarce or limited. From 2000 to 2008, the overall stroke incidence rates in low- to middle-income countries exceeded that in high-income countries by 20%.[50] In addition to having more strokes, the populations of developing countries have some of the highest stroke mortality rates in the world and account for more than two-thirds of stroke deaths worldwide.[51] Finally, ICH is more common in low- to middle-income coun-tries, likely due to poorly controlled hypertension.[50]

Proper management of patients with acute stroke symptoms greatly differs based on the pathologic stroke type. It is important to differentiate hemor-rhagic from ischemic stroke. As discussed previously, certain clinical factors can aid in the differentiation of ICH from ischemia, but these factors are not always reliable. CT is the most rapid, accessible, and reliable imaging modality for diagnosing ICH, but quick access to CT is not available in all settings.[51]

In those circumstances with a lack of access to brain imaging, clinical scores can be used to differ-entiate ICH from ischemic stroke. Two of the sim-plest are the Guy's Hospital Score and the Siriraj Score. Unfortunately, comparison of these scores in resource-poor settings shows that neither is highly accurate.[52]

Thrombolytics should not be given in the absence of neuroimaging, because of the risk of worsening hemorrhage. Further investigation on aspirin use and anticoagulation in stroke patients without a CT scan is necessary. Blood pressure should be managed according to local guidelines for critically ill patients. Given the limitations on the treatment of stroke in areas without brain imaging capabilities, health services should emphasize strategies to reduce the risk of stroke in these populations.[52]

Pearls and pitfalls

- All patients presenting with focal stroke symptoms must undergo urgent imaging with non-contrast CT or MRI (GRE) to diagnose or rule out ICH.
- Causes of secondary ICH should be considered in all patients with ICH, particularly in those who are young, have lobar hemorrhage or isolated IVH, or do not have a history of hypertension.
- Coagulopathy should be corrected rapidly.
- Though optimal treatment parameters remain investigational, acute hypertension in patients with ICH should be treated and monitored closely. Current recommended clinical guidelines for blood pressure management are listed in Table 3.2.
- Patients with ICH should undergo urgent specialty consultation and should be admitted to a stroke center.
- Patients with ICH should be managed aggressively early after onset and should be admitted to an intensive care unit.

References

1. Qureshi AI, Tuhrim S, Broderick JP, *et al.* Spontaneous intracerebral hemorrhage. *N Engl J Med* 2001; 344(19): 1450–60.

2. Broderick J, Connolly S, Feldmann E, *et al.* Guidelines for the management of spontaneous intracerebral hemorrhage in adults: 2007 update: a guideline from the American Heart Association/American Stroke Association Stroke Council, High Blood Pressure Research Council, and the Quality of Care and Outcomes in Research Interdisciplinary Working Group. *Stroke* 2007; 38(6): 2001–23.

3. Russell MW, Joshi AV, Neumann PJ, Boulanger L, Menzin J. Predictors of hospital length of stay and cost in patients with intracerebral hemorrhage. *Neurology* 2006; 67(7): 1279–81.

4. Woo D, Sauerbeck LR, Kissela BM, *et al.* Genetic and environmental risk factors for intracerebral hemorrhage: preliminary results of a population-based study. *Stroke* 2002; 33(5): 1190–5.

5. Sturgeon JD, Folsom AR, Longstreth WT Jr, *et al.* Risk factors for intracerebral hemorrhage in a pooled prospective study. *Stroke* 2007; 38(10): 2718–25.

6. Ariesen MJ, Claus SP, Rinkel GJ, Algra A. Risk factors for intracerebral hemorrhage in the general population: a systematic review. *Stroke* 2003; 34(8): 2060–5.

7. Arima H, Tzourio C, Anderson C, *et al.* Effects of perindopril-based lowering of blood pressure on intracerebral hemorrhage related to amyloid angiopathy: the PROGRESS trial. *Stroke* 2010; 41(2): 394–6.

8. Singer DE, Albers GW, Dalen JE, *et al.* Antithrombotic therapy in atrial fibrillation: the Seventh ACCP Conference on Antithrombotic and Thrombolytic Therapy. *Chest* 2004; 126(3 suppl): 429S–56S.

9. Steiner T, Kaste M, Forsting M, *et al.* Recommendations for the management of intracranial haemorrhage – part I: spontaneous intracerebral haemorrhage. The European Stroke Initiative Writing Committee and the Writing Committee for the EUSI Executive Committee. *Cerebrovasc Dis* 2006; 22(4): 294–316.

10. Rost NS, Greenberg SM, Rosand J. The genetic architecture of intracerebral hemorrhage. *Stroke* 2008; 39(7): 2166–73.

11. Goldstein JN, Gilson AJ. Critical care management of acute intracerebral hemorrhage. *Curr Treat Options Neurol* 2011; 13(2): 204–16.

12. Xi G, Keep RF, Hoff JT. Mechanisms of brain injury after intracerebral haemorrhage. *Lancet Neurol* 2006; 5(1): 53–63.

13. Vinters HV. Cerebral amyloid angiopathy: a critical review. *Stroke* 1987; 18(2): 311–24.

14. Lou M, Lieb K, Selim M. The relationship between hematoma iron content and perihematoma edema: an MRI study. *Cerebrovasc Dis* 2009; 27(3): 266–71.

15. Brott T, Broderick J, Kothari R, *et al.* Early hemorrhage growth in patients with intracerebral hemorrhage. *Stroke* 1997; 28(1): 1–5.

16. Kazui S, Naritomi H, Yamamoto H, Sawada T, Yamaguchi T. Enlargement of spontaneous intracerebral hemorrhage: incidence and time course. *Stroke* 1996; 27(10): 1783–7.

17. Dowlatshahi D, Demchuk AM, Flaherty ML, *et al.* Defining hematoma expansion in intracerebral hemorrhage: relationship with patient outcomes. *Neurology* 2011; 76(14): 1238–44.

18. Runchey S, McGee S. Does this patient have a hemorrhagic stroke?: clinical findings distinguishing hemorrhagic stroke from ischemic stroke. *JAMA* 2010; 303(22): 2280–6.

19. Morgenstern LB, Hemphill JC 3rd, Anderson C, *et al.* Guidelines for the management of spontaneous intracerebral hemorrhage: a guideline for healthcare professionals from the American Heart Association/American Stroke Association. *Stroke* 2010; 41(9): 2108–29.

20. Ginde AA, Foianini A, Renner DM, Valley M, Camargo CA Jr. Availability and quality of computed tomography and magnetic resonance imaging equipment in U.S. emergency departments. *Acad Emerg Med* 2008; 15(8): 780–3.

21. Chalela JA, Kidwell CS, Nentwich LM, *et al.* Magnetic resonance imaging and computed tomography in emergency assessment of patients with suspected acute stroke: a prospective comparison. *Lancet* 2007; 369(9558): 293–8.

22. Kidwell CS, Chalela JA, Saver JL, *et al.* Comparison of MRI and CT for detection of acute intracerebral hemorrhage. *JAMA* 2004; 292(15): 1823–30.

23. Singer OC, Sitzer M, du Mesnil de Rochemont R, Neumann-Haefelin T. Practical limitations of acute stroke MRI due to patient-related problems. *Neurology* 2004; 62(10): 1848–9.

24. Goldstein JN, Fazen LE, Snider R, *et al.* Contrast extravasation on CT angiography predicts hematoma expansion in intracerebral hemorrhage. *Neurology* 2007; 68(12): 889–94.

25. Wada R, Aviv RI, Fox AJ, *et al.* CT angiography "spot sign" predicts hematoma expansion in acute intracerebral hemorrhage. *Stroke* 2007; 38(4): 1257–62.

26. Zhu XL, Chan MS, Poon WS. Spontaneous intracranial hemorrhage: which patients need diagnostic cerebral angiography? A prospective study of 206 cases and review of the literature. *Stroke* 1997; 28(7): 1406–9.

27. Delgado Almandoz JE, Schaefer PW, Goldstein JN, *et al.* Practical scoring system for the identification of patients with intracerebral hemorrhage at highest risk of harboring an underlying vascular etiology: the Secondary Intracerebral Hemorrhage Score. *AJNR Am J Neuroradiol* 2010; 31(9): 1653–60.

28. Diringer MN, Edwards DF. Admission to a neurologic/neurosurgical intensive care unit is associated with reduced mortality rate after intracerebral hemorrhage. *Crit Care Med* 2001; 29(3): 635–40.

29. Becker KJ, Baxter AB, Cohen WA, *et al.* Withdrawal of support in intracerebral hemorrhage may lead to self-fulfilling prophecies. *Neurology* 2001; 56(6): 766–72.

30. Zahuranec DB, Brown DL, Lisabeth LD, *et al.* Early care limitations independently predict mortality after intracerebral hemorrhage. *Neurology* 2007; 68(20): 1651–7.

31. Gujjar AR, Deibert E, Manno EM, Duff S, Diringer MN. Mechanical ventilation for ischemic stroke and intracerebral hemorrhage: indications, timing, and outcome. *Neurology* 1998; 51(2): 447–51.

32. Gray CS, Hildreth AJ, Sandercock PA, *et al.* Glucose-potassium-insulin infusions in the management of post-stroke hyperglycaemia: the UK Glucose Insulin in Stroke Trial (GIST-UK). *Lancet Neurol* 2007; 6(5): 397–406.

33. Schwarz S, Hafner K, Aschoff A, Schwab S. Incidence and prognostic significance of fever following intracerebral hemorrhage. *Neurology* 2000; 54(2): 354–61.

34. Anderson CS, Huang Y, Wang JG, *et al.* Intensive blood pressure reduction in acute cerebral haemorrhage trial (INTERACT): a randomised pilot trial. *Lancet Neurol* 2008; 7(5): 391–9.

35. Antihypertensive Treatment of Acute Cerebral Hemorrhage (ATACH) Investigators. Antihypertensive treatment of acute cerebral hemorrhage. *Crit Care Med* 2010; 38(2): 637–48.

36. Goldstein JN, Rosand J, Schwamm LH. Warfarin reversal in anticoagulant-associated intracerebral hemorrhage. *Neurocrit Care* 2008; 9(2): 277–83.

37. Steiner T, Rosand J, Diringer M. Intracerebral hemorrhage associated with oral anticoagulant therapy: current practices and unresolved questions. *Stroke* 2006; 37(1): 256–62.

38. Skolnick BE, Mathews DR, Khutoryansky NM, Pusateri AE, Carr ME. Exploratory study on the reversal of warfarin with rFVIIa in healthy subjects. *Blood* 2010; 116(5): 693–701.

39. Watanabe M, Siddiqui FM, Qureshi AI. Incidence and management of ischemic stroke and intracerebral hemorrhage in patients on dabigatran etexilate treatment. *Neurocrit Care* 2012; 16(1): 203–9.

40. Eerenberg ES, Kamphuisen PW, Sijpkens MK, *et al.* Reversal of rivaroxaban and dabigatran by prothrombin complex concentrate: a randomized, placebo-controlled, crossover study in healthy subjects. *Circulation* 2011; 124(14): 1573–9.

41. Thompson BB, Bejot Y, Caso V, *et al.* Prior antiplatelet therapy and outcome following intracerebral hemorrhage: a systematic review. *Neurology* 2010; 75(15): 1333–42.

42. Guidelines for the management of severe traumatic brain injury. *J Neurotrauma* 2007; 24(suppl 1): S1–106.

43. Bladin CF, Alexandrov AV, Bellavance A, *et al.* Seizures after stroke: a prospective multicenter study. *Arch Neurol* 2000; 57(11): 1617–22.

44. Messe SR, Sansing LH, Cucchiara BL, *et al.* Prophylactic antiepileptic drug use is associated with poor outcome following ICH. *Neurocrit Care* 2009; 11(1): 38–44.

45. Hanley DF. Intraventricular hemorrhage: severity factor and treatment target in spontaneous intracerebral hemorrhage. *Stroke* 2009; 40(4): 1533–8.

46. Morgan T, Awad I, Keyl P, Lane K, Hanley D. Preliminary report of the Clot Lysis Evaluating Accelerated Resolution of Intraventricular Hemorrhage (CLEAR-IVH) clinical trial. *Acta Neurochir Suppl* 2008; 105: 217–20.

47. Mendelow AD, Gregson BA, Fernandes HM, *et al.* Early surgery versus initial conservative treatment in patients with spontaneous supratentorial intracerebral haematomas in the International Surgical Trial in Intracerebral Haemorrhage (STICH): a randomised trial. *Lancet* 2005; 365(9457): 387–97.

48. Hemphill JC 3rd, Bonovich DC, Besmertis L, Manley GT, Johnston SC. The ICH score: a simple, reliable grading scale for intracerebral hemorrhage. *Stroke* 2001; 32(4): 891–7.

49. Rost NS, Smith EE, Chang Y, *et al.* Prediction of functional outcome in patients with primary intracerebral hemorrhage: the FUNC score. *Stroke* 2008; 39(8): 2304–9.

50. Feigin VL, Lawes CM, Bennett DA, Barker-Collo SL, Parag V. Worldwide stroke incidence and early case fatality reported in 56 population-based studies: a systematic review. *Lancet Neurol* 2009; 8(4): 355–69.

51. Brainin M, Teuschl Y, Kalra L. Acute treatment and long-term management of stroke in developing countries. *Lancet Neurol* 2007; 6(6): 553–61.

52. Connor MD, Modi G, Warlow CP. Accuracy of the Siriraj and Guy's Hospital Stroke Scores in urban South Africans. *Stroke* 2007; 38(1): 62–8.

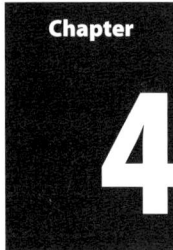

Aneurysmal subarachnoid hemorrhage

Jonathan A. Edlow

Headaches are exceedingly common. Most are categorized as migraine or tension type. Two percent of all emergency department (ED) patients have a chief complaint of headache; of those, 2 to 4% have a serious life-, limb-, brain-, or vision-threatening condition (Table 4.1).[1,2] One such condition is subarachnoid hemorrhage (SAH). Trauma is the leading cause of SAH. Of non-traumatic cases, ruptured intracranial aneurysms account for 80%. Of the remaining 20%, half are caused by non-aneurysmal venous "perimesencephalic" hemorrhages. Arteriovenous malformations, other vascular lesions, tumors, and other less common disorders account for the other half. This chapter will focus on aneurysmal SAH.

SAH is an uncommon cause of headache. Less than 1% of ED patients with headache have SAH; however, among patients with severe, abrupt-onset headache and normal neurologic examinations, 8 to 12% have SAH.[3–5] The initial bleed can be fatal, result in significant neurologic dysfunction, or produce relatively minor symptoms. Because early treatment is associated with improved outcomes, timely diagnosis is critical. Despite a straightforward diagnostic algorithm, misdiagnosis remains common. Mildly affected patients (who are most commonly misdiagnosed) have the best outcomes if the condition is correctly identified and treated.[6,7] Misdiagnosis of SAH may lead to medicolegal actions against physicians. National guidelines have been promulgated for the diagnosis and treatment of SAH.[8]

Incidence of aneurysms and effects of rupture

Intracranial aneurysms are common and are located on the large arteries of the circle of Willis and its

Table 4.1 "Cannot miss" causes of acute headache

- Subarachnoid hemorrhage.
- Meningitis or encephalitis.
- Cervical or cranial artery dissections.
- Temporal arteritis.
- Acute narrow angle-closure glaucoma.
- Hypertensive emergencies.
- Carbon monoxide poisoning.
- Idiopathic intracranial hypertension (pseudotumor cerebri).
- Spontaneous intracranial hypotension.
- Cerebral venous and dural sinus thrombosis.
- Acute stroke (hemorrhagic or ischemic).
- Pituitary apoplexy.
- Reversible cerebral vasoconstriction syndrome.
- Mass lesions.
  - Tumor.
  - Abscess.
  - Parameningeal infection.
  - Intracranial hematoma.
  - Colloid cyst of third ventricle.

branches. Autopsy series uncover them in 0.4 to 3.6% of individuals, and cerebral angiography documents incidental aneurysms in 3.7 to 6.0% of patients. Therefore, roughly 2% of all individuals harbor aneurysms. Approximately 80 to 85% of these lesions are in the anterior cerebral circulation; cerebral aneurysms are multiple in 25% of cases.[9]

The reasons for aneurysmal rupture are incompletely understood. Although local hemodynamic forces may initiate aneurysmal formation, the tensile stress in the aneurysm wall may be more important in rupture. Larger aneurysm size and aspect ratio (dome size/neck size) correlate independently with risk of rupture. Surface irregularities or multiple lobes on the aneurysm confer additive risk.

When an aneurysm does rupture, the intracranial pressure (ICP) rises precipitously. Cerebral perfusion may cease transiently, resulting in unconsciousness or death if the ICP is sufficiently high to cause

Vascular Emergencies, ed. Robert L. Rogers, Thomas Scalea, Lee Wallis, and Heike Geduld. Published by Cambridge University Press. © Cambridge University Press 2013.

Table 4.2 Common grading scales for subarachnoid hemorrhage (SAH)

(A) Hunt and Hess Severity Scale

Grade 1: Asymptomatic, mild headache

Grade 2: Moderate to severe headache, nuchal rigidity, no focal deficit other than cranial nerve palsy

Grade 3: Mild mental status change (drowsy or confused), mild focal neurologic deficit

Grade 4: Stupor or moderate to severe hemiparesis

Grade 5: Comatose or decerebrate rigidity

(B) World Federation of Neurological Surgeons

Grade 1: GCS score 15, no motor deficit

Grade 2: GCS score 13 or 14, no motor deficit

Grade 3: GCS score 13 or 14, motor deficit present

Grade 4: GCS score 7 to 12, motor deficit can be present or absent

Grade 5: GCS score 3 to 6, motor deficit can be present or absent

(C) Fisher Scale (CT appearance)

Group 1: No blood

Group 2: Diffuse deposits of SAH blood, no clots, no layers of blood >1 mm

Group 3: Local clots or vertical layers of blood ≥ 1 mm thick

Group 4: Diffuse or no SAH, but intracerebral or intraventricular clot

GCS, Glasgow Coma Scale.

irreversible structural damage or halt cerebral perfusion. SAH results in hemodynamic instability, metabolic disturbances, and neurocardiogenic injury, including ventricular dysfunction, cardiac enzyme leak, and electrocardiographic abnormalities. The mortality rates on the first day and during the first month after hemorrhage are approximately 12% and 40%, respectively.

The patient's clinical status at diagnosis is commonly measured by two metrics: the Hunt and Hess (H&H) grade and the World Federation of Neurosurgical Societies (WFNS) scale (Table 4.2). Hunt and Hess's original paper correlated clinical grade with death. Although commonly used, the H&H scale is somewhat subjective and is associated with significant interobserver variability. The more objective WFNS scale is based on the Glasgow Coma Scale (GCS) and the presence or absence of motor deficits. Other grading scales have been proposed but are not widely used. Their common thread is that higher scores indicate worse clinical condition and result in worse outcomes.

Epidemiology

The incidence of SAH, which has been stable over time, is roughly 10 per 100,000 of the population. SAH is more common in blacks and Hispanics than in whites. Women, especially those who are post-menopausal, are more frequently affected than men. Some studies suggest a rising incidence in elderly patients and a decreasing incidence in men.[10]

Given that the prevalence of aneurysms is approximately 200 times higher than the annual incidence of SAH, it is clear that most aneurysms do not rupture. Peak age at rupture is 50 years. Important risks for SAH include heavy alcohol use, cigarette smoking, hypertension, and possibly oral contraception use. The risk is also increased by a family or personal history of SAH and the use of cocaine. Disorders associated with SAH include autosomal dominant polycystic kidney disease, Ehlers–Danlos syndrome type IV, and neurofibromatosis type 1.[11]

Diagnosis

Which patients to evaluate?

Numerous studies over several decades document that SAH is misdiagnosed in approximately 25% of patients with the disorder (12–50%), even in this era of ready access to cranial computed tomographic (CT) scanning. These studies point to three recurring, preventable reasons for misdiagnosis: failure to consider the diagnosis, failure to perform (and correctly interpret) CT scans, and failure to perform (and correctly interpret the results of) lumbar puncture (LP) (Table 4.3).[6,7] One large study found that failure to obtain a CT scan was the most common error.[12] The largest and most recent report, from a Canadian population-based study, found a much lower rate of ED-attributable misdiagnoses (5.4%), and older studies include misdiagnoses attributable to patients, primary care physicians, and specialists.[13] The misdiagnosis rate might be decreasing, but methodological differences across these studies preclude a firm conclusion.

The first decision emergency physicians must make when evaluating patients with headache is whether to pursue diagnostic studies beyond the history and physical examination. Patients with SAH have a typical presentation – the abrupt onset of the worst headache of the person's life (a "thunderclap" headache) during exercise or the Valsalva maneuver, associated

Table 4.3 Reasons for misdiagnosis of SAH

- Failure to know the spectrum of presentations of subarachnoid hemorrhage.
- Not evaluating patients with unusual (for the patient) headaches.
  - Is the onset abrupt?
  - Is the quality different from previous headaches?
  - Is the severity greater than previous headaches?
- Are there associated symptoms that have been absent with prior headaches (such as vomiting, diplopia, syncope, or seizure)?
- Failure to appreciate that the headache can improve spontaneously or with non-narcotic analgesics.
- Over-reliance on the classic presentation, leading to misdiagnosis of the following:
  - Viral syndrome, viral meningitis, and gastroenteritis.
  - Migraine and tension-type headache.
  - Sinus-related headache.
  - Neck pain (rarely, back pain).
  - Psychiatric diagnoses.
- Focus on the secondary head injury (resulting from syncope and fall or a car crash).
- Focus on the electrocardiographic abnormalities.
- Focus on the elevated blood pressure.
- Lack of knowledge of presentations of the unruptured aneurysm.
- Failure to understand the limitations of computerized tomographic (CT) scans.
- CT scans are less sensitive with increasing time from onset of headache.
- CT scan can be falsely negative with small-volume bleeds (spectrum bias).
- Interpretation factors (expertise of the physician reading the scan).
- Technical factors. (Have thin cuts been taken at the base of the brain? Is motion artifact present?)
- CT can be falsely negative for blood at a hematocrit of less than 30%.
- Failure to perform lumbar puncture and correctly interpret cerebrospinal fluid findings.
- Failure to perform lumbar puncture in patients with negative, equivocal, or suboptimal CT scans.
- Failure to recognize that xanthochromia may be absent very early (<12 hours) and very late (>2 weeks).
- Failure to understand the limitations of xanthochromia measurement.
- Failure to properly distinguish a traumatic tap from true subarachnoid hemorrhage.

with transient syncope and vomiting – which facilitates the diagnosis. Evaluation of patients with headache who also have cognitive impairment, new focal abnormalities, or meningismus is also clear-cut.[6,7]

Less clear is when to evaluate patients with milder symptoms and normal neurologic examinations. One well-done, prospective (but as yet not validated) study identified high-risk characteristics in headache patients that suggest evaluation for SAH is needed.[14] The high-risk findings include higher age, elevated blood pressure (SBP > 100 mmHg and DBP > 100

mmHg), vomiting, loss of consciousness, neck pain or stiffness, onset on exertion, and arrival by ambulance.

Until these data are validated, we believe that four elements of the history best identify most patients for whom diagnostic testing is warranted: onset, severity, quality, and associated symptoms. The onset is usually sudden, and the patient usually describes the headache's severity as "the worst of my life." Since headaches are so common, comparing the quality of the index headache with any previous ones is important. Patients usually describe the headache from SAH as clearly different from other headaches. Ten percent of neurologically normal patients with abrupt-onset, severe, and unusual headaches have SAH. Half of all SAH patients present with atypical or mild features. Associated symptoms such as nausea, vomiting, neck pain, and stiffness are common. However, neck stiffness (meningismus) may be absent, especially in the early hours. Headache patients over the age of 50 are more likely to have SAH and other serious intracranial pathology.[2,15]

In many patients with SAH, the headaches begin at rest or during quiet activities. Presenting symptoms include vomiting, fever, headache, mild confusion, delirium, or severe neck pain, suggesting diagnoses such as a viral syndrome, gastroenteritis, psychiatric disorders, or neck strain. Undue focus on the associated findings, e.g., an abnormal electrocardiogram, arrhythmia, head injury (from syncope), or elevated blood pressure, can divert attention from the true cause of the symptoms. The headache may lessen or resolve with non-narcotic analgesics, including sumatriptan; therefore, no diagnostic significance should be ascribed to improvement with medications.[15,16] Headache from so-called warning (or sentinel) bleeds can remit spontaneously. On the other end of the spectrum, occasional patients with SAH who present in cardiac arrest can have excellent outcomes.

Understanding the full spectrum of the possible presentations of SAH is the best strategy to avoid misdiagnosis. Once the physician decides to perform a workup, the next steps – CT scanning and LP – are straightforward.

Computed tomography scanning

The standard first test, unenhanced cranial CT (Figure 4.1), is highly accurate but, like all tests, possesses limitations. First, its accuracy decays with time, because of the circulation of cerebrospinal fluid (CSF)

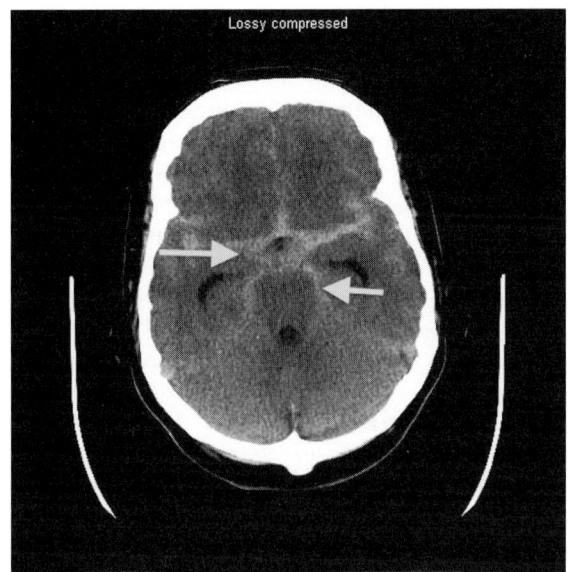

Figure 4.1 Non-contrast computed tomography scan shows an acute subarachnoid hemorrhage (SAH). The white areas in regions that normally contain cerebrospinal fluid (and are normally black) indicate an acute accumulation of blood. The blood is in the basal cisterns, a common location for aneurysmal SAH.

and the resultant dilution and catabolism of the blood. Studies using third-generation scanners demonstrate sensitivities in the range of 90 to 98% within the first 24 hours. A study of 953 neurologically intact patients with thunderclap headache who were scanned within six hours after headache onset (121 with SAH [12.7%]) found that CT was 100% sensitive (95% confidence interval, 97–100).[17] If this study can be replicated, it is possible that the workup can be limited to a CT scan if it is obtained within six hours after symptom onset. A recent retrospective report suggested that CT was 100% sensitive within three days after the headache. The incidence of SAH among these patients, who were referred to a neurosurgical unit, was 59%.[18] These results should not be extrapolated to the broad spectrum of ED patients with severe headache.

By three and seven days after the ictus, the sensitivity falls to 85% and 50%, respectively.[6,7] Aside from the issue of time, some investigators express hope that more modern scanners would make LP unnecessary. One study involving "fifth-generation" multidetector CT scanners showed that no SAH case was missed; however, the study was underpowered, and yielded a lower 95% confidence interval (CI) of only 61%.[19] Another study found the sensitivity of

modern CT scanners to be 91% in a group of neurologically intact patients.[20]

The second important limitation of CT is spectrum bias. In alert and awake patients (presumably with smaller-volume bleeds), the scans are less likely to show blood. Third, intracranial blood in anemic patients (with hematocrit < 30%) may appear isodense with brain and thus be more difficult to see. Last, many of these CT sensitivity studies relied on experienced neuroradiologists' interpretations; "real world" readings by general radiologists, neurologists, and emergency physicians are less accurate. False-positive CT scans for SAH are rare but have been reported with intravenous contrast neurotoxicity, purulent meningitis, spontaneous intracranial hypotension, isodense subdural hematomas, confusion with normal dural structures, and diffuse cerebral edema.[7] Whenever meningitis is a strong possibility, intravenous antibiotics should be administered rapidly.

Until more convincing data confirm the 100% sensitivity of ultra-early or ultra-modern CT scanning in SAH, our belief is that all patients being evaluated for SAH whose CT scans are normal, technically inadequate, or non-diagnostic, should undergo LP.

Lumbar puncture

CSF analysis also has limitations. Traumatic taps – the release of red blood cells (RBCs) from needle trauma – occur in 10 to 15% of procedures.[21] Fluoroscopically guided LP may decrease this incidence but is not routinely available. None of the methods of distinguishing traumatic taps from SAH are foolproof.[22] Like the accuracy of computed tomography, CSF findings evolve over time from onset of symptoms.

Blood from ruptured aneurysms rapidly disseminates throughout the subarachnoid space, and large numbers of RBCs appear in the lumbar theca within two to four hours. The development of xanthochromia, the yellowish hue resulting from hemoglobin catabolism into oxyhemoglobin, methemoglobin, and bilirubin, requires more time. The presence of xanthochromia indicates that the CSF contains blood that has undergone *in vivo* enzymatic degradation to bilirubin, implying true SAH. However, oxyhemoglobin can form *in vitro* and discolor the fluid in traumatic taps.

Xanthochromia can be measured visually or by spectrophotometry, the latter being clearly more sensitive. Vermeulen recommends using spectrophotometry exclusively, based on a study of 111 patients with CT-proven SAH, in which all subjects had spectrophotometrically measured xanthochromia from 12 hours to 2 weeks after the onset of headache.[23] Gunawardena and colleagues studied the more clinically relevant population of CT-negative patients. Of 463 patients, CSF spectrophotometry led to the diagnosis of SAH in 2% of patients in whom CT was negative.[24] Unfortunately, this retrospective chart review did not report the percentage of patients with visually measured xanthochromia, the timing of the LP, or the CSF RBC counts, making firm conclusions difficult.

One important problem with spectrophotometry is that, in series of unselected patients, false positives are very common, indicating that many patients without SAH are subjected to unnecessary diagnostic testing.[25] Furthermore, more than 99% of hospital laboratories in North America measure xanthochromia visually.[26] A recent comparison between the two methods found that, in CSF samples that clinicians deemed to be colorless, none contained bilirubin, as measured by spectrophotometry.[27]

However it is assessed, xanthochromia takes time to develop: up to 12 hours by spectrophotometry. Unfortunately, no well-performed clinical studies have been performed to establish false-negative rates for xanthochromia at specific time intervals from the bleed. To assess for xanthochromia, the CSF should be centrifuged rapidly and (in the case of spectrophotometry) stored in darkness. When measured visually, the CSF should be compared with an identical tube filled with an equal volume of tap water against a neutral white background. Spectrophotometric measurement should focus on the presence of bilirubin.[7]

Patients who present early usually have abnormal CT scans, and even those without xanthochromia all have large amounts of RBCs in the CSF. The rare exceptions (intraparenchymal or subdural rupture or spinal block) have positive CT scans. Two other useful, albeit imperfect, methods to distinguish traumatic taps from true bleeds are the "three-tube" test and measurement of the opening pressure of the CSF. In the former, one looks for diminishing numbers of RBCs from the first to the last tube, trending toward zero. This last detail is crucial. Older literature cautions that a "decrease" (undefined) does not discriminate between traumatic tap and true SAH, so this is not a perfect method of discrimination. A simple decrease is insufficient to exclude SAH. The RBC count in the last tube should approach zero. When bloody fluid is identified, wasting several milliliters of CSF to increase the gap

between the first and last tubes improves the odds that the last tube RBC count will approach zero. There is no specific number of RBCs that serves as a threshold amount, and the rate of RBC clearance is variable.

The opening pressure should be measured. This value is elevated in two-thirds of SAH patients and is normal in traumatic taps. Elevated pressure suggests the alternative diagnosis of cerebral venous sinus thrombosis or idiopathic intracranial hypertension. Abnormally low pressure suggests spontaneous intracranial hypotension.[7]

Diagnostic issues

Primary use of CT angiography for diagnosis of SAH

Computed tomography angiography (CTA) is very sensitive in detecting aneurysms, even those as small as 3 mm in size.[28] With the increasing availability of multidetector CT scanners, some have recommended the use of CTA to diagnose SAH.[29] For example, Carstairs and associates[29] studied a group of 116 patients with symptoms suggestive of SAH. Aneurysm was detected by CTA in six (5.1%). Of the six, three had a positive CT or CSF results; that is, these patients would have been identified by the standard workup. Three had positive CTA with normal CT scans and CSF. If one looks at their outcomes, it is very likely that they had asymptomatic aneurysms with a headache of another benign cause. As with spectrophotometry, a strategy of primary CTA for diagnosis of SAH would subject many patients to unnecessary workups, procedures, and angiographic contrast material. This strategy, which seems to be gaining momentum, has significant negative downstream implications.[30]

Magnetic resonance for primary diagnosis of SAH

The traditional view that magnetic resonance imaging (MRI) is not sensitive enough to detect acute blood is incorrect. MRI technology is constantly advancing. However, although fluid-attenuated inversion recovery (FLAIR) and T2 gradient-echo (GRE) MRI may be better than CT for detection of chronic subarachnoid blood and possibly equivalent for intraparenchymal hemorrhage, false-positive results have been documented in acute SAH with both techniques.[7]

In a series of 13 patients with positive CT scans who were tested within 12 hours after symptom onset by MRI (FLAIR and proton-density weighted), all were positive for SAH.[31] However, another study showed that of 12 patients with SAH (and negative CT scans), only the two with the highest RBC counts had FLAIR MRI findings positive for SAH, showing that spectrum bias exists with MR as well.[32] No large studies of the use of MRI to diagnose unselected headache patients have been reported. Therefore, CT, which is quicker, cheaper, more readily available, and easier to interpret, remains the diagnostic study of choice. If MRI is chosen for this diagnostic purpose, communication with a radiologist is critical to ensure acquisition of the correct sequences.

Lumbar puncture – first strategy

Some clinicians have advocated an LP-first strategy in patients with severe acute headache and normal vital signs and physical examination findings.[33] The rationale is that, in practice, physicians evaluating patients for SAH often omit LP after a negative CT scan. An LP-first strategy forces the LP to be done and therefore consumes fewer resources. This strategy may be particularly useful in an environment without access to CT.

An LP-first strategy may be safe, even in H&H grade 2 and 3 patients who have meningismus and are drowsy. However, this practice can be dangerous, since collecting CSF from patients with SAH may precipitate rebleeding or herniation from an unrecognized intracranial hematoma, which can occur in the absence of localizing neurologic findings.[34] Most of the patients who deteriorated in the two studies mentioned in this section had neck stiffness and were H&H grades 1 through 3 (mostly grade 2), although one patient did not exhibit meningismus.

An LP-first strategy is likely safe in carefully selected patients who are neurologically normal and without signs of elevated ICP. On the other hand, this approach is contraindicated in patients with any kind of neurologic abnormalities on examination and in those with symptoms or signs of high ICP. Unfortunately, no clinical trials have been conducted to assist clinicians in selecting patients for this approach, so CT followed by LP remains the standard diagnostic sequence.

When to stop the workup

Is further evaluation necessary in patients with acute, severe headache and normal neurologic examinations, CT scans, and CSF analysis? The vast majority of such patients have excellent outcomes. In a pooled analysis of seven studies involving 813 patients with thunderclap headache and normal CT and LP, none was found to have experienced sudden death or SAH in follow-up studies (six months to three years).[35] This evidence strongly suggests that most patients with normal CT and CSF examinations do not require angiography.

The occasional patients whose clinical presentation suggests cranial artery dissection, cerebral venous sinus thrombosis, reversible cerebrovascular constriction syndrome, or pituitary apoplexy may require further imaging. Some others with an exceptionally high pretest risk for SAH may require vascular imaging.

"Warning" or "sentinel" symptoms

Some patients with SAH report unusual, severe headaches in the weeks preceding their SAH diagnosis – a phenomenon loosely described in the literature as "warning bleeds" or "sentinel headaches." Such headaches occur in 10 to 43% of cases of SAH.[36] Possible explanations for these episodes include: (1) the initial misdiagnosis of a true SAH (missed recognition by the patient or missed diagnosis by the physician, (2) recall bias of patients being admitted for a serious neurologic problem, or (3) pain from symptomatic but unruptured aneurysms. The most likely explanation, supported by histologic evidence in one case, is that most instances represent small undiagnosed SAHs. Data supporting this hypothesis are mixed, some showing no worse outcomes in patients returning after a "warning" event and others showing worse outcomes. Whatever the explanation, aggressive evaluation of patients with severe headache of acute onset should reduce the number of delayed or missed diagnoses.

Symptomatic unruptured aneurysms

The vast majority of unruptured aneurysms are asymptomatic, but some patients have thunderclap headache from intact aneurysms that are acutely expanding, dissecting, or thrombosing.[37] Other symptoms of unruptured aneurysms include transient cerebral ischemia, gradual-onset headache, seizure, or mass

Table 4.4 Management issues to be addressed when SAH is diagnosed

- Airway management.
- Specialist consultation and arranging an angiogram.
- Arrangement for transfer to a neurovascular center.
- Treatment of hypertension.
- Volume status and intravenous fluids.
- Seizure prophylaxis.
- Acute treatment of hydrocephalus, extra-axial or intracerebral hematomas.
- Nimodipine administration for vasospasm prophylaxis.
- Short-term antifibrinolytics to prevent rebleeding.
- Cardiac telemetry.
- Analgesia.
- Intracranial pressure.

When SAH is diagnosed, rapidly consult with a cerebrovascular expert. This discussion should consider the points above on a case-by-case basis.

effect. The classic mass lesion is a third cranial nerve palsy.[38] Symptomatic unruptured aneurysms should be treated.

Initial management considerations

Once the diagnosis of SAH is established, the priority shifts to definitive therapy, prevention of complications, and consultation with a skilled cerebrovascular specialist.[7] The discussion between specialist and emergency physician should address several issues, including airway control, treatment of acute hydrocephalus, blood pressure control, seizure, and vasospasm prophylaxis (Table 4.4). In this age of endovascular treatment, the disposition of patients with SAH needs to be re-evaluated, since data suggest that SAH patients do better when treated in high-volume centers that offer surgical and endovascular approaches.[39–41]

Airway management

Patients with SAH often have altered sensorium and poor airway reflexes. When they are transferred from one facility to another in a supine position, they become prone to aspiration. Once a neurologic examination is done, patients with a decreased level of consciousness should be intubated, if necessary. Rapid-sequence intubation with adequate preoxygenation and pharmacologic therapy to prevent acute spikes in blood pressure should be performed. An orogastric tube should be placed immediately after intubation to prevent aspiration.

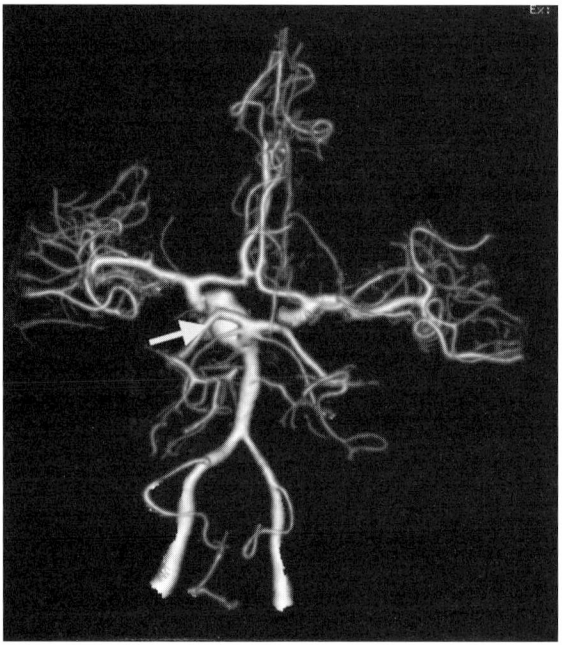

Figure 4.2 Reconstruction of a computed tomography angiogram, demonstrating a basilar artery aneurysm.

Cerebrovascular imaging

Upon diagnosis of SAH, cerebrovascular imaging should be obtained as soon as possible after stabilization. A high-quality, four-vessel cerebral digital subtraction angiogram (DSA) usually elucidates the cause of the SAH. Angiograms may be negative in patients with perimesencephalic hemorrhage, thrombosed aneurysms, or severe parent vessel spasm, which can interfere with aneurysmal filling.[7] In the case of intracranial aneurysm, 2D or 3D angiography demonstrates the size and location of the aneurysm very well. Modern DSA is very safe: one prospective series of nearly 3000 procedures revealed a complication rate of only 1.3%, and more than half of those cases were transient or reversible.[42] In the hands of an interventionalist, DSA also provides the means for endovascular treatment. Digital subtraction angiograms fail to identify a source of hemorrhage in 20 to 25% of patients with SAH. In this group, follow-up angiography after one week will identify a source in another 1 to 2% of patients.

Although DSA remains the gold standard, multidetector CTA (Figure 4.2) demonstrates high sensitivity and specificity. Four studies have evaluated a strategy of using only CTA to plan the surgical approach in large numbers of patients with SAH.[43–46] Other investigators have accumulated experience with surgical planning based exclusively on MRA. Occasionally, both CTA and MRA miss small aneurysms. Evidence suggests that neuroradiologists' interpretations may be superior to others. As of this writing, in 2012, the choice of cerebrovascular imaging study is evolving and should be left to the discretion of the consultant.

Rebleeding and blood pressure control

Rebleeding, an important cause of poor outcomes, is common in the hours to days after the initial bleed. In the first two weeks, about 25% of patients will rebleed if the aneurysm is not secured.[47] Those who rebleed tend to have higher H&H grades, larger aneurysms, and worse outcomes.[48] Therefore, strategies to reduce rebleeding are critical.

Although few data suggest that aggressively lowering blood pressure prevents rebleeding, most treating physicians insert an arterial catheter and use intravenous agents to maintain adequate cerebral perfusion in the patient with elevated ICP and in elderly patients with pre-existing atherosclerosis or hypertension. The limited data available seem to indicate that maintaining a systolic pressure below 150 to 160 is protective with regard to rebleeding. These steps are generally initiated in the intensive care unit. As there is no high-quality evidence to suggest the proper target blood pressure, this choice is generally left to the consultant. The most common antihypertensive agents used are labetalol, nicardipine, esmolol, and nitroprusside. No head-to-head clinical trials have been done to compare these agents. Nitroprusside, a vasodilator that can increase ICP, is generally best avoided. Treatment of pain and anxiety may also reduce elevated blood pressure. Conversely, hypotension should be avoided, as it will reduce cerebral perfusion, especially in situations where the ICP is elevated.

In the past, when surgery was delayed by weeks, antifibrinolytics (ε-aminocaproic acid and tranexamic acid) were used to reduce rebleeding. Current trends toward early aneurysm obliteration have reduced the need for long-term antifibrinolytic use. However, there is emerging interest in using short-term antifibrinolytics from the time of diagnosis to the time of definitive treatment, even if this interval is only several hours. A randomized, prospective, multicenter trial using short-term tranexamic acid suggested this strategy reduced rebleeding without increasing vasospasm or clinically significant cerebral ischemia.[49]

Hydrocephalus

Hydrocephalus occurs in one-third of all patients with SAH and is more likely to occur with larger volume hemorrhages.[50] Acute (early) hydrocephalus from intraventricular blood that occludes the foramen of Monro, magendic or Luschka, obstructing CSF outflow, occurs, in approximately 20% of patients. This cause of coma after SAH is reversible by treatment with emergent ventriculostomy.

Vasospasm, delayed cerebral ischemia, and seizure prophylaxis

Cerebral vasospasm typically develops several days after the initial SAH, peaking 7 to 10 days after the hemorrhage and lasting up to two weeks. The risk of developing vasospasm is related to the density of blood at the time of initial ictus, which is graded objectively using the Fisher Scale. Vasospasm may be an asymptomatic angiographic phenomenon, or it may lead to symptomatic delayed cerebral ischemia (DCI), which is an important cause of morbidity after SAH.[51] The resulting infarctions might be asymptomatic and can occur distant from the site of the offending aneurysm.[52] Emergency physicians should be aware of this fact since some patients present during this phase.

Prophylactic use of oral nimodipine improves outcomes, although its mechanism remains unclear.[53] Preliminary data suggest that intravenous magnesium sulfate may reduce the incidence of DCI and poor outcomes, but further research is needed to confirm these findings.[54]

If vasospasm is confirmed or suspected in the presence of neurologic deterioration, "triple H" therapy (hypertension, hemodilution, and hypervolemia) can be instituted.[55] Although a recent Cochrane Review concluded that there is no convincing evidence supporting it, triple H therapy is commonly used in practice.[56] If medical therapy fails, various endovascular strategies can be employed. These therapies underscore the advantages of a high-volume neurovascular center.

Fewer than 20% of patients with SAH have seizures.[57] Actual seizures should be treated with anticonvulsants. National guidelines recommend "considering" prophylactic anticonvulsants[8] since they pose some potential risk.[58]

Aneurysm obliteration

Early treatment of a ruptured aneurysm is the accepted strategy at most centers.[59] Occasionally, extenuating circumstances such as an unstable medical condition or a high classification grade and poor prognosis preclude surgery and delay treatment. However, the goal in most patients is to obliterate the aneurysm within one to three days after the hemorrhage with either microsurgical aneurysm clipping or endovascular coil embolization.

Intracranial microsurgical clipping is a technique that has evolved considerably since its introduction in the 1970s. Its development was made possible by the advent of the stereoscopic high-magnification microscope. Using microsurgical techniques, the neurosurgeon opens the dura, identifies the parent vessel and the ruptured aneurysm, and then clips the aneurysm to exclude it from the circulation. The durability of successful surgical clipping is high, with a follow-up study showing an aneurysm recurrence rate of 2 to 3%.

Endovascular coiling uses a microcatheter, which is threaded through a guide catheter to the origin of the ruptured aneurysm. Once inside the aneurysm, platinum coils are gently inserted into the sac in a sequential outside-in multilayered fashion until the aneurysm is densely packed (Figure 4.3). This process relies on a critical volume of embolization and requires that the aneurysm inflow zone be occluded securely to deflect blood from entering the aneurysm. Although wide-necked aneurysms were initially considered poor candidates for coil embolization, newer techniques have expanded the pool of endovascular candidates.

Patients treated with coil therapy require serial monitoring and follow-up cerebrovascular imaging to detect coil compaction or aneurysm recanalization, which occurs occasionally in larger wide-necked or poorly packed aneurysms. After the initial treatment, up to 70% of patients experience 95 to 100% occlusion of the aneurysm. However, complete obliteration is not achieved in 25 to 30% of patients, and recanalization can occur.[60]

The decision to proceed with open surgical clipping or endovascular treatment of an intracranial aneurysm after SAH rests on aneurysm-specific factors (location, size, morphology, and presence of thrombus) and patient-specific factors (age, density of SAH, patient

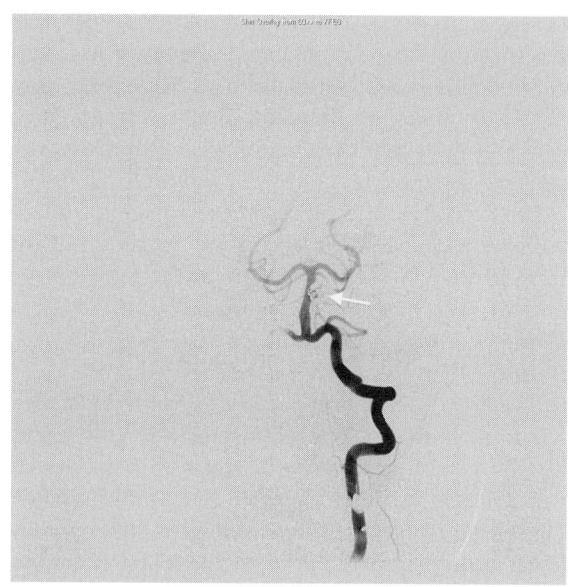

Figure 4.3 The response to coiling, showing the ghost of the aneurysm and the platinum coils within it.

preference, and medical comorbidities). The International Subarachnoid Aneurysm Trial (ISAT) randomized 2,143 SAH patients whose aneurysms were judged to be equally suitable for surgical clipping or endovascular coiling.[61] Because of the selection criteria, patients were typically in good pretreatment condition and had a preponderance of anterior circulation aneurysms. Using a modified Rankin Scale at one year as the outcome measure, the ISAT demonstrated a statistically significant relative risk reduction of 22.6% and an absolute risk reduction of 6.9% in favor of the endovascular procedure. Follow-up (one to seven years) revealed the durability of these outcomes.[62] The endovascularly treated patients had fewer seizures but more rebleeding. Similar results have been obtained in other studies.

The superiority of endovascular procedures is more evident in patients older than 65 years and in those with posterior circulation aneurysms. Retrospective studies based on the National Inpatient Sample database demonstrate that endovascular procedures result in less peri-procedural morbidity and mortality in patients with unruptured aneurysms. Nationwide, a greater proportion of ruptured aneurysms are being treated with endovascular procedures. Although higher recanalization rates in coiled aneurysms lead to a higher risk of rebleeding, the rates of rebleeding have been less than 1% and still do not negate the initial benefit over clipping. Emergency physicians need to be aware that a coiled aneurysm can recanalize and become symptomatic, for example, as SAH or diplopia. Since platinum coils produce artifact on CTA, the imaging modality of choice to detect recanalized aneurysms would be MRA.

Ideally, high-quality endovascular and surgical techniques will be available at a neurovascular center, allowing the best treatment decisions to be made on a case-by-case basis. Whether treated with an endovascular or a surgical procedure, patients should be monitored closely for blood pressure and for cardiac, renal, and respiratory function by a multidisciplinary team, with close neurologic monitoring to detect DCI. Table 4.5 lists various guidelines that are available.

Limited resources

In a location without CT availability, one could diagnose SAH with a lumbar puncture. This is probably safe in an alert conscious patient, but could be dangerous in those headache patients with focal or global neurologic abnormalities. The presence of bloody or xanthochromic CSF would suggest the diagnosis. In this situation, one could lower the blood pressure as above. However without the ability to define the vascular lesion and its location, there is not much more definitive care that could be accomplished, apart from transfer to a center that has these capabilities.

Critical actions

1. Evaluate patients with thunderclap headache thoroughly to exclude subarachnoid hemorrhage.
2. Remember that the sensitivity of diagnostic studies for subarachnoid hemorrhage changes with time from the onset of headache.
3. After diagnosing a subarachnoid hemorrhage, next steps include defining the causative vascular lesion, monitoring for, preventing, and treating complications, and prompt referral to a neurovascular specialist.

Pearls and pitfalls

The most serious pitfall in diagnosing SAH is not thinking about it; misdiagnosis still occurs. It is vital that emergency clinicians know that many patients with SAH are awake, alert, and have normal neurologic examinations. Although CT is very sensitive, especially in the first hours after the bleed, LP is

Table 4.5 Statements based on American College of Emergency Physicians (ACEP) and AHA guidelines for ED patients with headache and subarachnoid hemorrhage

(A) 2008 ACEP Clinical Policy on Acute Headache (evidence-based recommendations)

1. Emergent head CT **IS** the initial diagnostic study recommended in the diagnosis of any new, sudden-onset, severe headache or suspected case of SAH.

2. Lumbar puncture **IS** recommended for patients with suspected SAH after negative non-contrast head CT.

3. Angiography is **NOT** recommended in patients with sudden-onset, severe headache who have negative findings on head CT, normal opening pressure, and negative CSF findings.

4. Patients with a negative workup including negative CT and normal LP **CAN** be safely discharged from the ED with outpatient follow-up recommended.

5. Response to analgesia should **NOT** be used as the sole indicator of the cause of an acute headache.

(B) Additional guidelines (evidence and expert consensus-based recommendations)

Diagnostic recommendations

1. Although one guideline recommends spectrophotometry over visual inspection for CSF analysis, this practice is controversial (spectrophotometry is unavailable in the vast majority of North American clinical laboratories).

2. Once SAH is diagnosed, urgent cerebral angiography (CTA or MRA) **IS** needed to detect the underlying cerebral aneurysm.

Management recommendations

1. Control of elevated blood pressure **IS** recommended to balance the risk of stroke and rebleeding and for maintenance of cerebral perfusion pressure.

2. Oral nimodipine **IS** strongly recommended to reduce poor outcome from vasospasm.

3. Prophylactic anticonvulsant therapy **MAY** be considered in the immediate post-hemorrhage period.

4. Early surgery **IS** recommended for the majority of patients.

Disposition recommendations

1. Patients with SAH should be managed in an intensive care unit setting with cardiac and blood pressure monitoring.

2. Early referral to high-volume centers with cerebrovascular surgeons and endovascular services **IS** recommended.

still recommended in cases where the CT is non-diagnostic. The major pearls and pitfalls are summarized in Table 4.3. Once the diagnosis is made, the next steps are well defined.

Conclusions

Emergency physicians must be vigilant in evaluating patients with symptoms consistent with SAH or otherwise symptomatic aneurysms. The evaluation must take place with an understanding of the limitations of the available diagnostic tests. Attention to early complications and prompt referral to centers where there are teams with cerebrovascular expertise will maximize the options available to these patients.

References

1. Goldstein JN, Camargo CA Jr, Pelletier AJ, Edlow JA. Headache in United States emergency departments: demographics, work-up and frequency of pathological diagnoses. *Cephalalgia* 2006; 26(6): 684–90.

2. Ramirez-Lassepas M, Espinosa CE, Cicero JJ, *et al.* Predictors of intracranial pathologic findings in patients who seek emergency care because of headache. *Arch Neurol* 1997; 54(12): 1506–9.

3. Landtblom AM, Fridriksson S, Boivie J, *et al.* Sudden onset headache: a prospective study of features, incidence and causes. *Cephalalgia* 2002; 22(5): 354–60.

4. Morgenstern LB, Luna-Gonzales H, Huber JC Jr, *et al.* Worst headache and subarachnoid hemorrhage: prospective, modern computed tomography and spinal fluid analysis. *Ann Emerg Med* 1998; 32(3 Pt 1): 297–304.

5. Perry JJ, Spacek A, Forbes M, *et al.* Is the combination of negative computed tomography result and negative lumbar puncture result sufficient to rule out subarachnoid hemorrhage? *Ann Emerg Med* 2008; 51(6): 707–13.

6. Edlow JA, Caplan LR. Avoiding pitfalls in the diagnosis of subarachnoid hemorrhage. *N Engl J Med* 2000; 342(1): 29–36.

7. Edlow JA, Malek AM, Ogilvy CS. Aneurysmal subarachnoid hemorrhage: update for emergency physicians. *J Emerg Med* 2008; 34(3): 237–51.

8. Bederson JB, Connolly ES Jr, Batjer HH, *et al.* Guidelines for the management of aneurysmal subarachnoid hemorrhage: a statement for healthcare professionals from a special writing group of the Stroke Council, American Heart Association. *Stroke* 2009; 40(3): 994–1025.

9. Schievink WI. Intracranial aneurysms [published erratum appears in *N Engl J Med* 1997; 336(17): 1267]. *N Engl J Med* 1997; 336(1): 28–40.

10. The ACROSS Group. Epidemiology of aneurysmal subarachnoid hemorrhage in Australia and New Zealand: incidence and case fatality from the Australasian Cooperative Research on Subarachnoid Hemorrhage Study (ACROSS). *Stroke* 2000; 31(8): 1843–50.

11. Schievink WI, Michels VV, Piepgras DG. Neurovascular manifestations of heritable connective tissue disorders: a review. *Stroke* 1994; 25(4): 889–903.

12. Kowalski RG, Claassen J, Kreiter KT, *et al.* Initial misdiagnosis and outcome after subarachnoid hemorrhage. *JAMA* 2004; 291(7): 866–9.

13. Vermeulen MJ, Schull MJ. Missed diagnosis of subarachnoid hemorrhage in the emergency department. *Stroke* 2007; 38(4): 1216–21.

14. Perry JJ, Stiell IG, Sivilotti ML, *et al.* High risk clinical characteristics for subarachnoid haemorrhage in patients with acute headache: prospective cohort study. *BMJ* 2010; 341: c5204.

15. Edlow JA, Panagos PD, Godwin SA, *et al.* Clinical policy: critical issues in the evaluation and management of adult patients presenting to the emergency department with acute headache. *Ann Emerg Med* 2008; 52(4): 407–36.

16. Pope JV, Edlow JA. Favorable response to analgesics does not predict a benign etiology of headache. *Headache* 2008; 48(6): 944–50.

17. Perry JJ, Stiell IG, Sivilotti ML, *et al.* Sensitivity of computed tomography performed within six hours of onset of headache for diagnosis of subarachnoid haemorrhage: prospective cohort study. *BMJ* 2011; 343: d4277.

18. Cortnum S, Sorensen P, Jorgensen J. Determining the sensitivity of computed tomography scanning in early detection of subarachnoid hemorrhage. *Neurosurgery* 2010; 66(5): 900–3.

19. Boesiger BM, Shiber JR. Subarachnoid hemorrhage diagnosis by computed tomography and lumbar puncture: are fifth generation CT scanners better at identifying subarachnoid hemorrhage? *J Emerg Med* 2005; 29(1): 23–7.

20. Byyny RL, Mower WR, Shum N, *et al.* Sensitivity of noncontrast cranial computed tomography for the emergency department diagnosis of subarachnoid hemorrhage. *Ann Emerg Med* 2008; 51(6): 697–703.

21. Shah KH, Richard KM, Nicholas S, Edlow JA. Incidence of traumatic lumbar puncture. *Acad Emerg Med* 2003; 10(2): 151–4.

22. Shah KH, Edlow JA. Distinguishing traumatic lumbar puncture from true subarachnoid hemorrhage. *J Emerg Med* 2002; 23(1): 67–74.

23. Vermeulen M. Subarachnoid haemorrhage: diagnosis and treatment. *J Neurol* 1996; 243(7): 496–501.

24. Gunawardena H, Beetham R, Scolding N, Lhatoo SD. Is cerebrospinal fluid spectrophotometry useful in CT scan-negative suspected subarachnoid haemorrage? *Eur Neurol* 2004; 52(4): 226–9.

25. Perry JJ, Sivilotti ML, Stiell IG, *et al.* Should spectrophotometry be used to identify xanthochromia in the cerebrospinal fluid of alert patients suspected of

having subarachnoid hemorrhage? *Stroke* 2006; 37(10): 2467–72.

26. Edlow JA, Bruner KS, Horowitz GL. Xanthochromia. *Arch Pathol Lab Med* 2002; 126(4): 413–15.

27. Linn FH, Voorbij HA, Rinkel GJ, *et al.* Visual inspection versus spectrophotometry in detecting bilirubin in cerebrospinal fluid. *J Neurol Neurosurg Psychiatry* 2005; 76(10): 1452–4.

28. Menke J, Larsen J, Kallenberg K. Diagnosing cerebral aneurysms by computed tomographic angiography: meta-analysis. *Ann Neurol* 2011; 69(4): 646–54.

29. Carstairs SD, Tanen DA, Duncan TD, *et al.* Computed tomographic angiography for the evaluation of aneurysmal subarachnoid hemorrhage. *Acad Emerg Med* 2006; 13(5): 486–92.

30. Edlow JA. What are the unintended consequences of changing the diagnostic paradigm for subarachnoid hemorrhage after brain computed tomography to computed tomographic angiography in place of lumbar puncture? *Acad Emerg Med* 2010; 17(9): 991–7.

31. Wiesmann M, Mayer TE, Yousry I, *et al.* Detection of hyperacute subarachnoid hemorrhage of the brain by using magnetic resonance imaging. *J Neurosurg* 2002; 96(4): 684–9.

32. Mohamed M, Heasly DC, Yagmurlu B, *et al.* Fluid-attenuated inversion recovery MR imaging and subarachnoid hemorrhage: not a panacea. *AJNR Am J Neuroradiol* 2004; 25(4): 545–50.

33. Schull MJ. Lumbar puncture first: an alternative model for the investigation of lone acute sudden headache. *Acad Emerg Med* 1999; 6(2): 131–6.

34. Baraff LJ, Byyny RL, Probst MA, *et al.* Prevalence of herniation and intracranial shift on cranial tomography in patients with subarachnoid hemorrhage and a normal neurologic examination. *Acad Emerg Med* 2010; 17(4): 423–8.

35. Savitz SI, Levitan EB, Wears R, Edlow JA. Pooled analysis of patients with thunderclap headache evaluated by CT and LP: is angiography necessary in patients with negative evaluations? *J Neurol Sci* 2009; 276(1–2): 123–5.

36. Polmear A. Sentinel headaches in aneurysmal subarachnoid haemorrhage: what is the true incidence? A systematic review. *Cephalalgia* 2003; 23(10): 935–41.

37. Raps EC, Rogers JD, Galetta SL, *et al.* The clinical spectrum of unruptured intracranial aneurysm. *Arch Neurol* 1993; 50: 265–8.

38. Woodruff M, Edlow JA. Evaluation of third nerve palsy in the emergency department. *J Emerg Med* 2008; 35: 239–46.

39. Bardach NS, Zhao S, Gress DR, *et al.* Association between subarachnoid hemorrhage outcomes and number of cases treated at California hospitals. *Stroke* 2002; 33(7): 1851–6.

40. Berman MF, Solomon RA, Mayer SA, *et al.* Impact of hospital-related factors on outcome after treatment of cerebral aneurysms. *Stroke* 2003; 34(9): 2200–7.

41. Cross DT 3rd, Tirschwell DL, Clark MA, *et al.* Mortality rates after subarachnoid hemorrhage: variations according to hospital case volume in 18 states. *J Neurosurg* 2003; 99(5): 810–17.

42. Willinsky RA, Taylor SM, TerBrugge K, *et al.* Neurologic complications of cerebral angiography: prospective analysis of 2,899 procedures and review of the literature. *Radiology* 2003; 227(2): 522–8.

43. Boet R, Poon WS, Lam JM, Yu SC. The surgical treatment of intracranial aneurysms based on computer tomographic angiography alone – streamlining the acute mananagement of symptomatic aneurysms. *Acta Neurochir (Wien)* 2003; 145(2): 101–5.

44. Caruso R, Colonnese C, Elefante A, *et al.* Use of spiral computerized tomography angiography in patients with cerebral aneurysm: our experience. *J Neurosurg Sci* 2002; 46(1): 4–9.

45. Hoh BL, Cheung AC, Rabinov JD, *et al.* Results of a prospective protocol of computed tomographic angiography in place of catheter angiography as the only diagnostic and pretreatment planning study for cerebral aneurysms by a combined neurovascular team. *Neurosurgery* 2004; 54(6): 1329–42.

46. Pechlivanis I, Schmieder K, Scholz M, *et al.* 3-Dimensional computed tomographic angiography for use of surgery planning in patients with intracranial aneurysms. *Acta Neurochir (Wien)* 2005; 147(10): 1045–53.

47. Ohkuma H, Tsurutani H, Suzuki S. Incidence and significance of early aneurysmal rebleeding before neurosurgical or neurological management. *Stroke* 2001; 32(5): 1176–80.

48. Naidech AM, Janjua N, Kreiter KT, *et al.* Predictors and impact of aneurysm rebleeding after subarachnoid hemorrhage. *Arch Neurol* 2005; 62(3): 410–16.

49. Hillman J, Fridriksson S, Nilsson O, *et al.* Immediate administration of tranexamic acid and reduced incidence of early rebleeding after aneurysmal subarachnoid hemorrhage: a prospective randomized study. *J Neurosurg* 2002; 97(4): 771–8.

50. Germanwala AV, Huang J, Tamargo RJ. Hydrocephalus after aneurysmal subarachnoid hemorrhage. *Neurosurg Clin N Am* 2010; 21(2): 263–70.

51. Crowley RW, Medel R, Dumont AS, *et al.* Angiographic vasospasm is strongly correlated with cerebral infarction after subarachnoid hemorrhage. *Stroke* 2011; 42(4): 919–23.

52. Rabinstein AA, Weigand S, Atkinson JL, Wijdicks EF. Patterns of cerebral infarction in aneurysmal subarachnoid hemorrhage. *Stroke* 2005; 36(5): 992–7.

53. Dorhout Mees SM, Rinkel GJ, Feigin VL, *et al.* Calcium antagonists for aneurysmal subarachnoid haemorrhage. *Cochrane Database Syst Rev* 2007; (3): CD000277.

54. Suarez JI. Magnesium sulfate administration in subarachnoid hemorrhage. *Neurocrit Care* 2011; 15(2): 302–7.

55. Sen J, Belli A, Albon H, *et al.* Triple-H therapy in the management of aneurysmal subarachnoid haemorrhage. *Lancet Neurol* 2003; 2(10): 614–21.

56. Rinkel G, Feigin V, Algra A, Gijn J. Circulatory volume expansion therapy for aneurysmal subarachnoid haemorrhage. *Cochrane Database Syst Rev* 2004; (4): CD000483.

57. Lin CL, Dumont AS, Lieu AS, *et al.* Characterization of perioperative seizures and epilepsy following aneurysmal subarachnoid hemorrhage. *J Neurosurg* 2003; 99(6): 978–85.

58. Naidech AM, Kreiter KT, Janjua N, *et al.* Phenytoin exposure is associated with functional and cognitive disability after subarachnoid hemorrhage. *Stroke* 2005; 36(3): 583–7.

59. Mahaney KB, Todd MM, Torner JC. Variation of patient characteristics, management, and outcome with timing of surgery for aneurysmal subarachnoid hemorrhage. *J Neurosurg* 2011; 114(4): 1045–53.

60. Raymond J, Guilbert F, Weill A, *et al.* Long-term angiographic recurrences after selective endovascular treatment of aneurysms with detachable coils. *Stroke* 2003; 34(6): 1398–403.

61. Molyneux A, Kerr R, Stratton I, *et al.* International Subarachnoid Aneurysm Trial (ISAT) of neurosurgical clipping versus endovascular coiling in 2143 patients with ruptured intracranial aneurysms: a randomised trial. *Lancet* 2002; 360(9342): 1267–74.

62. Molyneux AJ, Kerr RS, Birks J, *et al.* Risk of recurrent subarachnoid haemorrhage, death, or dependence and standardised mortality ratios after clipping or coiling of an intracranial aneurysm in the International Subarachnoid Aneurysm Trial (ISAT): long-term follow-up. *Lancet Neurol* 2009; 8(5): 427–33.

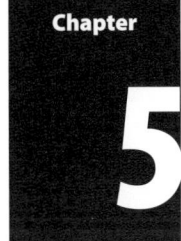

Chapter

5

Blunt and penetrating injuries to the neck

Niels K. Rathlev and Joseph C. Schmidt

The goal of this chapter is to provide a practical, evidence-based update of the evaluation and management of vascular injuries of the neck. Blunt and penetrating trauma to the neck may result in a spectrum of vascular injuries, ranging from minor to catastrophic. They frequently demand immediate attention and intervention on the part of the trauma team, including the emergency physician and trauma surgeon. The risk of devastating morbidity and mortality is significant because of the proximity of airway, neurologic, digestive, and major vascular structures in the fascial compartments of the neck.

Arterial injuries cause significant morbidity and mortality in association with neck trauma. Major arterial structures that may be involved include the subclavian, the vertebral, and the internal, external, and common carotid arteries. Injuries to these structures may cause exsanguinating hemorrhage or thrombosis. They are a major source of morbidity and account for up to 50% of all deaths resulting from penetrating neck trauma.[1]

Securing a stable definitive airway is a priority in patients with severe external hemorrhage or an expanding hematoma of the neck. Familiarity with multiple approaches to securing a definitive airway is required to ensure successful management of patients with vascular injuries; successful placement and maintenance of an appropriate airway is not assured with any single technique or modality. Accordingly, intubation through a neck wound and establishment of a surgical airway are procedural skills necessary for the successful management of victims of neck trauma.

Pathophysiology

The surface anatomy has been divided into three zones for the purpose of describing wounds of the anterior neck (Figure 5.1). Zone I comprises the thoracic outlet at the base of the neck from the sternal notch to the cricoid cartilage. It contains the subclavian artery, the great vessels of the superior mediastinum, the trachea, and the esophagus. Zone I injuries are considered high risk because of concern for injury to critical thoracic and mediastinal vascular structures. This area is not easily accessible to surgical exploration. Zone II is located between the cricoid cartilage and the angle of the mandible; the common and internal carotid arteries and the internal jugular vein are located close to the skin surface in this region and are easily accessible for surgical exposure and methods of vascular control. The pharynx, larynx, and upper portions of the trachea and esophagus are also located in this zone. Zone III extends from the angle of the mandible to the base of the skull. It contains the vertebral and distal internal and external carotid arteries as well as the upper segments of the jugular veins. The internal carotid artery courses cephalad behind the body of the mandible, which obviously complicates efforts to achieve proximal and distal vascular control. For the purpose of surgical repair, part of the mandible may have to be partially dislocated and repositioned anteriorly in order to gain adequate exposure to the internal carotid artery above the level of C2.

The neck is divided into anterior and posterior triangles by the sternocleidomastoid muscle. The anterior triangle contains the carotid sheath, which envelops important vascular structures such as the common and internal carotid arteries and internal jugular vein; it extends from the midline to the anterior aspect of the sternocleidomastoid muscle. The posterior triangle is located posterior to the sternocleidomastoid muscle, extending to the anterior border of the trapezius muscle. The posterior triangle is considered a lower-risk region of injury due to the

Vascular Emergencies, ed. Robert L. Rogers, Thomas Scalea, Lee Wallis, and Heike Geduld. Published by Cambridge University Press. © Cambridge University Press 2013.

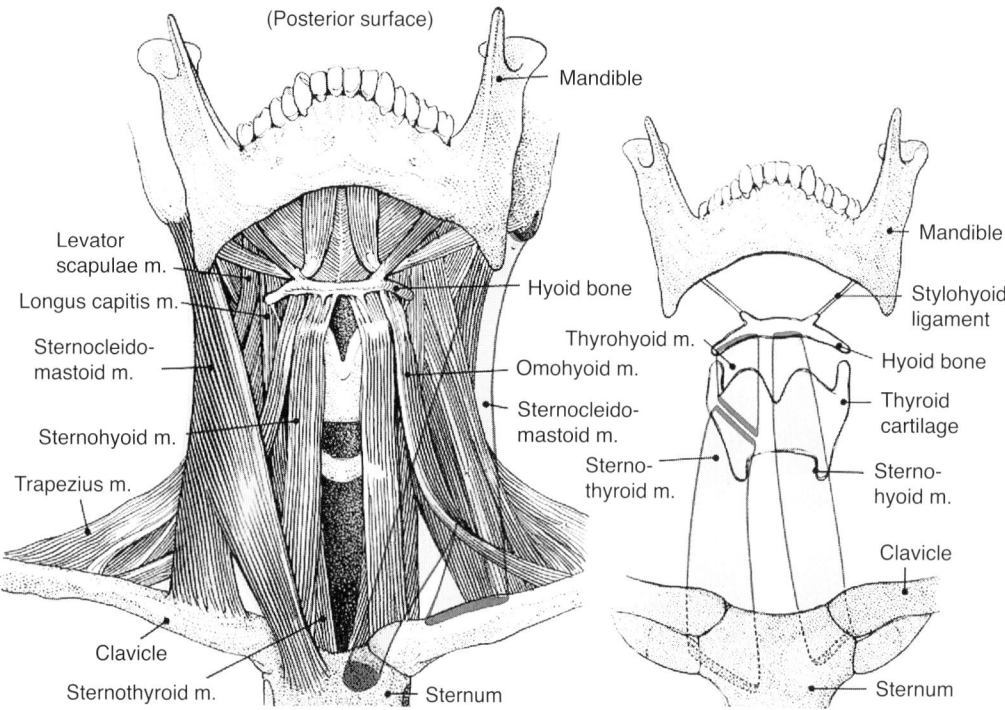

(Posterior surface)

Mandible

Levator scapulae m.

Longus capitis m.

Sternocleido-mastoid m.

Sternohyoid m.

Trapezius m.

Clavicle

Sternothyroid m.

Hyoid bone

Thyrohyoid m.

Omohyoid m.

Sternocleido-mastoid m.

Sterno-thyroid m.

Clavicle

Sternum

Mandible

Stylohyoid ligament

Hyoid bone

Thyroid cartilage

Sterno-hyoid m.

Clavicle

Sternum

Figure 5.1 Surface anatomy of the anterior neck; m., muscle. (From Legome and Shockley, p. 127, Figure 9.2.[2])

relative paucity of critical vascular structures. The three-zone nomenclature of anterior neck wounds does not apply to the posterior triangle. The vertebral arteries enter a bony canal known as the foramen transversarium, created by the transverse processes of the vertebrae of the cervical spine, starting proximally at C6. The arteries continue cephalad within this well-protected bony canal until they exit from this foramen at C2, entering the skull through the foramen magnum. Serious injuries to the vertebral arteries are rare because of this bony protection. Conversely, fractures involving the foramen transversarium and facet joint dislocations, caused by either penetrating or blunt trauma, should raise suspicion for vertebral artery injury.[3]

In the neck, vital structures are located near each other and are confined to compartments enclosed by relatively rigid and inflexible layers of fascia. The superficial and deep cervical fascial layers envelop these structures and offer protection against injury and excessive movement. The superficial fascia covers the platysma, a muscle that is only a couple of millimeters in width and located just below the skin surface. The platysma is located between the superficial

and deep cervical fascia and covers the entire antero-lateral neck. It is an important landmark in the management of neck trauma because penetration of this muscle should raise suspicion of injury to deeper structures. Historically, violation of the platysma was considered an indication for admission and observation in the absence of signs and symptoms of injury to vital structures.

The deep cervical fascia consists of several layers. The fascia surrounds the muscles of the neck circumferentially and envelops the sternocleidomastoid and trapezius muscles. The pre-tracheal fascia adheres to the thyroid gland, cricoid and thyroid cartilages, trachea, and esophagus. It courses behind the sternum and inserts caudally into the pericardium. This fascial plane is clinically important because of its connection to the anterior mediastinum. Perforation of the esophagus, larynx, or trachea leads to spillage of luminal contents, including air and undigested food, into adjacent spaces. The anatomic connections of the deep fascial compartment allow these contents to enter the anterior mediastinum, resulting in chemical and, eventually, infectious mediastinitis. Finally, the pre-vertebral fascia covers the muscles that stabilize

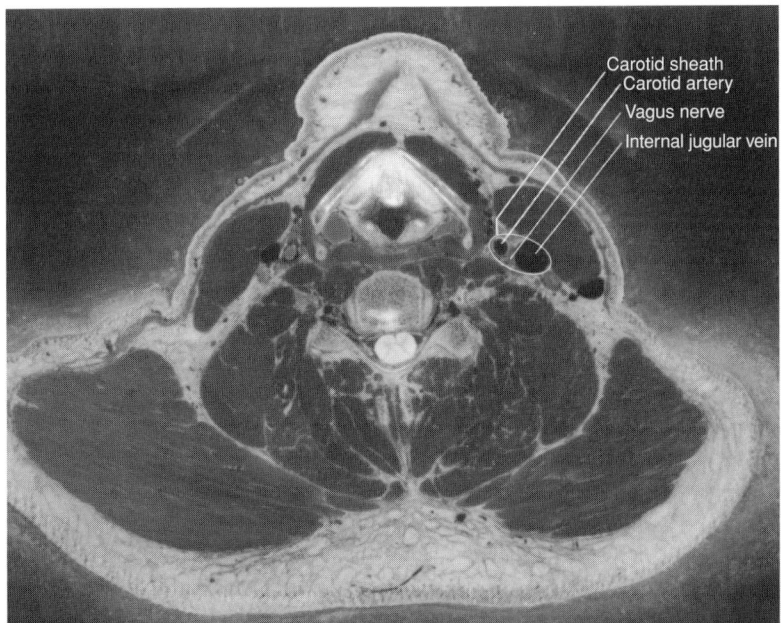

Carotid sheath
Carotid artery
Vagus nerve
Internal jugular vein

Figure 5.2 Cross-section of the neck at C7. (From Legome and Shockley, p. 129, Figure 9.3.[2])

the vertebrae and forms the axillary sheath that surrounds the subclavian artery.

The carotid sheath envelops the common and internal carotid arteries, internal jugular vein, and vagus nerve (Figure 5.2). In one case report, the carotid sheath deflected a low-speed projectile (a bullet from a handgun), thereby preventing damage to critical vascular and neurologic structures.[4] Because of the anatomic proximity of the airway and major arterial structures, hemorrhage from a significant, adjacent vascular injury may distort and externally compress the larynx and trachea. An expanding neck hematoma can quickly cause tracheal deviation and ultimately obstruct the airway. Accordingly, the size of a traumatic neck hematoma must be reassessed carefully at regular time intervals, and a definitive airway should be established early if continued expansion is noted. This dramatic phenomenon can occur over a period of only minutes.

Both penetrating and blunt vascular trauma can result in the formation of pseudoaneurysms, arteriovenous fistulas (AVFs), complete transections, and occlusions resulting from thrombus formation. Traumatic dissection is increasingly recognized as a primary injury to the vessel wall. In blunt trauma, injury to the cervical arteries is believed to be caused by rapid deceleration associated with distraction plus hyperextension or hyperflexion and rotation.[3] By

these mechanisms, vascular structures are stretched across bony prominences of the spine, and the resulting shearing forces create intimal tears in the vessel wall. Stroke resulting from occlusive thrombus or embolus formation is a devastating consequence in these patients.[5]

Epidemiology

Most penetrating neck injuries are caused by knives and low-energy gunshot wounds. Fortunately, these weapons impart a lower level of kinetic energy to tissues in comparison to military rifles and shotguns. The current mortality rate from civilian penetrating injuries to the neck is approximately 3 to 6%.[6] During the Korean and Vietnam conflicts, the mortality rates related to high-energy projectiles were significantly higher. Recent data from the wars in Iraq and Afghanistan document a significantly higher rate of vascular injury than in previous wars,[7] presumably related to higher-energy mechanisms of injury in modern warfare. Vascular reconstruction is now performed in nearly half of battlefield injuries. The mortality rate in civilians has not changed appreciably in recent years, despite continued improvement in diagnostic and therapeutic techniques.[6] This may reflect our continued inability to successfully change the outcome in a critical subset of spinal cord and major arterial injuries despite advances in diagnostic imaging and surgical intervention. In the hospital setting, attempts at central venous line placement are another cause of iatrogenic vascular injury and subsequent thrombosis. Factors that adversely affect mortality include gunshot wounds, Zone I entry or exit wounds, spinal cord injury, shock from uncontrolled hemorrhage, and missed vascular injuries. In total, 50% of all deaths from penetrating neck trauma are caused by arterial or venous injury. In addition, acute renal failure, stroke, air embolus, adult respiratory distress syndrome, severe brain injury, laryngotracheal trauma, and airway obstruction by hematoma also contribute as causes of death.[1]

The demographic characteristics of victims mirror the experience from penetrating trauma in general. Patients are primarily young men with injuries sustained as a result of interpersonal violence. Civilian series published between 1963 and 1990 reported the frequency of these injuries among a combined 2,495 patients with penetrating neck trauma caused primarily by gunshot and stab wounds.[1] Approximately 51% of patients had significant injuries to vascular, airway, and digestive tract structures. The compiled data demonstrated that the common and internal carotid arteries were the most frequently involved structures, accounting for almost 7% of all injuries. Approximately one-third of patients with penetrating injuries to the common and internal carotid arteries present with a concomitant neurologic deficit related to cerebrovascular ischemia and thrombus formation. In descending order of frequency, internal and common carotid artery injuries (6.7%) were followed by damage to the subclavian (2%), external carotid (2%), and vertebral (1.3%) arteries. The internal jugular vein was injured in 9% of all victims, making it the most frequently injured vein.

The most common mechanism of blunt trauma to the neck occurs during motor vehicle collisions.[8] This type of injury typically results from rapid acceleration and deceleration or direct blows to the anterior neck by the steering column or dashboard, which crushes the trachea at the cricoid ring and compresses the esophagus against the cervical vertebrae. Injuries can also occur from increased intrathecal pressure against a closed glottis, induced by improper seatbelt use.

Strangulation results from hanging, ligature suffocation, and manual choking. The usual mechanism of death in hangings is external pressure on the jugular veins, preventing venous return to the heart. This eventually results in loss of consciousness from edema of the brain. The unconscious patient falls with all of his or her weight against the ligature, compressing the trachea and restricting airflow to the lungs. Irreversible asphyxiation follows in minutes.[9] Choke holds typically generate even greater force and are no longer promoted in police training. Although reported, carotid artery occlusion and dissection is fortunately quite rare after strangulation.[10]

Clothesline injuries occur in various sports, such as football, martial arts, and the use of all-terrain vehicles, motorcycles, and snowmobiles. Direct blows by fists, feet, and weapons and excessive cervical manipulation account for the remainder of blunt vascular injuries.[11,12]

Significant vascular injuries to the neck occur in approximately 1 to 3% of all major blunt trauma victims.[13–16] High-speed motor vehicle crashes cause the majority of these injuries; other mechanisms include motorcycle crashes, pedestrians struck by motor vehicles, falls, and assaults involving direct blows to the neck.[17,18] Frequently associated injuries include intra-oral trauma as well as basilar skull and cervical spine fractures. Although vascular injuries are rare following blunt trauma, the morbidity and mortality rates are significantly higher than for penetrating trauma. The overall mortality related to blunt vascular injuries is 20 to 30%; in addition, 40 to 60% of these patients develop permanent neurologic deficits as a result of central nervous system ischemia.[19]

Diagnosis

For the purpose of discussion, the emergency department (ED) evaluation and treatment have been divided by mechanism of injury, i.e., penetrating and blunt vascular injuries of the neck. Basic trauma laboratory studies such as complete blood count and initial blood-bank studies are indicated but not helpful in making a diagnosis.

Penetrating trauma

The ED evaluation of penetrating injuries to the neck begins with the search for compelling evidence of vascular compromise. Patients with injuries that violate the platysma and exhibit "hard" signs of vascular injury (Table 5.1) require emergent surgical intervention. Injuries to Zones I and III often are not accessible

Table 5.1 "Hard" and "soft" signs of vascular injury

Hard signs

Pulse deficit

Bruit or thrill

Pulsatile or expanding hematoma

Pulsatile or severe hemorrhage

Soft signs

Stable, non-pulsatile hematoma

Hypotension and shock

Central or peripheral nervous system ischemia

Proximity to a major vascular structure

Table 5.2 Signs and symptoms of blunt cerebrovascular injury

- Arterial hemorrhage from neck, nose, or mouth.
- Expanding cervical hematoma.
- Cervical bruit in patients less than 50 years old.
- Focal neurologic deficit or neurologic deficit inconsistent with CT or MRI.
- Ischemia on CT or MRI.

and require endovascular modalities. Stable patients with a high clinical suspicion of injury or "soft" signs (Table 5.1) require further evaluation. In the past, Zone II injuries were all surgically explored. The relatively high number of negative surgical explorations led to the search for a more selective approach.

Traditionally, the physical examination has been considered unreliable in ruling out vascular injuries following penetrating trauma. More recently, several authors concluded that the physical examination can reliably eliminate vascular injuries requiring surgical repair in asymptomatic patients.[20,21] However, caution should be employed when applying this finding, as some injuries were missed and a prolonged period of observation may be required.

Historically, patients requiring imaging underwent conventional angiography. A search for a less invasive and resource-intense option has garnered support for both ultrasound (US) and computed tomography angiography (CTA). Early studies by Demetriades *et al.* demonstrated a sensitivity > 90% for Doppler ultrasound in the detection of penetrating vascular injuries of the neck.[22,23] The operator-dependent nature of ultrasound, coupled with its limitations in evaluating the vertebral vasculature as well as associated injuries, has led investigators to turn to CTA. Support for multidetector CTA (MDCTA) as a screening tool has grown with a body of evidence and improved image quality. Several studies have demonstrated CTA's reliability in finding significant vascular injuries.[24,25] This body of evidence led to a 2008 clinical practice guideline from the Eastern Association for the Surgery of Trauma (EAST), which states "CT angiography or duplex US can be used in lieu of conventional arteriography to rule out an arterial injury in penetrating injuries to zone II of the neck."[26]

In summary, patients with "hard" signs of vascular trauma require emergent intervention. Patients with high-risk mechanisms or "soft" signs should undergo further imaging, with MDCTA being the primary modality. Observation is a reasonable approach in asymptomatic patients with low-risk mechanisms.

Blunt trauma

Blunt carotid artery injuries (BCI) and blunt vertebral artery injuries (BVI) – referred to as blunt cerebrovascular injuries (BCVI) – are often evaluated together. Traditionally, these injuries were thought to be rare, but recent studies have found a consistent prevalence of BCVI in 1 to 2% of victims of significant blunt trauma.[27,28] The potentially devastating neurologic consequences of cerebrovascular injuries have prompted significant study of diagnostic and treatment modalities. It has been demonstrated that broad screening of patients at risk for BCVI can identify additional injuries and that early intervention can improve outcomes.[29] Although the merits of broad screening continue to be debated, screening for BCVI is cost effective, because of the devastating costs of missed injury.[30,31] The optimal modalities for evaluation and treatment remain controversial.

The ED evaluation of patients with blunt cervical trauma begins with a search for signs and symptoms indicating BCVI. Table 5.2 represents a combination of signs and symptoms derived from consensus statements produced by the Western Trauma Association (WTA)[32] and the Eastern Association for the Surgery of Trauma (EAST).[33]

Patients with signs and symptoms consistent with BCVI clearly require further evaluation, as they have a substantial rate of significant injuries.[5] Although controversial, some consensus has developed around high-risk screening criteria for BCVI in blunt trauma victims without signs and symptoms of vascular injury (Table 5.3).[32,33]

Conventional angiography remains the widely accepted reference standard in the evaluation of BCVI. However, because angiography is invasive and

Table 5.3 High-risk criteria for blunt cerebrovascular injuries (BCVI). Modified Denver Screening Criteria

- Basilar skull fracture.
- Cervical spine fracture.
- C1–C3 fracture, involvement of foramen transversarium, subluxation, severe hyperextension-rotation or hyperflexion mechanism.
- LeFort II and III facial fractures.
- Diffuse axonal injury with Glasgow Coma Scale score < 8.
- Focal neurologic deficit unexplained by neuroimaging.
- Signs or symptoms of TIA or brain ischemia.
- Seatbelt contusion or hematoma of the neck.
- Hemorrhage from mouth, nose, ears, or neck wound.
- Cervical bruit in patients less than 50 years of age.
- Hanging attempt with anoxic brain injury.
- Injury Severity Score > 16.

resource intense and has the potential for significant complications, several alternative imaging modalities have been investigated. Duplex ultrasonography, widely utilized for imaging the carotid arteries in non-trauma situations, thus far has failed to demonstrate sufficient sensitivity and specificity to be a useful screening tool in BCVI.[34] Similarly, MRA has not proved to be a useful screening modality.[35,36] Initial evaluations of early generation CTA were also disappointing.[35,36] Several authors studying the improved technology of CTA with 16 or more detector rows (16 slices) demonstrated significant improvement in accuracy. Eastman *et al.*, utilizing 16-slice CTA, found a sensitivity of 100% for carotid injuries and 96% for vertebral injuries.[37] Other authors had less impressive results, which was partially explained by missed initial readings of the angiogram[38] or a substantial learning curve, demonstrated by significant improvement in results over the course of the study.[39] Based on the available evidence, the WTA and the EAST, in 2009 and 2010, respectively, endorsed the incorporation of CTA (16 slice or higher) in the screening evaluation of patients at risk for BCVI.[32,33] This endorsement, however, has not ended the controversy. Three subsequent studies from groups lead by Sliker, Goodwin, and DiCocco, utilizing 16-slice or higher CTA, failed to demonstrate adequate sensitivity and specificity to support BCVI screening with CTA.[40–42]

In summary, the evaluation of BCVI begins with a thorough general trauma evaluation and resuscitation. Unstable patients require emergent surgical or endovascular intervention. Findings suspicious of BCVI (summarized in Tables 5.2 and 5.3) should prompt further imaging. Duplex ultrasonography and MRA are generally not useful. CTA can be considered

as a screening modality, understanding its potential lack of accuracy, particularly in institutions with limited experience with the technique. Consequently, conventional angiography remains the reference standard in the evaluation of BCVI.

Emergency department management

Patients with injuries to the vascular structures contained within the neck have a substantial rate of associated trauma to other critical structures. This mandates that the initial ED evaluation of these patients should focus on the stability of airway, breathing, circulation, and neurologic function. These patients should undergo a thorough trauma evaluation and resuscitation to identify the extent of their injuries, following the basic principles of emergency medical care. In addition to a primary and secondary survey, patients with cervical trauma should have a detailed physical examination of the head and neck. Appropriate and timely assessment of potential vascular injuries of the neck is crucial to patient outcomes. The natural inclination of care providers is to immobilize the cervical spine for victims of blunt and penetrating neck trauma. Although evidence supports this practice in the former, immediate management of the airway and hemorrhage control of the victim of a penetrating neck wound should take precedence over cervical spine stabilization in alert patients with no neurologic deficits.

There are no reports of unstable cervical spine injuries caused by penetrating trauma secondary to stabbings. Conversely, these injuries have been documented as a consequence of gunshot wounds to the neck. To create an unstable cervical spine fracture, the anterior and posterior columns must both be fractured. Consequently, the injury must traverse the spinal cord to cause this injury, and the patient will invariably present with neurologic signs and symptoms. A retrospective study of 19 patients sustaining gunshot wounds to the face and neck found that all of those with unstable cervical spine fractures also presented with neurologic deficits; they were either comatose due to hemorrhagic shock or anoxic brain injury or demonstrated paraplegia or quadriplegia upon presentation.[43] In this study, three awake and neurologically intact individuals presented with gunshot wounds to the face, which resulted in stable cervical spine fractures. Another series found no cervical spine injuries in 174 patients with gunshot wounds to the head.[44] Unstable cervical spine injuries were found in 0.4% (4 / 1,069) of patients with penetrating neck injury and all were related to gunshot wounds.[45] Based on these results, emergent treatment of a penetrating neck wound, such as hemorrhage control or airway management, should take precedence over cervical spine stabilization in alert patients with no neurologic deficits. This may involve removing the cervical collar to gain access to the injury. Once these immediate priorities have been addressed in the emergency setting, the collar may be replaced for stabilization. In "non-judicial" hanging attempts, the risk of an unstable cervical spine fracture is extremely low.[46] Moreover, a cervical collar may impede venous outflow from the head, leading to an increase in intracranial pressure.

Patients with progressive subcutaneous or mediastinal emphysema, uncontrolled hemorrhage, or an expanding hematoma require early airway intervention. This may be life-saving for patients with severe airway or vascular injuries because of potential progressive distortion of normal, recognizable tissues and landmarks. It is far preferable that an experienced emergency physician semi-electively intubates a patient with relatively normal anatomy rather than wait to perform a surgical airway in an emergency situation. Patients who require intubation for definitive airway control can be managed safely with in-line stabilization to minimize movement of the neck during the procedure. Standard procedure using direct laryngoscopy with a Macintosh or Miller laryngoscope blade causes minimal movement (10–11°) of the cervical spine in healthy patients positioned on a rigid board prior to intubation.[47] Providers must be aware that attempts at orotracheal intubation have resulted in extension of partial lacerations and complete transaction of the trachea, with disastrous consequences.[48] They must therefore be skilled in alternative methods of securing the airway.

Patients in hemorrhagic shock must be managed by stopping external bleeding and administering fluid resuscitation. External hemorrhage or a rapidly expanding hematoma of the neck must be controlled with uninterrupted, forceful, direct pressure. Intraoral bleeding can be controlled with gauze packing of the oropharynx once a definitive airway has been established. Rapidly increasing the blood pressure before bleeding is controlled can promote further bleeding and cause a transient or minimal response to resuscitation. Balancing the dual goals of maintaining organ perfusion and minimizing the risk of

Table 5.4 Critical actions for initial ED evaluation and treatment

- In awake and neurologically intact patients, airway management and hemorrhage control take precedence over cervical spine stabilization.
- Observe for expanding neck hematoma and manage the airway early.
- Prepare for difficult airway using various approaches, including surgical airway and intubation through accessible wound.
- Control hemorrhage with direct pressure.
- Patients with "hard" signs of vascular injury should go to the operating room for definitive repair.
- Patients with no "hard" signs of injury and hemodynamic stability should undergo the following:
  · careful observation for patients with a low-risk mechanism of injury and the absence of signs and symptoms;
  · angiography (conventional versus computed tomography) plus triple endoscopy or barium swallow (depending on the zone of injury) for patients with a high-risk mechanism or the presence of signs or symptoms.

rebleeding can be difficult. The strategy of accepting a lower than normal blood pressure while maintaining perfusion to vital organs is called "controlled" or "hypotensive" resuscitation.[49]

Pearls and pitfalls

The "pearls and pitfalls" of the initial ED diagnostic evaluation and management are summarized in Table 5.4. Failure to perform the critical actions listed here can have disastrous effects on the ultimate outcome.

Definitive treatment

Penetrating trauma

All patients with penetrating injuries involving the cervical vasculature require admission. In addition, asymptomatic patients being observed may require admission, based on the anticipated amount of time needed to conclude that a vascular injury is not present. Injuries in Zones I and III typically require an endovascular approach, as surgical approaches do not allow both proximal and distal control. Most Zone II arterial injuries are surgically explored and repaired. Venous injuries can be repaired or, more often, are ligated. In addition, some evidence suggests that certain internal jugular injuries can be managed nonoperatively.[50]

Table 5.5 Grading scale for blunt cerebrovascular injury

Grade	Angiographic findings
1	Intimal irregularity or dissection, < 25% narrowing of luminal diameter
2	Dissection, raised intimal flap, thrombus, > 25% narrowing of luminal diameter
3	Pseudoaneurysm
4	Total occlusion
5	Transection or extravasation

Blunt trauma

All patients with significant risk of BCVI should be admitted for observation and further evaluation. Treatment of BCVI varies according to injury severity. Much of the available literature references a grading scale described by Biffl and colleagues (Table 5.5).[32]

Treatment options fall into four categories: surgical repair, endovascular intervention, anticoagulation, or antiplatelet therapy and observation. Untreated BCVI demonstrate a significant rate of subsequent neurovascular ischemic events; therefore, observation alone should be used only in patients with contraindications to the other modes of therapy.[32] Antithrombotic agents, either heparin or antiplatelet agents, are currently the recommended mainstay for injuries categorized as grades 1 through 4.[32,33] Heparin remains first-line strategy, although several recent studies demonstrated similar event rates with antiplatelet agents alone.[51,52] Hemorrhagic complications are relatively common with heparin infusions, so close monitoring of partial thromboplastin times (PTTs), with a therapeutic goal of 40 to 50 seconds, has been recommended.[28] Endovascular interventions for severe stenosis and pseudoaneurysm remain controversial: some authors found a reasonable safety profile,[49] but others concluded that the high complication rate of acute intervention outweighs the benefits.[52] Surgery, or endovascular intervention for inaccessible lesions, remains the primary modality for grade 5 lesions, with revascularization as the goal.[32] Of note, however, patients with dense neurologic deficits before intervention have a poor prognosis regardless of which treatment modality is employed.[33] Follow-up imaging, preferably at approximately seven days, is recommended and leads to a change in treatment plan in up to 61% of patients.[28]

Clinical approach when resources are limited

In resource-limited areas, selective ligation of vascular structures remains an important management option, especially for venous and minor or distal arterial injuries. Ligation of the common and internal carotid arteries is associated with a high incidence of brain ischemia and stroke and should be undertaken only as a heroic life-saving maneuver when no other options are available.

Selective evaluation and mandatory exploration have similar diagnostic accuracy for Zone II injuries of the neck.[26] The former requires careful, repeated physical examinations, an approach that in isolation has a 95% sensitivity for detecting injuries that require intervention. In addition, either conventional or CT angiography is required to assess for cerebrovascular injury. Clearly, selective evaluation is a resource-intensive approach in terms of both the time and intensity of observation as well as necessary technology. This approach may not be feasible in resource-limited arenas where the volume of patients exceeds the ability of providers to actively observe them. Required equipment for conventional angiography may also not be available. Consequently, an approach of routine or mandatory exploration of patients with Zone II injuries is often the norm under these circumstances. Zone I and III injuries require a more sophisticated exploratory approach. Local resources and surgical protocols should determine whether transfer to a more advanced referral center is required.

References

1. McConnell DB, Trunkey DB. Management of penetrating trauma to the neck. *Adv Surg* 1994; 27: 97–127.

2. Legome E, Shockley LW, eds. *Trauma: A Comprehensive Emergency Medicine Approach*. Cambridge: Cambridge University Press; 2011.

3. Inamasu J, Guiot BH. Vertebral artery injury after blunt cervical trauma: an update. *Surg Neurol* 2006; 65(3): 238–45.

4. May M, Tucker HM, Dillard BM. Penetrating wounds of the neck in civilians. *Otolaryngol Clin North Am* 1976; 9(2): 361–91.

5. Biffl WL, Moore EE, Offner PJ, *et al.* Blunt carotid arterial injuries: implications of a new grading scale. *J Trauma* 1999; 47: 845–53.

6. Carducci B, Lowe RA, Dalsey W. Penetrating neck trauma: consensus and controversies. *Ann Emerg Med* 1996; 15(2): 208–15.

7. White JM, Stannard A, Burkhardt GE, *et al.* The epidemiology of vascular injury in the wars in Iraq and Afghanistan. *Ann Surg* 2011; 253: 1184–9.

8. Levy D. Neck trauma. Last updated December 7, 2010. Available at www.emedicine.com/emerg/topic331.htm. Accessed on March 6, 2012.

9. Hawley DA, McClane GE, Strack GB. Violence: recognition, management, and prevention. A review of 300 attempted strangulation cases. Part III: injuries in fatal cases. *J Emerg Med* 2001; 21(3): 317–22.

10. Clarot F, Vaz E, Papin F, Proust B. Fatal and non-fatal carotid artery dissection after manual strangulation. *Forensic Sci Int* 2005; 149(23): 143–50.

11. Bernat RA, Zimmerman JM, Keane WM, Pribitkin EA. Combined laryngotracheal separation and esophageal injury following blunt neck trauma. *Facial Plast Surg* 2005; 21(3): 187–90.

12. Dittrich R, Rohsbach D, Heidbreder A, *et al.* Mild mechanical traumas are possible risk factors for cervical artery dissection. *Cerebrovascular Dis* 2007; 23(4): 275–81.

13. Fabian TC, Patton JH, Croce MA, *et al.* Blunt carotid injury: importance of early diagnosis and anticoagulant therapy. *Ann Surg* 1996; 223: 513–25.

14. Kerwin AJ, Bynoe RP, Murray J, *et al.* Screening for blunt carotid and vertebral artery injuries is justified. *J Trauma* 2001; 51: 308–14.

15. Biffl WL, Moore EE, Ryu RK, *et al.* The unrecognized epidemic of blunt carotid arterial injuries: early diagnosis improves neurologic outcome. *Ann Surg* 1998; 228: 462–70.

16. Rozycki GS, Tremblay L, Feliciano DV, *et al.* A prospective study for the detection of vascular injury in adult and pediatric patients with cervicothoracic seat belt signs. *J Trauma* 2002; 52: 618–24.

17. Biffl WL, Moore EE, Offner PJ, *et al.* Optimizing screening for blunt cerebrovascular injuries. *Am J Surg* 1999; 178: 517–22.

18. Biffl WL, Moore EE, Elliott JP, *et al.* The devastating potential of blunt vertebral artery injuries. *Ann Surg* 2000; 231: 672–81.

19. Miller PR, Fabian TC, Croce MA, *et al.* Screening for blunt cerebrovascular injuries: analysis of diagnostic modalities and outcomes. *Ann Surg* 2002; 236: 386–95.

20. Azuaje RE, Jacobson LE, Glover J, *et al.* Reliability of physical examination as a predictor of vascular injury after penetrating neck trauma. *Am Surg* 2003; 69: 804–7.

21. Gonzalez RP, Falimirski M, Holevar MR, *et al.* Penetrating zone II neck injury: does dynamic computed tomographic scan contribute to the diagnostic sensitivity of physical examination for surgically significant injury? A prospective blinded study. *J Trauma* 2003; 54: 61–4.

22. Demetriades D, Theodorou D, Cornwell E III, *et al.* Penetrating injuries of the neck in patients in stable condition: physical examination, angiography, or color flow Doppler imaging. *Arch Surg* 1995; 130: 971–5.

23. Demetriades D, Theodorou D, Cornwell E, *et al.* Evaluation of penetrating injuries of the neck: prospective study of 223 patients. *World J Surg* 1997; 21: 41–8.

24. Munera F, Soto JA, Palacio D, *et al.* Diagnosis of arterial injuries caused by penetrating trauma to the neck: comparison of helical CT angiography and conventional angiography. *Radiology* 2000; 216: 356–62.

25. Ofer A, Nitecki SS, Braun J, *et al.* CT angiography of the carotid arteries in trauma to the neck. *Eur J Vasc Endovasc Surg* 2001; 21: 401–7.

26. Tisherman SA, Bokhari F, Collier B, *et al.* Clinical practice guideline: penetrating zone II neck trauma. *J Trauma* 2008; 64: 1392–405.

27. Goodwin RE, Beery PR, Dorbish RJ, *et al.* Computed tomographic angiography versus conventional angiography for the diagnosis of blunt cerebrovascular injury in trauma patients. *J Trauma* 2009; 67(5): 1046–50.

28. Biffl WL, Ray CE, Moore EE, *et al.* Treatment-related outcomes from blunt cerebrovascular injuries: importance of routine follow-up arteriography. *Ann Surg* 2002; 235(5): 699–706.

29. Cothren CC, Moore EE, Biffl WL, *et al.* Anticoagulation is the gold standard therapy for blunt carotid injuries to reduce stroke rate. *Arch Surg* 2004; 139(5): 540–6.

30. Cothren CC, Moore EE, Ray CE Jr, *et al.* Screening for blunt cerebrovascular injuries is cost-effective. *Am J Surg* 2005; 190(6): 845–9.

31. Kaye D, Brasel KJ, Neideen T, *et al.* Screening for blunt cerebrovascular injuries is cost-effective. *J Trauma* 2011; 70(5): 1051–7.

32. Biffl WL, Cothren CC, Moore EE, *et al.* Western Trauma Association critical decisions in trauma: screening for and treatment of blunt cerebrovascular injuries. *J Trauma* 2009; 67: 1150–3.

33. Bromberg WJ, Collier BC, Diebel LN, *et al.* Blunt cerebrovascular injury practice management guidelines: the Eastern Association for the Surgery of Trauma. *J Trauma* 2010; 68(2): 471–7.

34. Mutze S, Rademacher G, Matthes G, *et al.* Blunt cerebrovascular injury in patients with blunt multiple trauma: diagnostic accuracy of duplex Doppler US and early CT angiography. *Radiology* 2005; 237: 884–92.

35. Miller PR, Fabian TC, Croce MA, *et al.* Prospective screening for blunt cerebrovascular injuries: analysis of diagnostic modalities and outcomes. *Ann Surg* 2002; 236: 386–95.

36. Biffl WL, Ray CE Jr, Moore EE, *et al.* Noninvasive diagnosis of blunt cerebrovascular injuries: a preliminary report. *J Trauma* 2002; 53: 850–6.

37. Eastman AL, Chason DP, Perez CL, *et al.* Computed tomographic angiography for the diagnosis of blunt cervical vascular injury: is it ready for primetime? *J Trauma* 2006; 60: 925–9.

38. Utter GH, HollingworthW, Hallam DK, *et al.* Sixteen-slice CT angiography in patients with suspected blunt carotid and vertebral artery injuries. *J Am Coll Surg* 2006; 203(6): 838–48.

39. Malhotra AK, Camacho M, Ivatury RR, *et al.* Computed tomographic angiography for the diagnosis of blunt carotid/vertebral artery injury: a note of caution. *Ann Surg* 2007; 246(4): 632–43.

40. Sliker CW, Shanmuganathan K, Mirvis SE. Diagnosis of blunt cerebrovascular injuries with 16-MDCT: accuracy of whole-body MDCT compared with neck MDCT angiography. *AJR* 2008; 190(3): 790–9.

41. Goodwin RB, Beery PR 2nd, Dorbish RJ, *et al.* Computed tomographic angiography versus conventional angiography for the diagnosis of blunt cerebrovascular injury in trauma patients. *J Trauma* 2009; 67(5): 1046–50.

42. DiCocco JM, Emmett KP, Fabian TC, *et al.* Blunt cerebrovascular injury screening with 32-channel multi-detector computed tomography: more slices still don't cut it. *Ann Surg* 2011; 253: 444–50.

43. Medzon R, Rothenhaus T, Bono CM, *et al.* Stability of the cervical spine after gunshot wounds to the head and neck. *Spine* 2005; 30(20): 2274–9.

44. Lanoix R, Gupta R, Leak L, *et al.* C-spine injury associated with gunshot wounds to the head: retrospective study and literature review. *J Trauma* 2000; 49(5): 860–3.

45. Lustenberger T, Talving P, Lam L, *et al.* Unstable cervical spine fracture after penetrating neck injury: a rare entity in an analysis of 1,069 patients. *J Trauma* 2001; 70: 870–2.

46. Vander Krol L, Wolfe R. The emergency department management of near hanging victims. *J Emerg Med* 1994; 12: 285–92.

47. Hastings RH, Duong H, Burton DW, *et al.* Cervical spine movements during laryngoscopy with the Bullard, Macintosh, and Miller laryngoscopes. *Anesthesiology* 1995; 82(4): 859–69.

48. O'Connor PJ, Sasaki R, Masuda A, *et al.* Anesthetic implications of laryngeal trauma. *Anesth Analg* 1998; 87: 1283–4.

49. Bickell WH, Wall MJ Jr, Pepe PE, *et al.* Immediate versus delayed fluid resuscitation for hypotensive patients with penetrating torso injuries. *NEJM* 1994; 331(17): 1105–9.

50. Inaba K, Munera F, McKenney MG, *et al.* The nonoperative management of penetrating internal jugular vein injury. *J Vasc Surg* 2006; 43: 77–80.

51. Edwards NM, Fabian TC, Claridge JA, *et al.* Antithrombotic therapy and endovascular stents are effective treatment for blunt carotid injuries: results from longterm followup. *J Am Coll Surg* 2007; 204: 1007–15.

52. Cothren CC, Moore EE, Ray CE Jr, *et al.* Carotid artery stents for blunt cerebrovascular injury: risks exceed benefits. *Arch Surg* 2005; 140: 480–6.

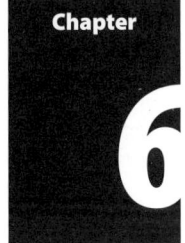

Cervical artery dissection

Bo E. Madsen and Selim H. Magdy

Cervical artery dissection is one of the most common causes of stroke in the young and middle-aged, arbitrarily defined as 15 to 45 years old. In those age groups, it represents 18.8 to 24% of all strokes.[1–4] Among the elderly, it accounts for approximately 2.5% of strokes.

Dissections can involve the vertebral artery (VA) or the internal carotid artery (ICA). They can be unilateral or bilateral and, in rare cases, involve multiple arteries. The most common location for cervical artery dissections is at the level of the first and second cervical vertebrae.

While the outcomes are generally good, a minority of patients experience severe disability or death.[1] Strokes, even when mild, have a profound effect on young people's lives in terms of job loss, divorce, and impairment of healthy behaviors.[1]

Although this disease entity is much better understood today than when the first case of internal carotid artery dissection was described by Jentzer in 1954,[5] it is still a condition with a highly variable presentation, course, and outcome. The purpose of this chapter is to review the pathophysiology, epidemiology, clinical presentation, diagnosis, and management of cervical artery dissection.

Pathophysiology

A dissection can be spontaneous or traumatic. The course and outcome are similar for both categories. Spontaneous dissection may occur during minor physical activity, including lunging for a ball, twisting the neck to avoid a falling tree branch, turning the neck abruptly while backing up a car, chiropractic manipulation, working out, and weight-lifting, or

following dental procedures associated with prolonged neck hyperextension. A case of vertebral artery dissection has even been described following an ordinary neurologic examination.[6] Many patients consider these activities irrelevant when they present with a dissection. Traumatic cases may be related to severe trauma, such as physical assault or motor vehicle accidents, or minimal trauma that the patient may not even recall, leading to a diagnosis of spontaneous dissection. Many different mechanisms have been described, including horseback riding accidents, horse attack, and motor vehicle accidents.[7–11] The presentation following major trauma can resemble the presentation associated with spontaneous dissections. Symptoms can develop gradually over minutes to days or the patient can present with devastating symptoms. Cervical artery dissection associated with major trauma is not discussed further in this chapter and is generally managed in the context of the coexisting injuries.

Regardless of the inciting event, once a tear occurs in one of the cervical arteries, blood enters between the layers of the arterial wall, creating an intramural hematoma. If the tear occurs between the intima and media, the hematoma can lead to stenosis and occlusion, which can lead to cerebral hypoperfusion, ischemia, or embolism. While ischemic symptoms and stroke often occur within hours to days after the dissection, stroke and transient ischemic attack (TIA) have been reported months after the initial insult without an intervening trauma.[12] If the tear occurs between the media and adventitia, aneurysmal dilatation (pseudoaneurysm) is typical.[13] Pseudoaneurysms can exert mass/pressure effects, resulting in local symptoms, or rupture, resulting in hemorrhage.

Vascular Emergencies, ed. Robert L. Rogers, Thomas Scalea, Lee Wallis, and Heike Geduld. Published by Cambridge University Press. © Cambridge University Press 2013.

Epidemiology

Incidence

Older community-based studies have reported an incidence of internal carotid artery dissection (ICAD) of 2.6 to 2.9 / 100,000 population.[14,15] A more recent study in one of the same populations found an incidence of 1.72 to 1.89 / 100,000.[16] The incidence of vertebral artery dissection (VAD) was found to be 0.97 to 1.12. Although the incidence of vertebral artery dissections remains lower than that of carotid artery dissections, it was found to be increasing during the second half of the study. This increase likely reflects better diagnostic abilities. The true incidence of cervical artery dissections is unknown, as many mild cases go undetected.

Risk factors

See Table 6.1.

Cardiovascular risk factors. In terms of traditional risk factors for ischemic stroke, a large multinational study found that patients with cervical artery dissection more frequently are hypertensive than the referent population. At the same time they have a lower prevalence of other risk factors for ischemic stroke, i.e., diabetes mellitus, hypercholesterolemia, smoking, and obesity.[17]

Spinal manipulation therapy. Several case reports and studies have found a temporal relation between spinal manipulation therapy, usually from chiropractic treatment, and dissection, particularly of the vertebral artery.[18–20] A case-control study of patients presenting with VAD found an odds ratio (OR) of 6.6 for having had spinal manipulation therapy within the past 30 days. Even after controlling for cervical pain before the stroke/TIA, the OR was elevated for an association between spinal manipulation therapy and VAD.[21] As a result of this study's findings, it is recommended that patients undergoing spinal manipulation therapy should be asked to give consent for the procedure, acknowledging the risk of vascular injury and stroke. In addition, the authors suggested that any significant increase in neck pain after therapy should lead to "immediate medical evaluation."[21]

Table 6.1 Patient characteristics and risk factors for cervical artery dissection

Risk factors	Internal carotid artery dissection (ICAD)	Vertebral artery dissection (VAD)
Men	38–73% [12,16,22,23,24,25]	51–67% [12,16,22,24, 26]
Age (yr)	44–50.5% [12,16,22,23,24,25,27]	34.6–50.5% [12,16,22,24, 26,27]
Hypertension	OR 1.56 (1.19–2.05) [17]	OR 1.73 (1.21–2.46) [17]
Hypercholesterolemia	OR 0.57 (0.42–0.78) [17]	OR 0.48 (0.30–0.78) [17]
Diabetes mellitus	OR 0.30 (0.12–0.75) [17]	OR 0.94 (0.39–2.28) [17]
Smoking	OR 1.17 (0.91–1.51) [17] OR 1.83 [24]	OR 1.39 (1.02–1.89) [17]
Migraine	18–41% [16,22,27,28]	7–24% [16,22,26,28]
Migraine with aura	OR 5.17 for women, 4.05 for men [24]	
Trauma	16–29.2% [12,22,23,29]	16–36.5% [12,22] 30% minor, 7% major [26]
Spinal manipulation therapy	6% [29]	30% [29]
OR, odds ratio.		

Cervical trauma. Mild cervical trauma in the preceding month has been reported by 15 to 36.5% of patients presenting with cervical artery dissection. There is no clinically significant difference between the ICAD and VAD groups.[12,23,26,29] In addition, sports that pose a risk of neck trauma have been linked to cervical artery dissection.[30]

Migraine. Several studies have found an increased prevalence of migraine in patients with cervical artery dissections, compared with the general population as well as with patients with ischemic stroke.[16,22,24,27,28,31] In one study, 25% of patients with a history of migraine reported that the pain they experienced as part of their cervical artery dissection was similar to the pain they experience during migraine attacks.[32] Studies have found elevated serum elastase activity in migraineurs, providing a possible mechanistic link between migraine and cervical artery dissection.[33] **Connective tissue disorders**. Connective tissue disorders are presumed to predispose to cervical artery dissection. The reported prevalence of connective tissue disorders in case series ranges from 0 to 6%.[16] The number of cases in which a recognized connective tissue disorder has been found is limited. The best proven association between a monogenic connective tissue disorder and cervical artery dissection involves vascular Ehlers–Danlos syndrome (EDS), also called EDS type IV. It is found in less than 1% of all patients with cervical artery dissection.[34] Marfan's syndrome also has been implicated as a risk factor for cervical artery dissections through case reports. However, no cervical artery dissection has been documented in large series of Marfan's patients.[34] A large study of genetic risk factors for cervical artery dissection is underway.[35]

Morbidity and mortality

Morbidity and mortality associated with cervical artery dissection are linked to the incidence of embolization of intraluminal clots from the cervical arteries and the location and extent of subsequent cerebral infarction. Overall, the prognosis for patients with cervical artery dissection is good. Ischemic stroke is more prevalent among patients with VAD, but their functional outcome is better than in patients with ICAD.[12,16,24,26,29] Approximately, 90 to 94% of patients with strokes related to VAD, compared with 75 to 91% of patients with ICAD, achieve a modified Rankin Scale score of 0 to 2, i.e., functional independence.[12,16,24,29] Despite these low scores, stroke-specific quality-of-life scores have been found to be impaired in long-term survivors of cervical artery dissection.[36] This was also found to be true for patients with only local or transient symptoms without functional impairment.[36] Death is relatively rare.

Recurrence

Recurrent dissections are relatively uncommon. In a large multinational study, recurrence at three months was found to be 2.1%, with a trend of being more common among patients with ICAD than with VAD.[12] In general, patients with a first event of cervical artery dissection have a low risk of recurrence of dissection or ischemic events.[25]

Diagnosis

History

Patients with cervical artery dissection can present with a wide variety of local signs and symptoms, ischemic symptoms, or completed infarcts. The most suggestive presentation is cervical trauma accompanied by a severe unilateral headache of gradual onset, followed by cerebral ischemia hours to days after the onset of the headache. In order of declining frequency, the following local symptoms occur: headache, facial pain, neck pain, tinnitus, and visual disturbance. Horner's syndrome, lower cranial nerve palsies, and dysgeusia (distortion of the sense of taste) can occur with ICAD.

Patients typically delay their presentation to a healthcare facility for days after the onset of symptoms. A retrospective study of 126 patients found that, among the patients who suffered a stroke as a result of cervical artery dissection, 78% had warning symptoms, with a median time from symptom onset to the stroke of three days. Forty-four percent noticed symptoms from 12 hours to 14 days before the stroke occurred.[29]

General symptoms

Headache. Headache, the most common presenting symptom, is experienced by 44 to 92% of patients.[12,16,27,29,37,38] There is typically a delay (median, four days) from the onset of the headache to the emergence of other symptoms.[27] However, in some patients, other symptoms are the initial complaint, with headache following later. In the vast majority of cases, the location of the headache is ipsilateral to the dissection, but it can be bilateral (typically seen with bilateral dissection or concurrent ICAD and VAD).[32]

In patients with ICAD, the headache is most commonly focal, frontal, and unilateral, but less commonly it can be diffuse unilateral or diffuse bilateral.[38] It is uncommon for patients with ICAD to present with occipital headache.[27,38] The quality of the headaches is reported as being aching (66%), throbbing (25–40%), or sharp (7%).[28,32] Some patients have onset of "thunderclap" headache, suggesting subarachnoid

Table 6.2 Prevalence of symptoms of cervical artery dissection

Symptom	Internal carotid artery dissection (ICAD) (%)	Vertebral artery dissection (VAD) (%)
Headache	44–92 [12,16,27, 29,37,38]	50–69 [12,16,27,29]
Neck pain	19–49 [12,16,27,29, 37]	39–72 [12,16,27,29]
Tinnitus	9–16 [29,37]	0 [29]
Visual disturbance	14–34 [23,27]	25 [27]
Eye, ear, face pain	35–53 [23,27]	0 [27]

Table 6.3 Prevalence of ischemic symptoms associated with ICAD and VAD

	Internal carotid artery dissection (ICAD) (%)	Vertebral artery dissection (VAD) (%)
Multi-vessel	Bilateral 10 [12] Unilateral 93 [24] Two vessels 7 [24] Multiple dissections 15.7 [25]	Bilateral 15.6 [12]
Cerebral ischemia	59–73, 2 [12,16]	78–90, 2 [12,16]
Ischemic stroke	60, 4–71 [12,24,28,29] 28 [23] 41 [16]	77, 1–85 [12,16,24, 29]
Transient ischemic attack	13–36.5 [12,16,28,29]	11–21.4 [12,16,29]
Transient monocular blindness	8.2 [12]	0 [12]
Subarachnoid hemorrhage	1 [12]	0.3 [12]
Horner's syndrome	21–37 [16,23,29,37]	0–22 [16,29]
Lower cranial nerve palsy	10–12 [37,39]	*
Dysgeusia	2–9 [27,37]	

*Lower cranial nerve palsies from VAD can occur from infarcts in the medulla, but we found no studies reporting its prevalence.

hemorrhage. The severity of the pain is severe in 75% and mild to moderate in 25%.[32] In 25% of patients with a history of migraine and ICAD, the pain associated with the dissection is similar to the patient's typical migraine pain.[32]

Approximately 50 to 69% of patients with VAD have headache.[12,16,27,29] It is typically occipital and unilateral but can present as bilateral or diffuse as well.

Neck pain. The second most common symptom of cervical artery dissections is neck pain, which is the initial symptom in approximately 25% of the patients. As with headache, the cervical pain is most often gradual in onset; however, in approximately one-quarter of patients, the pain is sudden. Cervical pain is more prevalent in association with VAD (reported by 66% of patients) than with ICAD (reported by 39% of patients).[12] Cervical and facial pain is practically always ipsilateral to the dissection.[32]

Other symptoms. The prevalences of less common symptoms are listed in Table 6.2.

Cerebral ischemia

TIA and ischemic stroke. TIA/ischemic stroke can result from two distinct mechanisms in cervical artery dissection, most importantly from embolization of an intraluminal clot created by extension of the intramural hematoma. The resulting deficits vary according to the involved vascular territory. A less dominant mechanism of TIA/ischemic stroke is by dissection that produces severe stenosis or occlusion, leading to cerebral hypoperfusion. TIAs frequently occur more than once in the course of cervical artery dissection; most episodes occur within the first month after

symptom onset. Ischemic stroke can occur from minutes after symptom onset until weeks later; 82% of ischemic strokes occur within the first week after symptom onset.[12,28] Features of ICAD and VAD are presented in Table 6.3.

Cranial nerve palsies

Cervical artery dissection can affect the cranial nerves directly or as a result of cerebral ischemia and infarction. Cranial nerve palsies can be induced if the expanding artery causes local pressure or stretching, or alternatively by the expanding artery interrupting the nutrient vessels supplying the nerve.[39]

Dysgeusia without other cranial nerve involvement can occur by involvement of the chorda tympani nerve.

Horner's syndrome (miosis and ptosis) is a typical manifestation of carotid artery dissection. It occurs without facial anhydrosis, since the sweat glands are innervated by the sympathetic plexus surrounding the external carotid artery that is uninvolved in the dissection. Horner's syndrome can also manifest after VAD if it results in medullary or pontine infarctions.

Cranial nerve involvement due to cerebral embolization and ischemia varies depending on the affected arterial territory (ICA vs. VA) and the specific brain region affected.

Physical examination

The diagnosis of cervical artery dissection rests on the history, a high index of suspicion for the condition, a detailed neurologic examination, and the appropriate imaging study. Red flags that suggest dissection include the following:

- headache or neck pain;
- history of trauma or neck manipulation (if it can be elicited);
- Horner's syndrome (especially if ipsilateral to neck pain or headache);
- stroke symptoms in the young without obvious risk factors (especially in association with neck pain or headache).

The following laboratory tests should be requested during the emergency department evaluation:

- complete blood count; CHEM-7; calcium; magnesium; phosphorus; liver function tests; aPTT; PT/INR; consider drug screen, as warranted; electrocardiogram.

The following imaging should be considered as part of the emergency department evaluation:

- computed tomography angiography (CTA) or magnetic resonance angiography (MRA), or Doppler ultrasound (see Figures 6.1, 6.2 and 6.3 all taken from the same patient). (Angiography was once considered the gold standard, but its use has diminished with increasing access to CTA and MRA.)

The following diagnostic features can be elicited by CTA/MRA:

- a narrowed centric or eccentric lumen surrounded by a crescent-shaped mural thickening and an associated increase in the vessel's external diameter;
- an abrupt or tapered occlusive lumen and an associated increase in external diameter;

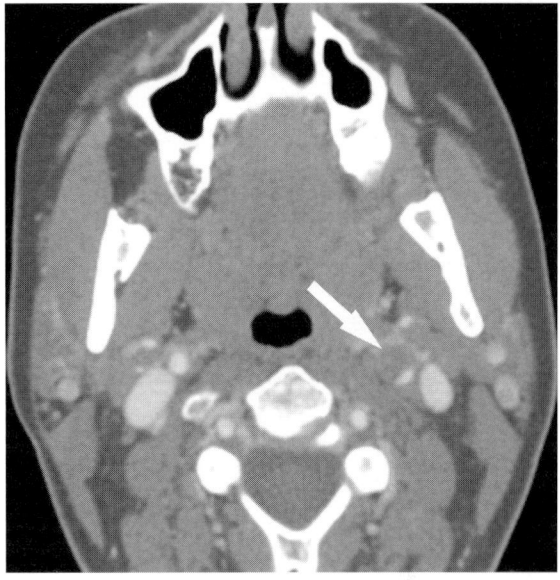

Figure 6.1 Axial image from CT angiogram demonstrates dissection and subtotal occlusion of the left internal carotid artery (white arrow) just proximal to the foramen lacerum (compare with contralateral side).

- a lumen dilated by an aneurysm or a dilated and narrowed lumen with or without crescent-shaped mural thickening;
- an intimal flap;
- lack of visualized flow;
- a mural hematoma.

Emergency department management

Initial assessment

As for any patient, initial attention is directed to the airway, breathing, and circulation, which are usually intact in patients with cervical artery dissection. If stroke is present, then the focus rapidly becomes defining the presence of infarction by obtaining relevant imaging according to locally available resources.

The differential diagnosis for patients presenting with headache and neck pain includes the following:

- migraine;
- subarachnoid hemorrhage;
- cluster headache;
- protracted headache due to venous sinus thrombosis;
- musculoskeletal neck pain.

Table 6.4 Critical actions to be taken in the emergency department

- Establish the diagnosis.
- Start antithrombotic therapy, as indicated (see discussion in text).
- Maintain adequate cerebral perfusion by avoiding hypotension and dehydration.
- Admit the patient to a monitored setting where frequent neurologic checks can be performed.

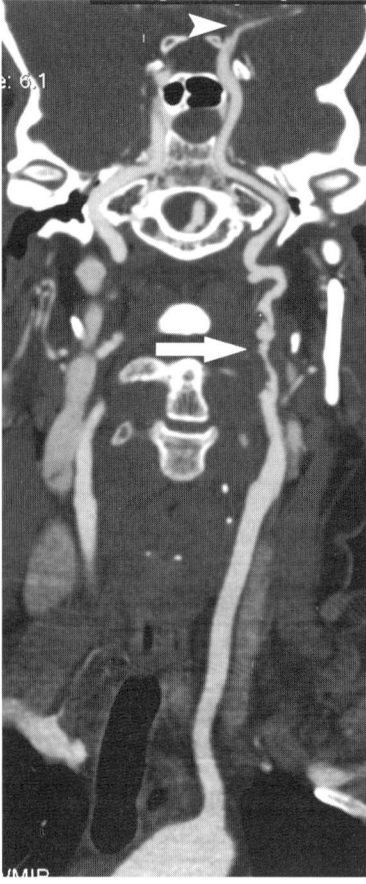

Figure 6.2 Curved planar reformatted image demonstrates a nearly occlusive circumferential thrombus at the proximal left internal carotid artery (ICA) (white arrow), with embolus noted at the left ICA terminus and proximal left middle cerebral artery (arrowhead).

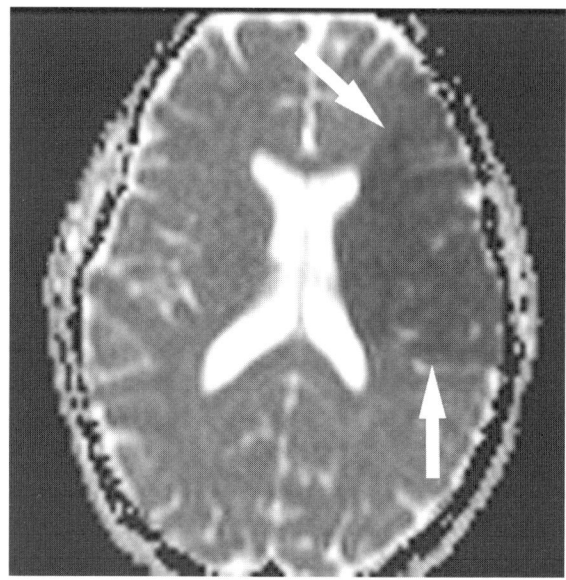

Figure 6.3 Apparent diffusion coefficient (ADC) map from subsequent MRI scan demonstrates the large territory of ischemia (between white arrows) in the left middle cerebral artery distribution.

Critical actions to be taken in the emergency department are listed in Table 6.4. The diagnosis is established with imaging. CTA and MRA both have a high sensitivity for detecting cervical artery dissection. Duplex ultrasonography may be useful for visualizing reduced flow or thrombus, but its sensitivity varies according to the vessel involved and the accompanying symptoms. In facilities where neither CT nor MR is available, duplex ultrasound or transcranial Doppler might be useful in suggesting the diagnosis.

Drug therapy

The informed choice of therapy suffers from a lack of randomized controlled trials comparing antiplatelet treatment with systemic anticoagulation. Several studies have found no difference between antithrombotic treatment and anticoagulation. One study of 298 consecutive patients found no difference in outcome between patients given aspirin and those who received systemic anticoagulation. Patients who presented with an ischemic event were more likely to have another ischemic event; this was however independent of the choice of treatment.[40] Meta-analyses have failed to find a difference in the incidence of stroke and death.[41,42] A non-randomized, observational, prospective study done in Germany found that 2% of patients treated with anticoagulation had a subsequent stroke during the first six months after discharge, whereas 16.7% of patients treated with antiplatelet agents had a stroke.[43] The difference was statistically significant. A meta-analysis from 2009, involving 1,033 patients, found that, for anticoagulation versus antiplatelet treatment, the rate of ischemic stroke was 2.3% versus 6.9%, and bleeding complications were reported in 0.7% versus 0 patients. Expressing reservations for methodologic flaws in the studies that were included, the authors concluded that "it cannot be excluded that there is net benefit from anticoagulant therapy in cervical dissection."[44] It is important to point out that anticoagulation may not be appropriate for patients with large infarcts, given the increased risk of hemorrhagic complications.

Stenting

Endovascular stenting has been found to be a feasible and safe therapeutic strategy for patients with cervical artery dissection who have failed medical therapy; i.e., those who continue to have fluctuating neurologic deficits despite adequate anticoagulation, blood pressure, and volume status.[45] A case series of eight patients with progressive or fluctuating neurologic deficits treated with self-expanding stents reported good outcomes: all were discharged with excellent functional status after presenting to the hospital with a National Institutes of Health Stroke Scale (NIHSS) score of 5 to 21.[46] Stents must be used on a case-by-case basis by cerebrovascular specialists with expertise in this area.

Thrombolysis

There are concerns regarding the use of thrombolysis in patients with dissection, as it could theoretically worsen the mural hematoma. However, the use of thrombolytic therapy in otherwise eligible patients presenting with acute stroke caused by cervical artery dissection is not contraindicated. In one study, 33 patients treated with intravenous (IV) thrombolysis for ICAD showed no new or worsened local signs, subarachnoid hemorrhage, pseudoaneurysm formation, or rupture of the internal carotid artery. An improvement of the NIHSS score at three months was seen in 26 / 33 (79%) patients.[47] A recent meta-analysis including individual patient data from 180 patients in case series and case reports found a rate of intracranial hemorrhage of 3% and an overall mortality of 8%.[48] This is very similar to the results for IV tissue plasminogen activator (tPA) for ischemic strokes.

Admission/level-of-care criteria

First few hours

Patients are generally started on some form of antithrombotic therapy and admitted for monitoring of neurologic status, blood pressure, and fluid status. Neurologic checks should be performed frequently, because these patients are at risk for developing an ischemic stroke.

Definitive treatment (outside the ED)

Various treatment modalities exist for cervical artery dissection, including antiplatelet treatment or anticoagulation, stenting, and IV and local intra-arterial thrombolytic treatment in acute stroke cases. Evidence indicating optimal therapy is sparse; however, for uncomplicated cases, there seems to be agreement that three to six months of antithrombotic treatment is a reasonable treatment strategy.[49]

Rationale for duration of therapy

A number of studies have investigated the pace of healing and recanalization. Lee and colleagues found a median time to healing, defined as complete recanalization or development of a fixed lesion, of 0.29 years. Eighty percent of patients healed after six months.[16] Arauz and associates reported that 46% of patients had achieved complete recanalization in three months and 62% in six months. They found only marginal benefit in extending treatment to 12 months, when 64% of the study group had achieved complete recanalization.[26] Based on a smaller study, following 38 patients, Caso *et al.* found that complete recanalization occurred in 42% of patients after six weeks and that no further recanalizations occurred beyond that point.[22] The authors of the last two of these studies concluded that neither the development nor degree of recanalization affected functional outcomes.[22,26]

Clinical approach when resources are limited

There are few good diagnostic options in resource-poor environments, especially those without access to CT or MR. If feasible, the patient should be transferred to a facility that has those resources. When the diagnosis is suggested by the history, transcranial Doppler, if available, might increase the likelihood of the diagnosis. A course of aspirin might be appropriate.

Inpatient care

If the condition of a patient with dissection worsens despite antithrombotic treatment, it is worthwhile considering blood pressure and fluid (normal saline) augmentation, especially if no new infarcts are seen on brain MRI. If symptoms persist, in the absence of infarction, arterial stenting might be an option.

Subarachnoid hemorrhage is a rare complication of the condition; it is seen in 1% of patients with ICAD and in 0.3% of those with VAD.[22] If a subarachnoid hemorrhage is detected, antithrombotic therapy should be stopped and reversed.

Disposition

Patients with new cervical artery dissection should be admitted for antithrombotic treatment. They should be admitted to a monitored setting where frequent neurologic checks can be performed.

Pearls and pitfalls

1. Patients with migraine are at an increased risk of developing cervical artery dissection. Their pain can often be similar to the pain experienced during migraine attacks. New neurological symptoms experienced during migraine attacks should lead to a consideration of cervical artery dissection, especially if accompanied by new or different neck pain.
2. Patients with neck dissections may not have had neck trauma, or it may have been trivial.
3. Patients with VAD may present with acute dizziness from small cerebellar strokes that can mimic an acute peripheral vestibular syndrome.

Conclusion

Cervical artery dissection is a common cause of stroke in the young. It can occur spontaneously or in the setting of often relatively trivial trauma. A typical presentation is cervical trauma accompanied by gradual onset of a severe unilateral headache, followed by cerebral ischemia hours to days after the onset of the headache. The diagnosis is usually confirmed with CTA or MRA. Antithrombotic treatment is typically initiated, but it is unclear if anticoagulation or antiplatelet therapy is superior. Outcomes are generally good with regard to functional level.

References

1. Leys D, Bandu L, Henon H, *et al.* Clinical outcome in 287 consecutive young adults (15 to 45 years) with ischemic stroke. *Neurology* 2002; 59(1): 26–33.
2. Kristensen B, Malm J, Carlberg B, *et al.* Epidemiology and etiology of ischemic stroke in young adults aged 18 to 44 years in northern Sweden. *Stroke* 1997; 28(9): 1702–9.
3. Nedeltchev K, der Maur TA, Georgiadis D, *et al.* Ischaemic stroke in young adults: predictors of outcome and recurrence. *J Neurol Neurosurg Psychiatr* 2005; 76(2): 191–5.
4. Blunt SB, Galton C. Cervical carotid or vertebral artery dissection. *BMJ* 1997; 314(7076): 243.
5. Jentzer A. Dissecting aneurysm of the left internal carotid artery. *Angiology* 1954; 5(3): 232–4.
6. Dittrich R, Nassenstein I, Bachmann R, *et al.* Can an ordinary neurological examination induce a dissection of the vertebral artery?: a case report. *J Neurol* 2007; 254(1): 118–19.
7. Abuzayed B, Aydin S, Bozkus H, *et al.* Traumatic carotid artery dissection and bilateral vertebral artery occlusion after a horse attack: an unusual combination and etiology. *J Neurol Surg A Cent Eur Neurosurg* 2012; 73(1): 53–55.
8. Brand S, Teebken OE, Bolzen P, *et al.* Traumatische Karotisdissektion nach Motorradunfall. [Traumatic dissection of carotid arteries caused by high energy motorcycle accident.] Unfallchirurg, September 1, 2011 [Epub ahead of print].
9. Busch T, Aleksic I, Sirbu H, *et al.* Complex traumatic dissection of right vertebral and bilateral carotid arteries: a case report and literature review. *Cardiovasc Surg* 2000; 8(1): 72–4.
10. Fletcher J, Davies PT, Lewis T, *et al.* Traumatic carotid and vertebral artery dissection in a professional jockey: a cautionary tale. *Br J Sports Med* 1995; 29(2): 143–4.
11. Knobloch K, Beil C, Wilhelmi M, *et al.* A catastrophic car crash: right main bronchial rupture with concomitant thrombosis of the right carotid artery, vertebral artery dissection, and dislocated cervical spine fracture. *J Trauma* 2009; 66(2): 587.
12. Debette S, Grond-Ginsbach C, Bodenant M, *et al.* Differential features of carotid and vertebral artery dissections. *Neurology* 2011; 77(12): 1174–81.
13. Schievink WI. Spontaneous dissection of the carotid and vertebral arteries. *N Engl J Med* 2001; 344(12): 898–906.
14. Giroud M, Fayolle H, Andre N, *et al.* Incidence of internal carotid artery dissection in the community of Dijon. *J Neurol Neurosurg Psychiatr* 1994; 57(11): 1443.
15. Schievink WI, Mokri B, Whisnant JP. Internal carotid artery dissection in a community. Rochester, Minnesota, 1987–1992. *Stroke* 1993; 24(11): 1678–80.
16. Lee VH, Brown RD, Mandrekar JN, *et al.* Incidence and outcome of cervical artery dissection. *Neurology* 2006; 67(10): 1809–12.

17. Debette SP, Metso T, Pezzini A, *et al.* Association of vascular risk factors with cervical artery dissection and ischemic stroke in young adults. *Circulation* 2011; 123(14): 1537–44.

18. Nadgir RN, Loevner LA, Ahmed T, *et al.* Simultaneous bilateral internal carotid and vertebral artery dissection following chiropractic manipulation: case report and review of the literature. *Neuroradiology* 2003; 45(5): 311–14.

19. Parenti G, Orlandi G, Bianchi M, *et al.* Vertebral and carotid artery dissection following chiropractic cervical manipulation. *Neurosurg Rev* 1999; 22(2–3): 127–9.

20. Lee KP, Cslini WG, McCormick GF, *et al.* Neurologic complications following chiropractic manipulation. *Neurology* 1995; 45(6): 1213–15.

21. Smith WS, Johnston SC, Skalabrin EJ, *et al.* Spinal manipulative therapy is an independent risk factor for vertebral artery dissection. *Neurology* 2003; 60(9): 1424–8.

22. Caso V, Paciaroni M, Corea F, *et al.* Recanalization of cervical artery dissection: influencing factors and role in neurological outcome. *Cerebrovasc Dis* 2004; 17(2-3): 93–7.

23. Rao AS, Makaroun MS, Marone LK, *et al.* Long-term outcomes of internal carotid artery dissection. *J Vasc Surg* 2011 4(2): 370–5.

24. Metso TM, Metso AJ, Salonen O, *et al.* Adult cervicocerebral artery dissection: a single-center study of 301 Finnish patients. *Eur J Neurol* 2009; 16(6): 656–61.

25. Touze E, Gauvrit JY, Moulin T, *et al.* Risk of stroke and recurrent dissection after a cervical artery dissection: a multicenter study. *Neurology* 2003; 61(10): 1347–51.

26. Arauz A, Márquez JM, Artigas C, *et al.* Recanalization of vertebral artery dissection. *Stroke* 2010; 41(4): 717–21.

27. Silbert PL, Mokri B, Schievink WI. Headache and neck pain in spontaneous internal carotid and vertebral artery dissections. *Neurology* 1995; 45(8): 1517–22.

28. Biousse V, D'Anglejan-Chatillon J, Touboul PJ, *et al.* Time course of symptoms in extracranial carotid artery dissections. A series of 80 patients. *Stroke* 1995; 26(2): 235–9.

29. Dziewas R, Konrad C, Drager B, *et al.* Cervical artery dissection – clinical features, risk factors, therapy and outcome in 126 patients. *J Neurol* 2003; 250(10): 1179–84.

30. Pary LF, Rodnitzky RL. Traumatic internal carotid artery dissection associated with taekwondo. *Neurology* 2003; 60(8): 1392–3.

31. Tzourio C, Benslamia L, Guillon B. Migraine and the risk of cervical artery dissection: a case-control study. *Neurology* 2002; 59(3): 435–7.

32. Biousse V, D'Anglejan-Chatillon J, Massiou H, *et al.* Head pain in non-traumatic carotid artery dissection: a series of 65 patients. *Cephalalgia* 1994; 14(1): 33–6.

33. Tzourio C, El Amrani M, Robert L, *et al.* Serum elastase activity is elevated in migraine. *Ann Neurol* 2000; 47(5): 648–51.

34. Grond-Ginsbach C, Debette S. The association of connective tissue disorders with cervical artery dissections. *Curr Mol Med* 2009; 9(2): 210–14.

35. Debette S, Metso TM, Pezzini A, *et al.* CADISP-genetics: an international project searching for genetic risk factors of cervical artery dissections. *Int J Stroke* 2009; 4(3): 224–30.

36. Fischer U, Ledermann I, Nedeltchev K, *et al.* Quality of life in survivors after cervical artery dissection. *J Neurol* 2009; 256(3): 443–9.

37. Baumgartner RW, Arnold M, Baumgartner I, *et al.* Carotid dissection with and without ischemic events: local symptoms and cerebral artery findings. *Neurology* 2001; 57(5): 827–32.

38. Mokri B, Sundt TM Jr, Houser OW, *et al.* Spontaneous dissection of the cervical internal carotid artery. *Ann Neurol* 1986; 19(2): 126–38.

39. Mokri B, Silbert PL, Schievink WI, *et al.* Cranial nerve palsy in spontaneous dissection of the extracranial internal carotid artery. *Neurology* 1996; 46(2): 356–9.

40. Georgiadis D, Arnold M, von Buedingen HC, *et al.* Aspirin vs anticoagulation in carotid artery dissection. *Neurology* 2009; 72(21): 1810–15.

41. Eddy SL. Treatment of carotid artery dissection. *Ann Emerg Med* 2005; 46(3): 294–5.

42. Menon R, Kerry S, Norris JW, *et al.* Treatment of cervical artery dissection: a systematic review and meta-analysis. *J Neurol Neurosurg Psychiatr* 2008; 79(10): 1122–7.

43. Weimar C, Kraywinkel K, Hagemeister C, *et al.* Recurrent stroke after cervical artery dissection. *J Neurol Neurosurg Psychiatr* 2010; 81(8): 869–73.

44. Kim Y-K, Schulman S. Cervical artery dissection: pathology, epidemiology and management. *Thromb Res* 2009; 123(6): 810–21.

45. Yin Q, Li Y, Fan X, *et al.* Feasibility and safety of stenting for symptomatic carotid arterial dissection. *Cerebrovasc Dis* 2011; 32(suppl 1): 11–15.

46. Jeon P, Kim BM, Kim DI, *et al.* Emergent self-expanding stent placement for acute intracranial or extracranial internal carotid artery dissection with significant hemodynamic

insufficiency. *AJNR Am J Neuroradiol* 2010; 31(8): 1529–32.

47. Georgiadis D, Lanczik O, Schwab S, *et al.* IV thrombolysis in patients with acute stroke due to spontaneous carotid dissection. *Neurology* 2005; 64(9): 1612–14.

48. Zinkstok SM, Vergouwen MD, Engelter ST, *et al.* Safety and functional outcome of thrombolysis in dissection-related ischemic stroke: a meta-analysis of individual patient data. *Stroke* 2011; 42(9): 2515–20.

49. Writing Committee Members, Brott TG, Halperin JL, *et al.* 2011 ASA/ACCF/AHA/AANN/AANS/ACR/ ASNR/CNS/SAIP/SCAI/SIR/SNIS/SVM/SVS Guideline on the Management of Patients with Extracranial Carotid and Vertebral Artery Disease. *Stroke* 2011; 42(8): e464–540.

Chapter

Acute aortic dissection

John A. Elefteriades and Samuel Youssef

There is no disease more conducive to clinical humility than aneurysm of the aorta.
Sir William Osler (Circa 1900)

Aortic dissection is one of the most challenging conditions that emergency physicians will face in their careers. This condition is very difficult to diagnose and is lethal if the diagnosis is delayed or missed. This combination of characteristics – difficulty in diagnosis and lethality – represents a virtual "Scylla and Charybdis" challenge for those on the front lines in the emergency department. In fact, only 50% of cases of aortic dissection are diagnosed accurately premortem – a vivid expression of the difficulty in diagnosis and inherent lethality of this disease process.[1]

Couple those issues with the fact that aortic dissection is a "needle in a haystack," in the sense that the emergency physician will see 100 primary cardiac causes of chest pain for each dissection, then there is great potential for error.[1] In addition, aortic dissection cases are highly litigated; hence, a high state of anxiety exists in their regard. Acute care practitioners on the front lines have a much harder job than aortic specialists; front-line physicians have to sense and select-out patients with acute aortic dissection from the hundreds seen each day in the emergency department. Complicating the situation is the fact that aortic dissection has a well-earned reputation as "the great masquerader" (see below), able to mimic or disguise itself as a disease of virtually any organ system in the body.[1] By the time the aortic specialist is consulted, the hard work of sifting out and identifying the acute dissection has already been done. Those of us who care for the thoracic aorta have a great deal of respect for the talented physicians charged with sorting out the cause of critical illness in the emergency department.

The best advice we can offer to those on the front lines is to keep aortic dissection in mind and to include it liberally in their differential diagnoses.

Definition and classification

Aortic dissection is a splitting of the aortic wall into two layers – an inner layer and an outer layer. The split occurs in mid-media, at varying depths into the medial lamellae (Figure 7.1). The split then propagates for varying distances longitudinally along the aorta. The most important distinction is between *ascending* (Type A) and *descending* (Type B) aortic dissection (Figure 7.2). Ascending dissection begins with a tear about a centimeter or two above the coronary ostea and propagates longitudinally along the aorta (usually to the aortic bifurcation or beyond). Ascending dissection requires urgent surgery in most cases. Descending aortic dissection begins with an intimal tear a centimeter or two beyond the origin of the left subclavian artery and propagates for various distances down the aorta, usually to the aortic bifurcation or beyond. Descending dissection usually is treated medically. Aside from the distinction of ascending versus descending, it is important to recognize that aortic dissection can take any of three morphologies:[2] *typical aortic dissection* (with the splitting of two layers as just described), *penetrating aortic ulcer* (in which an ulcer in the aortic wall permits entry of blood between the layers of the aorta), and *intramural hematoma* of the aorta (in which a crescentic layer of blood forms in the aortic wall, but without a frank separation of layers with an inner intimal flap) (Figure 7.3). All three can present with acute symptoms (see below) as what has recently been termed *acute aortic syndrome*. Penetrating ulcer is a disease of advanced age, almost invariably occurring in a heavily arteriosclerotic aorta; we

Vascular Emergencies, ed. Robert L. Rogers, Thomas Scalea, Lee Wallis, and Heike Geduld. Published by Cambridge University Press. © Cambridge University Press 2013.

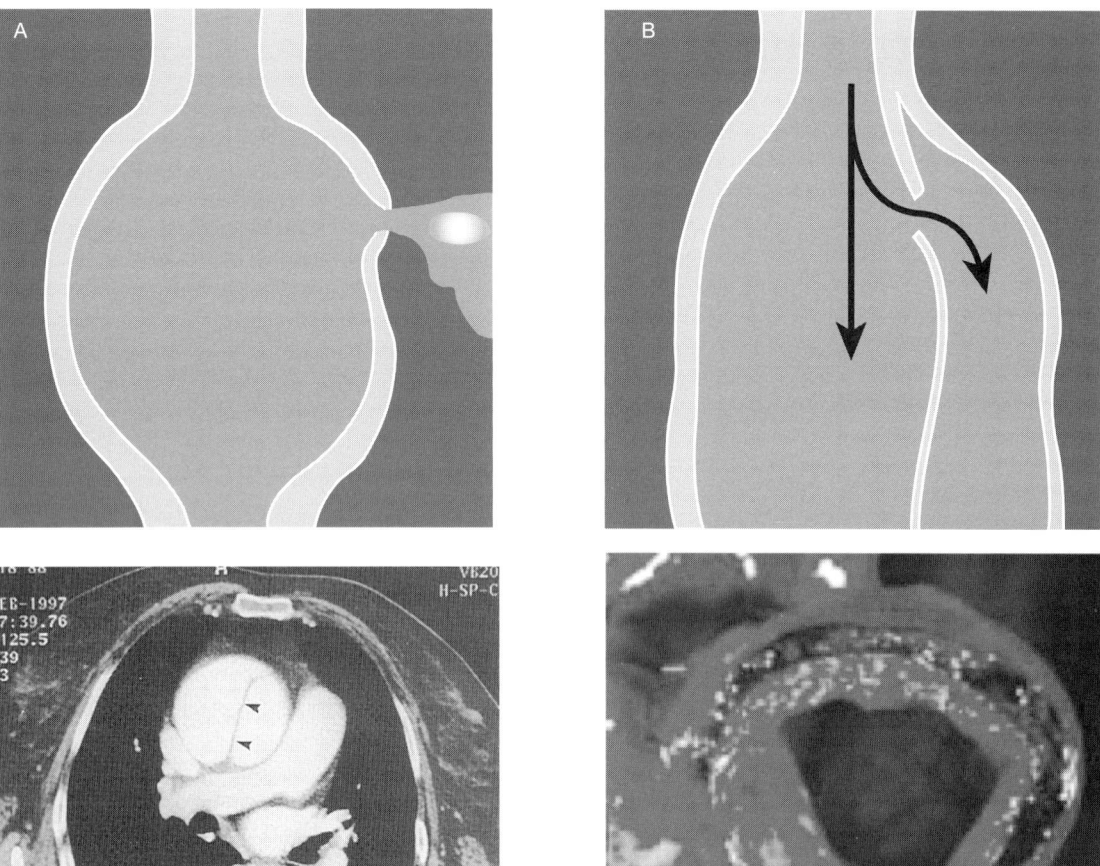

Figure 7.1 Artist's depiction of aortic dissection. Note the difference between (A) free rupture and (B) aortic dissection. (C) Note dissection in mid-media in this pathologic specimen. (D) Typical CT scan appearance of aortic dissection. Note flap in ascending and descending aorta. (Reproduced with permission from Elefteriades.[3])

almost always find, at surgery, many more ulcers than detected by even the most advanced imaging studies. Intramural hematoma is like a mild form of aortic dissection; it often progresses to frank typical aortic dissection, although, in select cases, it can heal completely spontaneously.

It is important to differentiate three conditions whose distinction and terminology are often confused (Figure 7.4). *Acute aortic transection* is an acute traumatic condition in which the aorta is torn to various depths. This occurs in normal, undiseased aortas subjected to the trauma of a motor vehicle crash or a fall from a great height. Aortic transection does not generally dissect (the layers of the aortic wall do not split

and propagate). *"Degenerative" aneurysm* is a chronic disorder leading to enlargement of the aorta, which is not usually an emergency condition, in the absence of rupture or dissection. *Acute aortic dissection*, the subject of this chapter, is a non-traumatic condition that occurs instantaneously in an aorta whose media is heavily diseased, usually due to an inherited condition.

Etiology

Aortic disease has long been thought to be a manifestation of arteriosclerosis. However, it is becoming increasingly clear that, for the ascending aorta

Type A

Type B

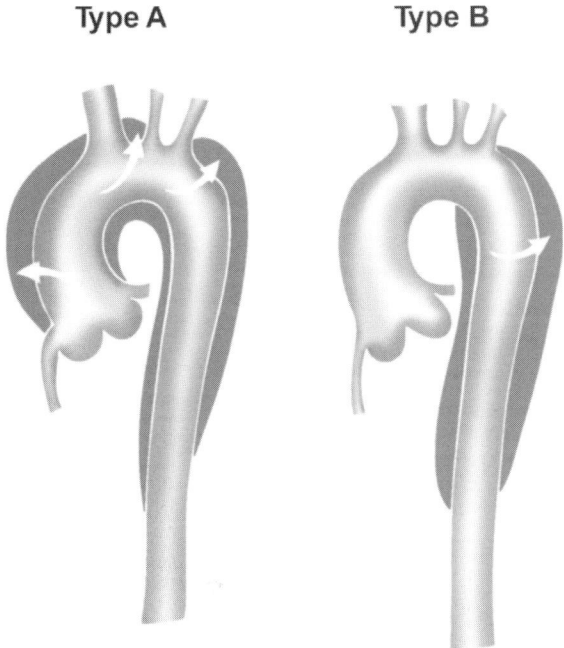

Figure 7.2 Classification system for aortic dissection: Type A (ascending) and Type B (descending). Treatment is predicated on type: ascending usually requires urgent surgical replacement of the aorta, whereas descending is usually treated medically. (Reproduced with permission from www.cedars-sinai.edu/Patients/Health-Conditions/Aortic-Dissection.aspx.)

especially, the development of aneurysm and dissection are not at all related to arteriosclerosis or to arteriosclerotic risk factors, but rather are manifestations of inborn, genetically mediated, connective tissue weakness (see Figure 11.2).[4–7] These disorders run strongly in families (see Figure 11.4).

Pathophysiology

We have been able to clarify the pathologic sequence that leads to acute aortic dissection.[4] This clarification has its origins in the recognition that aortic aneurysm and aortic dissection run strongly in families.[4–7] In addition, physical stress and acute emotional stress can trigger aortic dissection.[8–10] We first identified this factor in five healthy young weightlifters treated at our institution within a short period for acute ascending aortic dissection. These investigations led to the schema presented in Figure 7.5. First, an inherited predisposition leads to development of an aortic aneurysm. We now know that the matrix metalloproteinases (MMPs) participate actively in genetically induced degradation of the aortic wall, leading to aortic aneurysm formation. Then, in a patient with an aneurysm, a specific stress – physical or emotional – leads to acute severe hypertension, resulting in splitting of the diseased aortic wall into the layers that constitute an aortic dissection.

Acute aortic dissection can kill a patient quickly in four ways (Figure 7.6):

1. cardiac tamponade (from intrapericardial rupture of ascending aortic dissection);
2. acute aortic insufficiency (from unseating of the aortic valve; in contradistinction to chronic aortic insufficiency, which is well tolerated, acute aortic

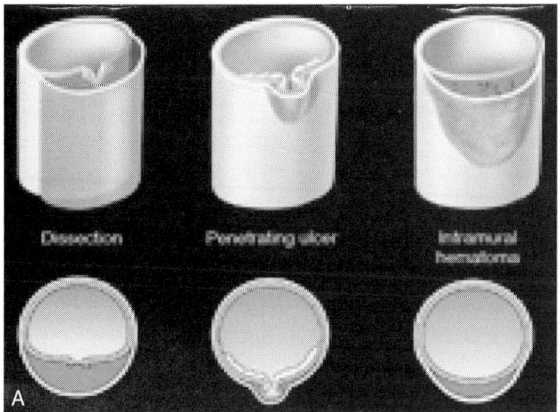
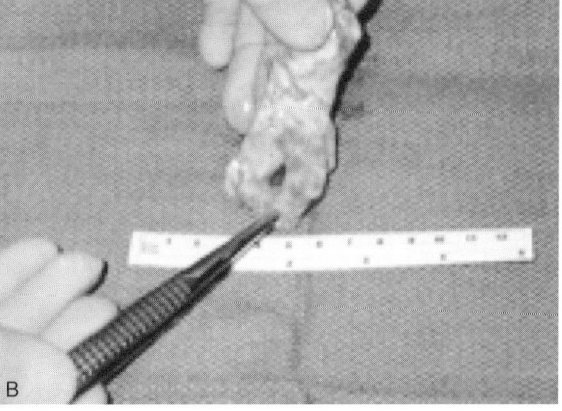

Figure 7.3 Types of aortic dissection phenomena. (A) Typical aortic dissection has a flap traversing the lumen. A penetrating ulcer permits entry of blood into the aortic wall at the base of the ulcer. Intramural hematoma involves a circumferential collection of blood in the aortic wall, but without a frank flap. (B) A penetrating ulcer of the aorta (surgical specimen shown) resembles a duodenal ulcer in its overall appearance. (Reproduced with permission from Elefteriades.[11])

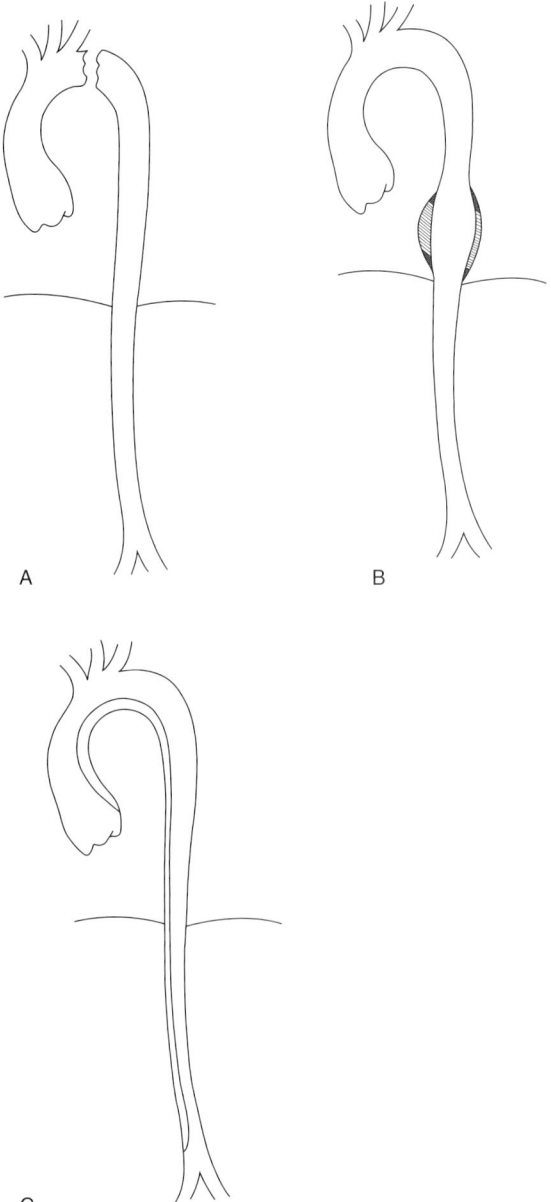

Figure 7.4 Differentiation of three commonly confused conditions, the terminology for which is often inappropriately applied: (A) aortic transection, (B) "degenerative" aortic ulcer, and (C) acute aortic dissection. See text. (Reproduced with permission from Elefteriades.[11])

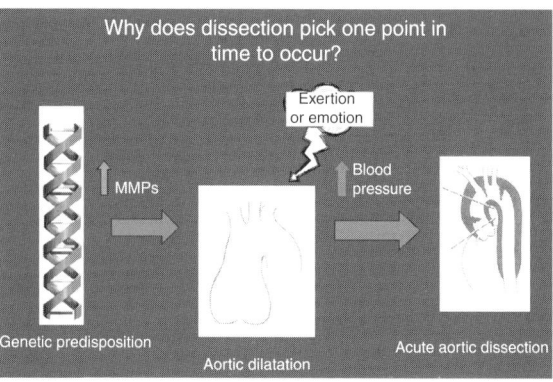

Figure 7.5 Schema of events leading to aortic dissection: from inborn genetics, through molecular pathology, to acute precipitating events. MMPs, matrix metalloproteinases. (Reproduced with permission from Elefteriades.[11])

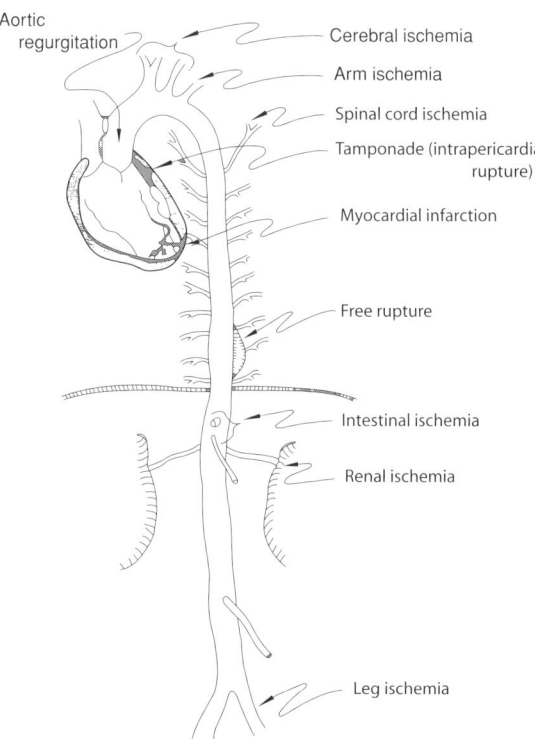

Figure 7.6 The four ways that aortic dissection can kill a patient in the early first hours: intrapericardial rupture with cardiac tamponade, acute aortic insufficiency, free rupture into the left pleural space, and ischemia related to any branch of the aorta (from coronary arteries to iliac vessels). See text. (From Elefteriades et al.[12])

insufficiency can produce immediate cardiogenic shock);

3. free rupture (usually into the left pleural space);
4. organ ischemia (any organ can be affected).

Epidemiology

Largely unappreciated, aortic aneurysm and aortic dissection constitute the 15th most common cause of death in humans, accounting for more loss of life than

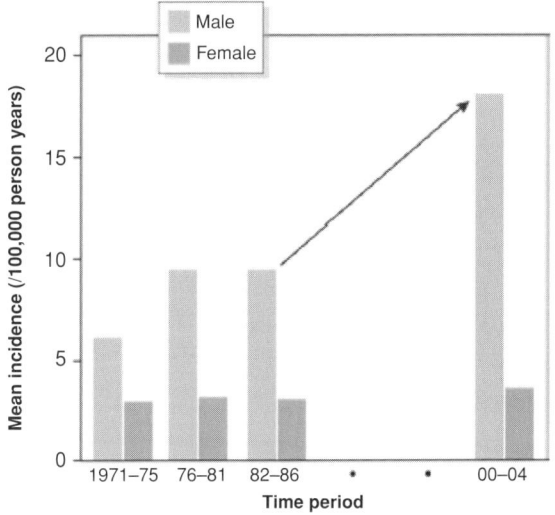

Figure 7.7 Increase in incidence of aortic aneurysm disease. (From Elefteriades.[13])

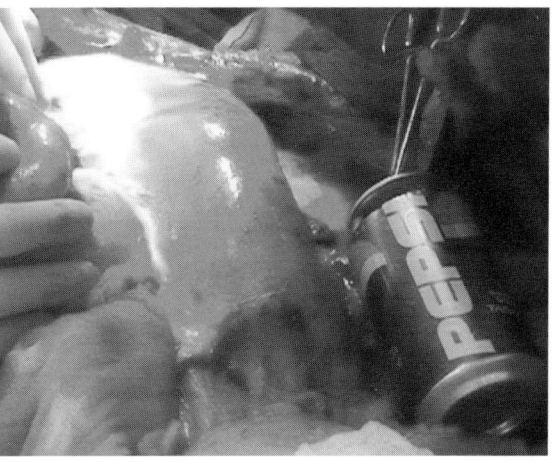

Figure 7.8 A "python-sized" thoracoabdominal aortic aneurysm, being resected surgically at the time of the photograph. The patient's head is to the upper left and his feet are to the lower right. If a patient's aorta is approaching the size of a soda can (~6 cm in diameter), it needs to be resected. (Reproduced with permission from Elefteriades.[11])

the better-appreciated diseases associated with infection with the human immunodeficiency virus.[14] Aortic dissection is even more common than databases show, as many cases are misdiagnosed as myocardial infarction. When a middle-aged male presents to the emergency department complaining of chest pain, and subsequently dies, the cause of death is generally presumed to be a myocardial infarction. Autopsy studies performed have shown that many of these patients have actually succumbed to aortic dissection. Aortic dissection is more common in winter (because blood pressure tends to be higher in the cold) and in the morning (because blood pressure tends be higher upon awakening in the morning). Aortic dissection is recognized throughout the world; no major countries are immune. The disease, and its intramural hematoma variant especially, appears to be less virulent in Japan. For reasons that are completely unclear, the incidence of aortic aneurysm is increasing, doubling every couple decades (Figure 7.7).[14] Studies have shown that this is a bona fide increase, not just an artifact from the increased availability of computed tomography (CT) scanning.

Based on concerted clinical epidemiologic study, we have now clarified when aortic dissection is likely to occur, based on aneurysm size (see Table 11.1).[15,16] For the ascending aorta, rupture or dissection occurs at about 6 cm diameter or more, so pre-emptive surgery at 5.0 to 5.5 cm almost always precludes rupture or dissection, safely preserving life. For descending aortic aneurysms, rupture and dissection occur at larger sizes, and we use a criterion of about 6.0 cm for pre-emptive surgical intervention. For practical purposes, if a patient's aorta is approaching the dimension of a soda can (6 cm), it needs to be removed prophylactically (Figure 7.8). Please remember that size criteria apply only for the asymptomatic aneurysm. *A symptomatic aneurysm (a painful one) needs to be removed regardless of size.*

Diagnosis

The diagnosis of aortic dissection is both difficult and of paramount importance, for the reasons mentioned in the opening section of this chapter. The quintessential symptom of aortic dissection is pain. The characteristics of the pain reflect vividly the nature of the disorder. It is described as the most severe pain possible (more than a kidney stone and more than childbirth). The pain has a tearing or knife-like quality. With ascending dissection, the pain originates and is maximal under the breastbone. With descending dissection, the pain typically originates between the shoulder blades in the upper thoracic back. The pain may migrate distally and the dissection splits the layers further, travelling toward the abdomen and the legs. The pain usually has an abrupt onset – virtually instantaneous. The pain is often preceded by acute physical exertion or an acute emotional event, and it behooves the physician to ask what was transpiring at the time of onset.

History

A detailed family history of aortic aneurysm, aortic valve disease, or premature sudden cardiac death should be obtained. This is considered basic information obtained in a medical history. An affirmative response should raise acute aortic dissection high into the differential diagnosis. If the patient or any family member has a bicuspid aortic valve the diagnosis should be considered, as presence of a bicuspid aortic valve is strongly associated with aortic dissection.

Physical examination

The physical examination may be normal in patients with acute aortic dissection. Occasionally, one can hear the murmur of aortic insufficiency, reflecting unseating of the aortic valve by an ascending aortic dissection. Less commonly, there may be an absent or reduced pulse, usually in the femoral artery or in the brachial or carotid artery. A difference in blood pressure between the two arms may be a clue that the branch arteries are being compromised. Patients may present in shock, usually indicating internal bleeding from rupture of the dissection or cardiac tamponade from intrapericardial rupture. In the latter case, jugular venous distention and grayish discoloration of the face may be found.

The patient who presents with sharp, extremely severe, substernal chest pain of sudden onset following strenuous exertion may be easy to recognize as having an acute ascending aortic dissection. On the other hand, as depicted in Figure 7.6, aortic dissection may masquerade as disease of virtually any organ of the body, because each organ receives its blood flow from a branch of the aorta – a branch that can be compromised or occluded by the dissection process. Thus, aortic dissection may present as a stroke, as arm ischemia, as myocardial infarction or pericarditis, as paraplegia from involvement of critical spinal arteries, as an abdominal catastrophe, or as extremity ischemia. The abdominal presentation is especially difficult to recognize. Aortic dissection is often misdiagnosed as anxiety attack, transient ischemic attack (TIA), lumbar disc disease, cholecystitis, or gastroenteritis.[1]

Aortic dissection can occur during pregnancy, either during parturition or for up to a week afterward.

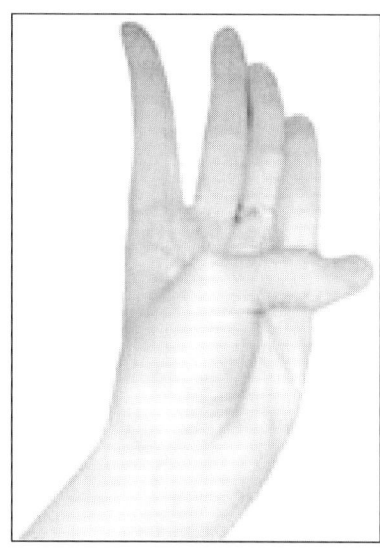

Figure 7.9 The "thumb-palm sign" for connective tissue disease. See text. (Reproduced with permission from Elefteriades.[11])

These cases are often missed in the emergency department.

Certain physical stigmata can be part of the overall appearance of patients with connective tissue disease. A tall, thin body build should be a clue, not only for Marfan's disease but also for non-Marfanoid connective tissue disease.[17] Pectus excavatum or carinatum is another sign of connective tissue disease, as is the thumb-palm sign (Figure 7.9), in which the thumb can stretch all the way beyond the flat palm. A history of "double jointedness" is another clue that the connective tissues are lax.

Laboratory tests

A full battery of blood tests will typically be conducted for these patients. The D-dimer can be a useful test in some circumstances.[18,19] D-dimer is released very quickly from the breakdown of thrombus that invariably forms in the space between the dissected layers. The D-dimer is more than 99% sensitive in detecting the clot associated with most cases of aortic dissection. The absolute value of the D-dimer reflects the length of the dissection and predicts the likelihood of death. In theory, if the D-dimer is negative, the patient does not have an acute aortic dissection. D-dimer may also be released in acute myocardial infarction and pulmonary embolism, so care should be taken and other diagnoses considered. D-dimer is sensitive, and it is this sensitivity that is of paramount value to the emergency physician. Caution should be exercised, however, because there is not an accepted cutoff level for D-dimer below which acute aortic dissection can be excluded. In addition, D-dimer may not be a useful test in the small subset of patients with the intramural hematoma variant of aortic dissection. Since there is not an intimal tear in cases of intramural hematoma, theoretically very little D-dimer would be released into the circulation. Despite concerted efforts, no other predictive (before the fact) or diagnostic (after the fact) blood markers for aortic dissection have come into clinical practice, although promising progress is being made.[20,21]

Imaging studies

The main advice to offer regarding imaging is to *image liberally*. Whenever aortic dissection is in the differential diagnosis – and it should be frequently, and for a wide range of presentations – an imaging study should be obtained. It has been shown repeatedly that echocardiography, CT, and MRI are all sensitive and specific for aortic dissection. MRI is usually more difficult to obtain, and advanced imaging facilities are often located remote from acute care areas. Echocardiography (ECHO) is available in many emergency departments and is frequently the study of choice, particularly when a CT scan cannot be obtained. More and more, emergency physicians are acquiring expertise in echocardiography and can perform their own examinations in the acute care setting. It is important to recognize that ECHO cannot "see" more than a few centimeters up the aorta from the aortic valve (see Figure 11.7). CT imaging is recommended for complete visualization of the aorta, especially the ECHO-inaccessible descending aorta.

Thus far, we have been discussing standard transthoracic echocardiography, which can usually diagnose an ascending aortic dissection. Transesophageal echocardiography (TEE) gives even more precise images and can certainly be employed as well. It is important to note that some patients may strain against the TEE probe. In some cases the stimulus of a probe or an endotracheal tube is just enough to rupture an ascending aortic dissection. Lastly, TEE is operator dependent, requires an experienced sonographer, and is not available in many emergency departments.

Between transthoracic echocardiography and CT scan, aortic dissection will essentially be ruled in or out – conclusively. The CT images will be of other benefit too. We often refer to the "triple rule-out CT scan."[1] This term recognizes that three conditions that usually present with chest pain commonly take the life of the acutely ill patient. All are ruled in or out by CT scanning. The first and perhaps most deadly is aortic dissection. Another is acute pulmonary embolism, which will be seen clearly in most cases on contrast CT scanning. The third is acute myocardial infarction; the CT will not visualize the infarct itself, but it may show the coronary calcification that leads to the infarction.

It is important to remember that plain chest radiography can give important clues about the aorta as well. The aortic contours can usually be discerned well (see Figures 11.5 and 11.6). The ascending aorta, if enlarged or dissected, will "peek out" beyond the right mediastinal shadow; the aortic knob, representing the aortic arch, will be enlarged if the arch is large or dissected; the straight paravertebral tissue plane representing the descending aorta will be enlarged and/or deviated if the descending aorta is enlarged or dissected. The emergency physician would do well to glean as much information from the aortic contour on the plain film as possible.

Emergency department management

The main goal in the emergency department is to consider and confirm the diagnosis of aortic dissection. The second goal is to begin medical management of the aortic dissection as rapidly as possible.[22,23] Initial management, regardless of type of dissection and irrespective of whether surgery is pending, entails "anti-impulse" therapy. Blood pressure must be decreased to lower the wall tension within the aorta. This is performed by straightforward means, usually with intravenous (IV) administration of nitroglycerin or nitroprusside. However, it is vital to recognize that, without concomitant β-blocking therapy, to decrease the strength of the cardiac impulse (*dp/dt*), lowering blood pressure will actually increase the stress on the aortic wall (see Figure 11.9). Thus, along with the afterload-reducing drug, we administer a β-blocker, usually esmolol by IV infusion. In order to prevent reflex tachycardia induced by the administration of a powerful afterload-reducing medication, β-blocker therapy should first be initiated. Labetalol, which has both β-blocking properties and α-receptor blocking properties, is an acceptable alternative to the two-drug combination. In patients with bronchospasm, in whom β-blockers are to be avoided, we often use a calcium channel blocker to decrease *dp/dt*. Table 7.1

Table 7.1 Intravenous agents for treatment of ascending dissection

Name	Category	Loading dose	Maintenance dose	Adverse effects	Caution
Sodium nitroprusside	Vasodilator	0.3–3 μg/kg·min; max. limit for an adult is 10 μg/kg·min for 10 min	1–3 μg/kg·min	Nausea, vomiting, agitation, muscle twitching, sweating, cutis anserina and cyanide toxicity, tachycardia	In patients with hepatic or renal dysfunction
Propranolol	β-Blocker	1–3 mg (given at 1 mg intervals over 1 min). Can be repeated in not less than every 4 hours	1–3 mg every 4 hours	Hypotension, nausea, dizziness, cold extremities, reversible hair loss, bradycardia	In patients with bradycardia or history of CHF and bronchospasm. Max. initial dose should not exceed 0.15 mg/h.
Esmolol	β-Blocker	500 μg/kg bolus	Continuous 50 μg/kg·min up to 200 μg/kg·min	Hypotension, nausea, dizziness, bronchospasm, dyspepsia, constipation; increases digoxin level	In patients with CHF or asthma or on concomitant CCB therapy
Labetalol	α- and β-Blockers	20 mg over 2 min, then 40–80 mg every 10–15 min (max. 300 mg)	Continuous IV at 2 mg/min and titrate up to 5–10 mg/min	Vomiting, nausea, scalp tingling, burning in throat, dizziness, heart CCB disease, block, orthostatic hypotension	In patients with concomitant therapy
Diltiazem	CCB	0.25 mg/kg, 5–10 mg/h by IV bolus continuous (up to 25 mg) infusion		Heart block, constipation, liver dysfunction	In patients with heart failure, concomitant β-blocker therapy
Enalapril	Vasodilator ACE inhibitor	0.625–1.25 mg bolus	0.625–5 mg every 6 hours	Precipitates fall in BP in high renin states, variable response, renal failure	In patients with high possibility of myocardial ischemia, renal dysfunction
Fenoldopam	Dopamine D1 receptor agonist	0.03–0.1 μg/kg·min initially	0.1–0.3 μg/kg·min, max. 1.6 μg/kg·min	Tachycardia, hypotension, headache, nausea, flushing, hypokalemia, elevation of IOP	In patients with glaucoma

CCB, calcium channel blocker; ACE, angiotensin-converting enzyme; IV, intravenous; BP, blood pressure; IOP, intraocular pressure; CHF, congestive heart failure.

gives a complete roster of therapeutic options for anti-impulse therapy.

In a patient with an acute aortic dissection, we usually aim to drop the systolic blood pressure to around 100–120 mmHg. In fact, acute aortic dissection is the one hypertensive emergency in which the goal of initial therapy is to cause a state of "relative hypotension" by lowering the mean arterial pressure by much more than the 25% recommended for most other hypertensive emergencies. Mentation and urine output should be carefully monitored. If such a low pressure produces mental changes or oliguria, we liberalize our blood pressure criterion mildly. Some patients with chronic hypertension and severe vascular disease may not be able to function at lower pressures, and we may have no alternative but to permit a blood pressure of 120 or 130 mmHg.

Definitive treatment

Definitive treatment depends on the location of the aortic dissection. Ascending aortic dissections, with a tear just above the coronary arteries, require urgent surgery because of the danger of death from rupture, tamponade, coronary ischemia, or aortic insufficiency. It has been estimated that patients in this circumstance die at a rate of about 1% per hour without surgical treatment. It is important to note that, if aortic dissection is diagnosed in a delayed fashion, as is often the case, the "eye of the storm" may have passed, and surgery may be done semi-electively. Specifically, if more than 48 to 72 hours have passed between onset of symptoms and correct diagnosis, we usually do not take patients to the operating room in the middle of the night. It is not uncommon for a late diagnosis of this type to be made, usually incidentally on an imaging study done for another purpose.

Descending aortic dissections are managed by a "complication-specific" approach. If there are no complications they are managed exclusively medically, with anti-impulse therapy, transitioned after several days to oral antihypertensive therapy. A repeat CT image is obtained in about 72 hours and then again before hospital discharge, to make certain there is no rapid early progression on medical therapy.

If complications of descending aortic dissection emerge, then surgery is required. For rupture, aortic replacement is performed. For organ ischemia, surgical fenestration is performed, taking the pressure off the true lumen and permitting resumption of organ flow (Figure 7.10). For persistent pain or rapid enlargement, surgical replacement is performed.

Interventional therapy with placement of an endovascular stent is beginning to find a role in the treatment of acute aortic dissection. Some ruptures and rapid aortic enlargements can be treated by stent deployment. Organ ischemia can be treated by stenting open the compromised vessel. A fenestration can be created by deliberate endovascular puncture or incision of the offending false membrane. These therapies have produced satisfactory early results. Although endovascular therapy of uncomplicated descending aortic dissection is often performed with the goal of "obliterating the false lumen," its efficacy is unproven and the procedure is potentially harmful. Retrograde dissection into the ascending aorta, a very serious complication, is seen in a percentage of patients subjected to routine stent placement for uncomplicated descending aortic dissection.

Summary

We advise the following:

- Emergency care providers should have a high index of suspicion for aortic dissection. It should be included in the differential diagnosis of every chest and/or back pain patient.
- Although D-dimer is being used by some as a screening tool (it is nearly 100% sensitive for aortic dissection in small studies), caution should be exercised since the cutoff for D-dimer value has not been established for acute aortic dissection.
- Remember that dissection is "the great masquerader" and can mimic disease of any organ.
- Most ascending aortic ruptures and dissections can be prevented by pre-emptive surgical extirpation of the aorta at a dimension of 5.0 to 5.5 cm.
- *Symptomatic* aneurysms require resection *regardless of size.*
- Remember that aortic dissection kills patients via:

  · rupture;
  · cardiac tamponade;
  · acute aortic insufficiency;
  · organ ischemia.

- Ask about acute physical exertion or severe emotion before the onset of pain.
- Inquire about a family history of aortic aneurysm or dissection or sudden cardiac death.
- Image liberally (usually by CT and ECHO).
- Remember the utility of the "triple rule-out CT" (can rule out dissection, coronary artery disease, and pulmonary embolism).
- Upon diagnosis, start "anti-impulse" therapy.
- Do not use unopposed afterload reduction (nitroglycerin or nitroprusside) without concomitant β-blockade to decrease dp/dt.
- Ascending aortic dissection requires urgent surgery.
- Descending aortic dissection is treated medically.

Aortic dissection is a virulent foe for those of us on the front lines in the emergency department and those of us doing later battle in the operating room. By following key principles, based on recent data, together we can combat this shrewd opponent. Although it is still a humbling disease, as it was for Osler 100 years

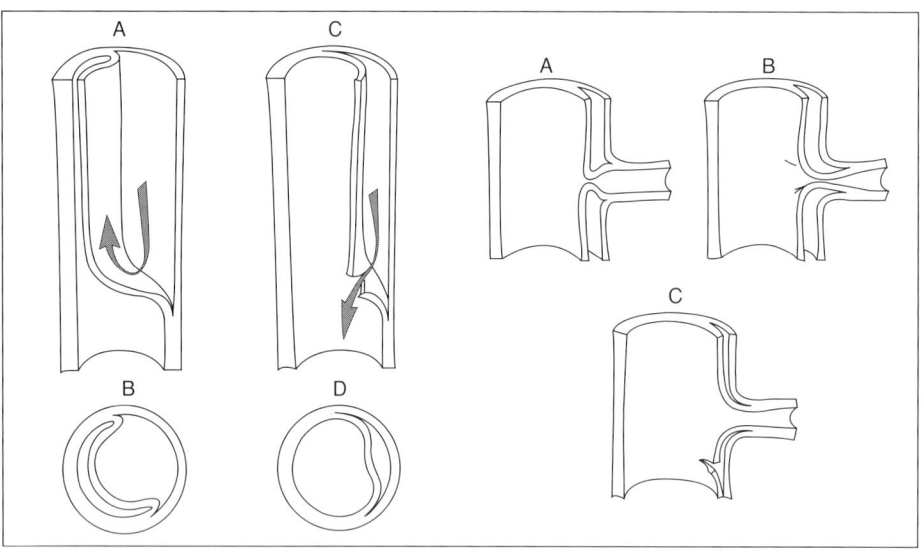

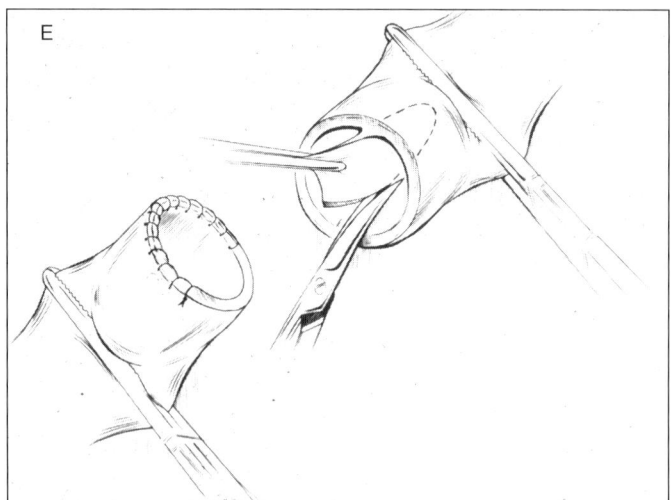

Figure 7.10 (A–D) Mechanism by which aortic dissection produces a false lumen under pressure, which compromises the true lumen. Relief of pressure in the false lumen ameliorates the situation. (E) Surgical technique of fenestration to produce relief schematized in A–D: transect the aorta at the infrarenal level via a flank incision. "Fenestrate" the upper aorta, cutting out a large window of the flap. Reconstitute the layers of the lower aorta with running suture. Sew the upper and lower aorta together. Fenestration can also be performed by endovascular approaches.

ago, aortic dissection is slowly yielding to thoughtful, evidence-based diagnosis and therapy.

References

1. Elefteriades JA, Barrett PW, Kopf GS. Litigation in nontraumatic aortic diseases – a tempest in the malpractice maelstrom. *Cardiology* 2008; 109: 263–72.

2. Tittle SL, Lynch RJ, Cole PE, *et al.* Midterm follow-up of penetrating ulcer and intramural hematoma of the aorta. *J Thorac Cardiovasc Surg* 2002; 123: 1051–9.

3. Elefteriades JA. Beating a sudden killer. *Sci Am* 2005; 293: 65–71.

4. Elefteriades JA, Farkas EA. Thoracic aortic aneurysm: clinically pertinent controversies and uncertainties. *J Am Coll Cardiol* 2010; 55: 841–57.

5. Coady MA, Davies RR, Roberts M, *et al.* Familial patterns of thoracic aortic aneurysms. *Arch Surg* 1999; 134: 361–7.

6. Albornoz G, Coady MA, Roberts M, *et al.* Familial thoracic aortic aneurysms and dissections – incidence,

modes of inheritance, and phenotypic patterns. *Ann Thorac Surg* 2006; 82: 1400–5.

7. Milewicz DM, Michael K, Fisher N, *et al.* Fibrillin-1 (FBN1) mutations in patients with thoracic aortic aneurysms. *Circulation* 1996; 94: 2708–11.

8. Elefteriades JA, Hatzaras I, Tranquilli MA, *et al.* Weight lifting and rupture of silent aortic aneurysms. *JAMA* 2003; 290: 2803.

9. Hatzaras I, Tranquilli M, Coady MA, *et al.* Weight lifting and aortic dissection: more evidence for a connection. *Cardiology* 2006; 107: 103–6.

10. Hatzaras IS, Bible JE, Koullias GJ, *et al.* Role of exertion or emotion as inciting events for acute aortic dissection. *Am J Cardiol* 2007; 100(9): 1470–2.

11. Elefteriades JA, ed. *Acute Aortic Disease.* New York: Informa Healthcare; 2007.

12. Elefteriades JA, Tribble C, Geha AS, Siegel M, Cohen LS. *House Officer Guide to ICU Care*, 3rd edition. New York: Cardiotext; 2012.

13. Elefteriades JA. Thoracic aortic aneurysm: reading the enemy's playbook. *Curr Probl Cardiol* 2008; 33: 203–7.

14. Elefteriades JA, Rizzo JA. Epidemiology. In Elefteriades JA, ed. *Acute Aortic Disease.* New York: Informa Healthcare; 2007: 89–97.

15. Coady MA, Rizzo JA, Hammond GL, *et al.* What is the appropriate size criterion for resection of thoracic aortic aneurysms? *J Thorac Cardiovasc Surg* 1997; 113: 476–91.

16. Davies RR, Gallo A, Coady MA, *et al.* Novel measurement of relative aortic size predicts rupture of thoracic aortic aneurysms. *Ann Thorac Surg* 2006; 81: 169–77.

17. Putnam EA, Zhang H, Ramirez F, Milewicz DM. Fibrillin-2 (FBN2) mutations result in the Marfan-like disorder, congenital contractural arachnodactyly. *Nat Genet* 1995; 11: 456–8.

18. Ohlmann P, Faure A, Morel O, *et al.* Diagnostic and prognostic value of circulating D-dimers in patients with acute aortic dissection. *Crit Care Med* 2006; 34: 1358–64.

19. Trimarchi S, Sangiorgi G, Sang X, *et al.* In search of blood tests for thoracic aortic diseases. *Ann Thorac Surg* 2010; 90(5): 1735–42.

20. Lemaire SA, McDonald ML, Guo DC, *et al.* Genome-wide association study identifies a susceptibility locus for thoracic aortic aneurysms and aortic dissections spanning FBN1 at 15q21.1. *Nat Genet* 2011; 43(10): 996–1000.

21. Wang Y, Barbacioru CC, Shiffman D, *et al.* Gene expression signature in peripheral blood detects thoracic aortic aneurysm. *PLoS One* 2007; 10: e1050.

22. Sanz J, Einstein J, Fuster V. Acute aortic dissection: anti-impulse therapy. In Elefteriades JA, ed. *Acute Aortic Disease.* New York: Informa Healthcare; 2007: 229–50.

23. Feldman M, Shah M, Elefteriades JA. Medical management of acute type A aortic dissection. *Ann Cardiovasc Thorac Surg* 2009; 15: 286–93.

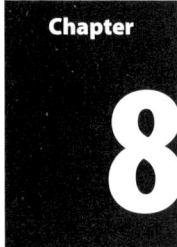

Acute aortic occlusion

8

Akhilesh Jain, Jeffrey Indes, John A. Elefteriades,
and Bart E. Muhs

Acute aortic occlusion is a relatively infrequent vascular emergency that can easily go unrecognized or can be misdiagnosed as an acute neurologic event. While there is a lack of contemporary series, the mortality in published literature has ranged from 30 to 70%, along with a high morbidity. The majority of patients with aortic occlusion develop this condition as a chronic phenomenon with an insidious onset of a symptom complex classically known as Leriche's syndrome. It has been described in male patients as a triad of the following symptoms: (1) claudication of the buttocks and thighs, (2) atrophy of the musculature of the legs, and (3) impotence.

In contradistinction to chronic aortic occlusion, acute aortic occlusion is a different clinical entity, with its own unique set of causes and clinical findings. This chapter will discuss acute aortic occlusions and how emergency care practitioners can provide expert care for patients with this deadly entity.

Pathophysiology

The absence of well-developed collaterals in acute occlusion is the key reason for both the acuity of symptoms and generally poor outcomes. In addition, patients with acute aortic occlusion are typically sicker at baseline, with multiple cardiopulmonary comorbidities, accounting for a poorer prognosis compared to chronic aortic occlusions. The acuity of clinical presentation is a function of the relative speed of onset of pathology (occlusion) resulting in an inability of the body to recruit compensatory collateral circulation. Therefore, patients with embolic occlusion generally present sooner and with more severe symptoms compared to patients with chronic aortic occlusions.

As would be suspected based on fluid dynamics, in any arterial tree, thrombosis generally starts distally at

Table 8.1 Causes of acute aortic occlusion

Common (> 90% of cases)

Aortic thrombosis in a setting of pre-existing aorto-iliac occlusive disease

Saddle embolus from the heart secondary to arrhythmias like atrial fibrillation

Structural heart disease leading to ventricular clot

Uncommon

Fungal endocarditis with embolism of a large vegetation (increasingly being reported)

Spontaneous thrombosis of a small aortic aneurysm

Migration and kinking of an aortic stent graft following EVAR (endovascular aneurysm repair)

Hypercoagulable state

Vasculitis

Traumatic injuries to the aorta

Chronic aortic dissection with thrombosis of the true lumen

True lumen compression by aortic dissection

Aortic trauma

a diseased branch point and progresses proximally up the arterial tree secondary to blood stasis. Thrombosis typically stops at the first proximal patent arterial branch. Thus, in a majority of cases of aortic thrombosis, the process generally starts around the diseased aortic bifurcation and ends just inferior to the renal arteries. Consequently, renal failure is not a common presentation of acute aortic thrombosis.

Causes

See Table 8.1.

A saddle embolus that develops at the aortic bifurcation and *in situ* aorto-iliac thrombosis are the two most common causes of acute aortic occlusions,

---

Vascular Emergencies, ed. Robert L. Rogers, Thomas Scalea, Lee Wallis, and Heike Geduld. Published by Cambridge University Press. © Cambridge University Press 2013.

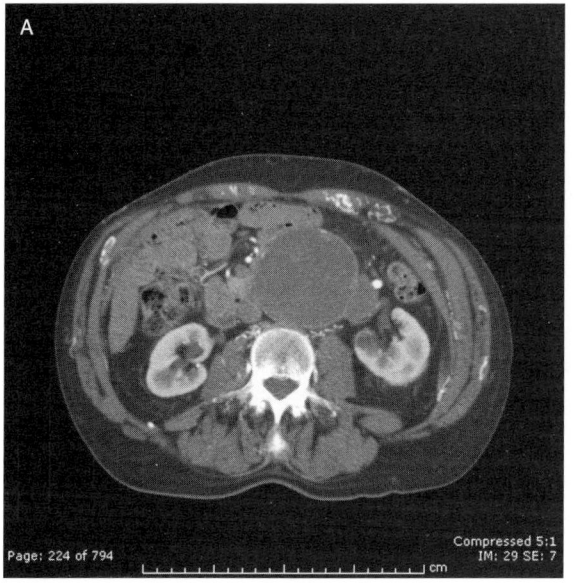
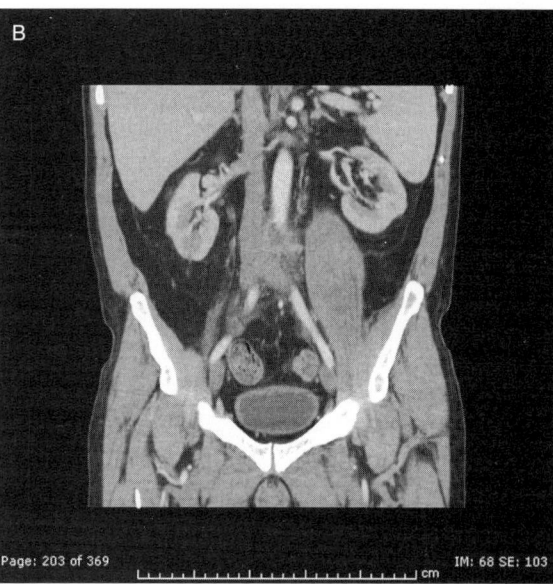

Figure 8.1 (A, B) A 56-year-old man presented with sudden onset of lower back pain and paresthesias in the buttocks and thighs. This was associated with worsening bilateral claudication of both legs for about five days prior to presentation to the emergency department. The patient had weak femoral pulses bilaterally and had undergone redo mitral valve replacement a month before for fungal endocarditis.

accounting for over 90% of cases.[1] Left atrial or ventricular clot in the setting of atrial fibrillation or structural heart disease is the commonest source of an occlusive embolus. Vasculitis and hypercoagulable states have also been suggested to be an infrequent cause of acute aortic occlusion, in which case the aorta is relatively healthy at baseline. Although acute thrombosis is a recognized complication of arterial aneurysms, it is rarely associated with abdominal aortic aneurysms (AAAs), with a reported incidence of 0.6 to 1.8% of AAA cases (Figure 8.1A).

Proposed mechanisms of such thromboses include the presence of pre-existing iliac occlusive disease, cardio-aortic embolization, a hypercoagulable state, shifting of intramural thrombus, or a combination thereof.[2] More contemporary publications have reported cases of aortic occlusion secondary to embolization of large vegetations from fungal endocarditis or due to a fungal ball in the setting of fungal aortitis.[3] As opposed to bacterial endocarditis, where vegetations are typically small, fungal endocarditis leads to large vegetations. Besides its cardiac and systemic implications, the most likely complication of fungal endocarditis is embolism leading to occlusion of large peripheral arteries (Figures 8.1B and 8.2A). With the increasing use of aortic stent grafts to treat infrarenal aortic

aneurysms, migration and kinking of an aortic stent graft leading to aortic thrombosis is another recently reported, though infrequent, cause to be considered (Figures 8.2B–C and 8.3).[4]

Clinical presentation and evaluation

The typical patient with acute aortic occlusion is in the sixth or seventh decade of his/her life. Almost 50% of patients with acute aortic occlusion do not have a pre-existing history of peripheral vascular disease. The etiology in this set of patients is more likely to be an embolus from a cardiac source. Patients with embolic occlusion are also more likely to be female and have a higher incidence of coexisting heart disease. A search for atrial fibrillation and structural valvular disease should therefore be carried out in all patients with a suspected embolus. A history of prosthetic cardiac valves or intravenous drug abuse is cause to suspect endocarditis, likely mycotic, leading to embolization of a large mass of vegetation.

As opposed to those with embolic occlusion, nearly 80% of patients presenting with acute aortic thrombosis have evidence of pre-existing peripheral vascular disease. Thrombosis in these patients is often precipitated by a low-flow state, caused by severe volume depletion, such as dehydration, aggressive

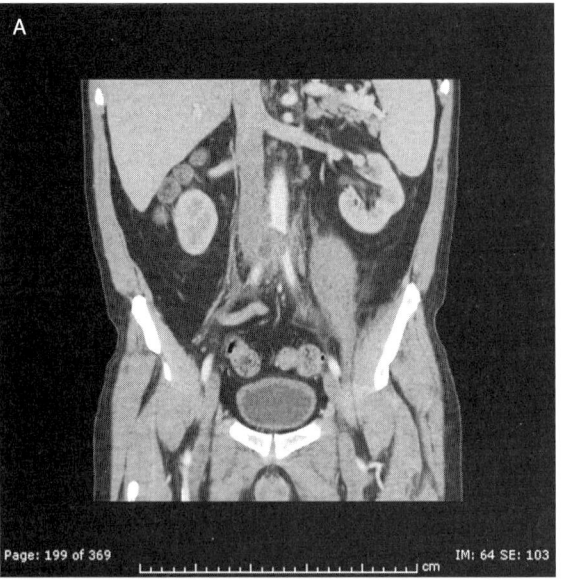
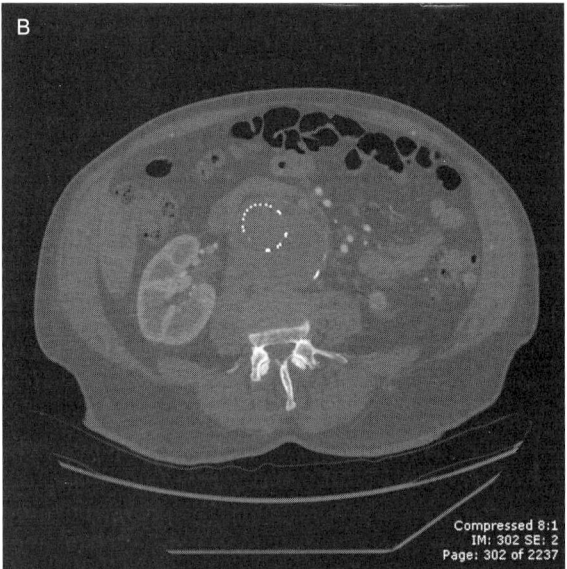
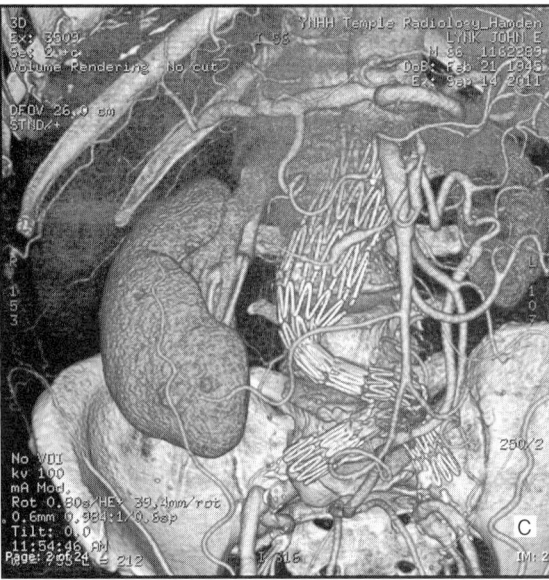

Figure 8.2 (A–C) A 66-year-old man had undergone emergent endovascular aneurysm repair for a ruptured infrarenal abdominal aortic aneurysm one year ago. He now presents with sudden onset of severe bilateral lower extremity claudication and rest pain. A CT angiogram demonstrated acute thrombosis of the stent graft. A careful review of images reveals interval distal displacement of the stent graft, resulting in kinking and consequent thrombosis of the stent, and presenting with acute limb ischemia.

diuresis, or sudden cardiac dysfunction. Thus an associated acute/subacute cardiac event, such as congestive heart failure, myocardial infarction, or arrhythmia, is not uncommon and should be actively investigated. Due to the minimally invasive nature of endovascular aneurysm repair, physical examination may not reveal a surgical scar, and specific inquiry into history of an endovascular aneurysm repair is useful. This can be an important pointer toward a migrated aortic endograft leading to kinking and subsequent thrombosis (Figures 8.1B and 8.2A).

Contrary to what might be expected, not all patients with acute aortic occlusion present with classic symptoms of acute lower extremity ischemia. A vast

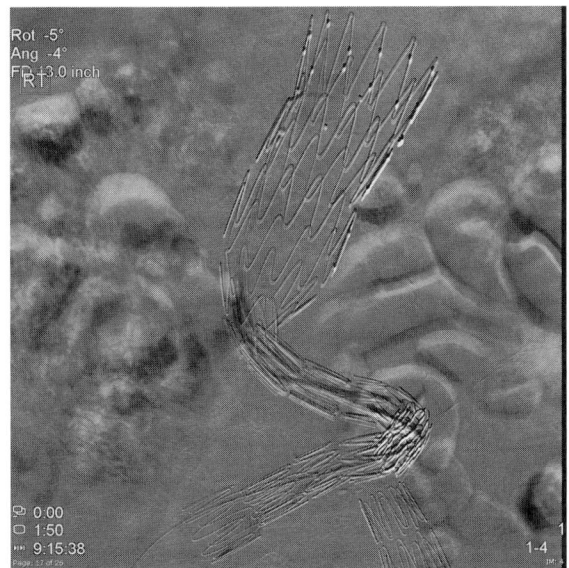

Figure 8.3 Thrombosed abdominal aortic aneurysm (AAA): An 80-year-old man presented with sudden onset of abdominal pain radiating to his back. He had similar pain a few weeks ago and was known to have a thrombosed infrarenal AAA, which was also diagnosed initially following abdominal pain. CT scan on this visit demonstrated interval expansion of his aneurysm with a chronic leak. The patient underwent successful repair of the aneurysm on a semi-emergent basis with an aortobifemoral bypass grafting with resolution of his symptoms.

majority, however, still presents with acute onset of bilateral lower extremity ischemia or a sudden exacerbation of pre-existing chronic vascular disease. Given the acuity of symptoms, patients with embolic occlusion, unlike *in situ* thrombosis, are more likely to present to the emergency department within 24 hours of onset of symptoms.

Five Ps of history and physical examination

Pain. Acute lower extremity pain is usually the first symptom of acute limb ischemia. The patient usually experiences sudden onset of low back, buttock, and bilateral lower extremity pain. However, in cases of aortic thrombosis, paralysis, not pain, may be the first and sometimes the only symptom. Once established, pain is severe and can be resistant to narcotics. This is markedly different from rest pain of chronic critical limb ischemia, which is often limited to the forefoot.

Paresthesia. Small myelinated nerve fibers carrying proprioception and light touch are the ones most sensitive to ischemia. Loss of proprioception and

light touch are hence the earliest findings in patients with acute limb ischemia and indicate deteriorating neurologic function. Loss of temperature and of pressure and pain sensation indicates prolonged and generally irreversible limb ischemia.

Paralysis. Paralysis is an ominous symptom and often the first symptom of lower extremity ischemia secondary to aortic occlusion. Bilateral lower extremity paresis/paralysis in association with sudden onset of back, buttock, and lower extremity pain and paresthesias can easily be confused for acute spinal cord pathology; for instance, an acute spinal cord compression syndrome. Batz and Brückner[5] reported that 84% of patients with acute aortic occlusion presented with paralysis. Only 14% had pain, and 55% had already been referred to a neurologist. Neurologic manifestations of acute aortic occlusion do not imply spinal cord infarction but severe ischemic neuropathy.

Pallor. Pallor indicates obstruction of arterial inflow to the extremity and is particularly pronounced with acute embolic phenomena due to absence of collateral circulation. This gives a marble white, waxy appearance to the legs with collapsed veins or "venous guttering." The consequent mottling of the limbs often extends up to the umbilicus, giving a cadaveric appearance. Capillary refill on blanching the skin indicates patent capillaries and a salvageable extremity. Thrombosis and rupture of capillaries leads to fixed staining indicative of a non-salvageable limb.

Pulselessness. Absent or feeble pulses are the hallmark of acute limb ischemia. This is one of the most important pointers toward a vascular catastrophe in a patient presenting with signs and symptoms that can otherwise easily be confused for acute spinal cord pathology. Absence of bilateral femoral pulses is an important distinguishing feature with such a presentation. Patients with a neurologic deficit have often been referred to a neurologist or a neurosurgeon, even with a physical finding of absent femoral pulses.[6]

Acute aortic occlusions typically do not involve the renal arteries; however, renal failure is a rare presentation in cases of acute aortic occlusion and generally indicates progression of thrombosis to the suprarenal aorta, with potential involvement of visceral vessels and a significantly worse prognosis. Acute renal failure is, however, a frequent clinical finding and one of the

Table 8.2 Criteria for limb viability

| | | Findings | | Doppler signal | |
Category	Description/prognosis	Sensory loss	Muscle weakness	Arterial	Venous
I – Viable	Not immediately threatened	None	None	Audible	Audible
II – Threatened					
IIa – Marginally	Salvageable if promptly treated	Minimal or none	None	Often inaudible	Audible
IIb – Immediately	Salvageable with immediate revascularization	More than toes, rest pain	Mild, moderate	Usually inaudible	Audible
III – Irreversible	Major tissue loss or permanent nerve damage inevitable	Profound, anesthetic	Profound, paralysis	Inaudible	Inaudible

From two articles by Rutherford et al.[7,8]

major causes of mortality following revascularization of a thrombosed aorta. Acute renal failure is caused by significant fluid shifts and reperfusion syndrome, leading to washout of oxygen free radicals into the systemic circulation.

Diagnosis

See Table 8.2.

Acute bilateral lower extremity ischemia is a hallmark of acute aortic occlusion. This, in association with bilateral lower extremity neurologic deficit (paresthesia, paresis, paralysis), can easily be confused for an acute spinal cord pathology such as acute compression syndrome. In various series, a diagnosis of acute neurologic catastrophe was entertained and pursued in almost 25 to 50% of patients with a neurologic deficit secondary to acute aortic occlusion, leading to a delayed diagnosis and treatment of the underlying pathology.[1,9,10] Since early heparinization and surgical intervention are crucial to improving outcome in this group of patients, an accurate diagnosis and correct referral from the emergency department has an impact on the prognosis. In the setting of bilateral lower extremity neurologic symptoms, an astute emergency physician will easily come to a diagnosis of acute aortic occlusion by a simple clinical finding of absent femoral pulses bilaterally. Thus the need to perform a simple vascular examination on any patient with a neurologic deficit in the lower extremities cannot be over-emphasized.

Imaging

Role of angiography. Traditional teaching in cases of limb ischemia suggests that investigations should not delay revascularization. Preoperative imaging, however, reduces operating time and allows a more focused and directed approach to revascularization. While a formal angiogram in the radiology suite is not always feasible secondary to institutional constraints, current generation CT scans allow fairly rapid and accurate evaluation of the vascular pathology. On-table angiograms are an alternative when a patient with stage IIb limb ischemia has to be rushed to the operating room prior to imaging.

Patients with suspected embolus to the bifurcation should be operated on without angiography. Patients with suspected *in situ* abdominal aortic thrombosis with clinically unclear renal or mesenteric arterial involvement (rare), however, benefit from preoperative angiography.

Cardiac evaluation. Patients with acute aorto-iliac occlusion frequently have associated cardiopulmonary comorbidities. An electrocardiogram is important to rule out arrhythmia, and a chest film aids in diagnosis and also in preoperative risk assessment. An echocardiogram is indicated to rule out a cardiac source of embolism; however, echo is frequently postponed until after the limbs are revascularized and thus falls outside the requirements of an emergency physician.

Management

Coexisting conditions should be aggressively investigated and treated. Cardiac disease is the most common form of comorbidity found in these patients (60%) and is primarily responsible for the high mortality rate in these patients.

Prognosis is time dependent; thus, early recognition, institution of supportive care, and prompt diagnosis (if possible) are essential elements of management. The treatment of acute aortic occlusion is surgical. The cause of occlusion is important because transfemoral embolectomy is likely to restore perfusion in patients with saddle embolus but is usually unhelpful in patients with *in situ* thrombosis. When the diagnosis is made, the patient should be heparinized immediately to prevent proximal and distal propagation of the thrombotic process. Bilateral transfemoral embolectomy is the first procedure of choice.

Aorto-iliac embolectomy via bilateral common femoral arteriotomies is carried out. If this fails to restore circulation, then bilateral axillo-femoral grafting should be performed. Severity of ischemia at presentation, rather than the duration of symptoms, is a better predictor of final outcome.

Clinical approach when resources are limited

In the case of limited resources, acute aortic occlusion can still be diagnosed on the basis of the findings discussed above. CT scanning can usually delineate the anatomy clearly. Initial heparinization can begin in any hospital setting. Therapeutic embolectomy or axillo-femoral grafting can be carried out at any center that performs vascular surgery. Thus, the diagnosis and treatment of this disorder do not usually require extremely advanced resources.

Pearls and pitfalls

- Look for the five Ps to make the diagnosis.
- Look for cardiac origin of emboli.
- Heparinize early to prevent further thrombosis in the small run-off vessels.
- Time is of the essence for diagnosis and treatment.
- Acute aortic occlusion can mimic a spinal cord lesion. Perform a careful examination of distal pulses in all cases.

Critical actions

The most critical actions are to make a diagnosis based on clinical grounds (as discussed above), to obtain imaging studies, to heparinize early, to look for cardiac embolic sources, and to call immediately for a vascular consultation (in order to avoid limb loss and to lessen the already high chance for a lethal outcome).

Conclusion

Acute aortic occlusion is a rare but catastrophic pathology resulting from thrombus formation, saddle embolism, false-lumen expansion in aortic dissection, aortic trauma, and other etiologies related to arteriosclerosis or hypercoagulability. Postoperative mortality is extremely high even if blood perfusion to the lower extremities is restored by emergent surgical intervention. Mortality rates are approximately 50%, with the most common causes of death being myocardial infarction and renal failure.[1,9,11] The causes of death are associated not only with major organ ischemia such as stroke, myocardial infarction, hepatic infarction, and mesenteric ischemia but also with severe respiratory failure, fatal arrhythmia, uncontrollable hyperkalemia, or renal failure secondary to myonecrosis. Studies have shown that the causes of death could be attributed to a wide range of pathologies, including respiratory failure (e.g., respiratory distress syndrome), mesenteric ischemia, fatal arrhythmia, myocardial infarction, stroke, hyperkalemia, or renal failure. Most patients who died after revascularization appear to have had fatal organ failure even without obvious arterial occlusion in major organs.

References

1. Surowiec SM, Isiklar H, Sreeram S, Weiss VJ, Lumsden AB. Acute occlusion of the abdominal aorta. *Am J Surg* 1998; 176: 193–7.

2. Hirose H, Takagi M, Hashiyada H, *et al.* Acute occlusion of an abdominal aortic aneurysm – case report and review of the literature. *Angiology* 2000; 51: 515–23.

3. Kraev AI, Shah G, Omerovic V, Itskovich A, Landis GS. Acute aortic occlusion from a Candida fungus ball. *J Vasc Surg* 2011; 54: 1475–7.

4. Thurley PD, Glasby MJ, Pollock JG, *et al.* Endovascular management of delayed complete graft thrombosis after endovascular aneurysm repair. *Cardiovasc Intervent Radiol* 2010; 33: 840–3.

5. Batz W, Brückner R. Symptoms and therapy of aortic bifurcation embolism. *Chirurg* 1985; 56(3): 166–9.

6. Meagher AP, Lord RSA, Graham AR, Hill DA. Acute aortic occlusion presenting with lower limb paralysis. *J Cardiovasc Surg* 1991; 32: 643–7.

7. Ad Hoc Committee on Reporting Standards, Society for Vascular Surgery/North American Chapter, International Society for Cardiovascular Surgery. Suggested standards for reports dealing with lower extremity ischemia. *J Vasc Surg* 1986; 4: 80–94.

8. Rutherford RB, Baker JD, Ernst C, *et al.* Recommended standards for reports dealing with lower extremity ischemia: revised version. *J Vasc Surg* 1997; 26(3): 517–38.

9. Babu SC, Shah PM, Nitahara J. Acute aortic occlusions – factors that influence outcome. *J Vasc Surg* 1995; 21: 567–75.

10. Bolduc ME, Clayson S, Madras PN. Acute aortic thrombosis presenting as painless paraplegia. *J Cardiovasc Surg* 1989; 30: 506–8.

11. Frost S, Jorden RC. Acute abdominal aortic occlusion. *J Emerg Med* 1992; 10: 139–45.

Ruptured abdominal aortic aneurysms

Matthew K. Folstein, Karan Chopra, and Kapil Gopal

An aneurysm is defined as focal dilatation of an arterial vessel to the extent that the vessel is at least 50% larger than its expected normal diameter.[1] The normal diameter of the infrarenal abdominal aorta is approximately 20 mm (2 cm), giving a general definition of an abdominal aortic aneurysm (AAA) as anything greater than or equal to 3 cm.[2] With the increasing of an endovascular approach for elective aneurysm repair, the overall incidence of ruptured AAA has decreased 30% over the past decade.[3,4] The overall mortality rate among patients with ruptured AAA who arrive at the hospital alive ranges between 40 and 70%. That rate has largely remained unchanged since 1954, when Cooley and DeBakey reported a 50% survival rate after repair of ruptured abdominal aortic aneurysm (RAAA).[3,5,6] When autopsy data are included, the mortality rate associated with RAAA approaches 90%.[6] Among patients whose aneurysm ruptures before they arrive at an emergency department, 50 to 65% die from sudden cardiovascular collapse. The survival rate decreases by 1% per minute prior to arrival. The survival rate is even lower among patients with comorbidities such as congestive heart failure, renal failure, and chronic obstructive pulmonary disease. It is imperative to have a high index of suspicion for AAA and to initiate appropriate care pathways to maximize survival after the patient arrives at the emergency facility.

Pathophyisology

It is critical to distinguish a ruptured from a symptomatic AAA. Ruptured AAA occurs when bleeding extends beyond the aortic wall, possibly into the retroperitoneum or the peritoneal cavity. Rupture into the retroperitoneum generally occurs toward the left side. The surrounding tissues can provide a tamponade effect to contain the bleeding and increase the chance of survival. Rupture into the peritoneal cavity has a worse prognosis, associated with more profound blood loss, as there is no surrounding tissue to give a tamponade effect.[6] Symptomatic aneurysms are painful and tender, signaling impending rupture. The pain can be of varying degrees and is related to rapid expansion, intramural hemorrhage, wall degeneration, or bleeding into the thrombus, which increases focal wall stress. Since symptomatic aneurysms have not ruptured, the patient does not have the associated hypotension. Patients with symptomatic AAA require urgent repair to prevent rupture and its associated morbidity and mortality.[7]

The pathophysiology of AAA with a degenerative or non-specific cause is a complex interplay of various factors, including enzymatic degradation pathways with matrix metalloproteinases, inflammatory cytokines, wall stress, and aneurysmal shape. These subjects are the focus of extensive ongoing research that is beyond the scope of this chapter. The approximate risks of rupture are imprecise because large numbers of patients with unruptured aneurysms have not been observed. In addition, patients with large aneurysms are treated, thereby causing calculations of the overall risk to be underestimates. By convention, the pathophysiology of rupture is most closely related to the diameter of the AAA. Several population-based studies have shown increasing rupture rates with increasing diameter (Table 9.1).[8] More recent randomized trials, such as the UK Small Aneurysm Trial and the Aneurysm Detection and Management Trial, illustrated that the annual risk of rupture was 6.5% at diameters of 5.0 to 5.9 cm. In contrast, smaller AAAs had an annual risk of rupture of 1.5% with diameters of 4.0 to 4.9 cm, and only 0.3% in those with diameters of

Vascular Emergencies, ed. Robert L. Rogers, Thomas Scalea, Lee Wallis, and Heike Geduld. Published by Cambridge University Press. © Cambridge University Press 2013.

Table 9.1 Abdominal aortic aneurysm (AAA) size and estimated annual risk of rupture

AAA diameter (cm)	Rupture risk (%/year)
<4	0
4–5	0.5–5
5–6	3–15
6–7	10–20
7–8	20–40
>8	30–50

Source: Gloviczki *et al.*[7]

3.9 cm and smaller.[9,10] Both trials support elective repair of AAAs at 5.5 cm.[9–11] A caveat is made for females, as gender was found to be an independent risk factor for increased incidence of rupture. This increase is thought to be related to the smaller diameter of the aortic vessels in females, creating more wall stress in comparison with aneurysms in men. Therefore, elective repair of AAA in women is advocated at a diameter of 5 cm.[6,9]

Epidemiology

The development of AAA has been studied extensively in relation to a complex array of risk factors: gender, genetic, tobacco use, and inflammatory factors. In the VA study by Lederle *et al.*, male gender (5.6-fold risk), tobacco use (5.1-fold risk), age (1.7-fold risk), and family history (1.9-fold risk) were independent markers for increased risk of having AAAs with a diameter of 4 cm or greater.[10] Other markers that conferred an increased risk of AAA were white race, chronic obstructive pulmonary disease, hypertension, hypercholesterolemia, and coronary artery disease. The strong association of smoking, gender, and age has been confirmed by several other studies.[12]

The true incidence of RAAA is difficult to determine because patients who die outside the hospital are excluded from population-based surveys. The incidence of RAAA in the United States Inpatient Sample decreased from 9,979 per year in 1993 to 6,921 per year in 2003.[13] As of 1999, AAA accounted for 15,810 deaths per year in the United States; 93% of them occurred in patients older than 55 and 83.5% in patients older than 65. In the United Kingdom, 2.1% of all deaths in men older than 65 are related to RAAA.[14] A significant gender-related concern has

emerged with the recent trials, illustrating a significantly greater decline in RAAA incidence among men than among women. Conversely, a greater proportion of women than men had rupture.[15,16] These differences could be related to the fact that the majority of patients in aortic aneurysm trials have been men. As stated above, the criterion for size at which to perform elective repair in women may need to be around 5 cm rather than 5.5 cm.

Diagnosis
Symptomatology and physical examination

In the group described by Akkersdijk and van Bockel, the classic triad of RAAA – severe abdominal or back pain, hypotension, and palpable pulsatile abdominal mass – was present in 34% of correctly diagnosed patients and in only 9% of misdiagnosed patients.[17] The sensitivity of finding an AAA on physical examination increases with size of the AAA and performing a focused examination. Seventy-five percent of AAAs with a diameter of 5 cm or larger were diagnosed with a focused physical examination.[18] Other factors such as the patient's body habitus and the skill and focus of the examiner can be confounding variables that decrease the sensitivity of examination. Furthermore, a thin patient can have prominent pulsations with an aorta of normal caliber. As a result, most AAAs are identified as incidental findings on abdominal imaging. Special attention should be paid to the patient's medical history, especially previous endovascular aneurysm repair, because patients with this history can present with RAAA if the aneurysm sac has become repressurized with an endoleak (Figure 9.1).

Other findings on the initial presentation of RAAA can be a constellation of signs and symptoms suggesting hypotension, mass affect, or from rupture of the AAA into the venous system through an aortocaval fistula, or arteriovenous fistula involving the iliac or renal veins. A history of syncopal episodes could be indicative of hypotension; sudden congestive heart failure with distension of neck veins or lower extremity edema could result from aneurysmal rupture into the venous system; increased intra-abdominal pressure from bleeding may result in groin pain, hematoma, groin hernia, or even painful scrotal mass. The differential diagnosis should include but not be limited to

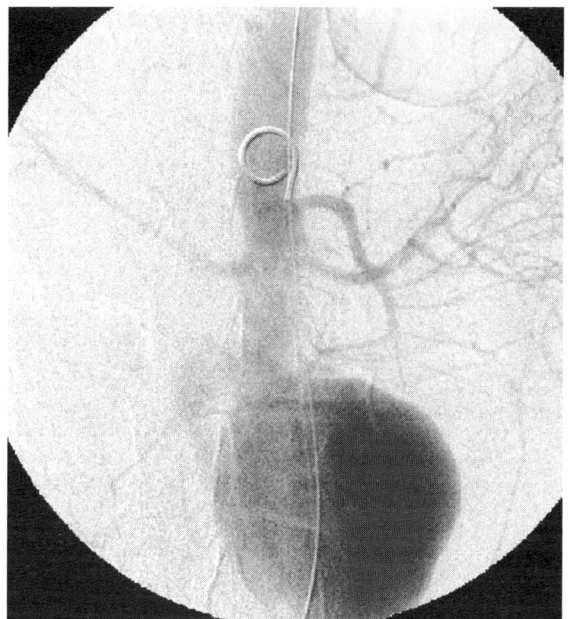

Figure 9.1 Aortogram of patient with acutely symptomatic AAA with previous endograft. The image demonstrates contrast accumulating in the AAA sac despite previous endovascular repair.

diverticulitis, pancreatitis, myocardial infarction, gastrointestinal hemorrhage, and perforated ulcer. Misdiagnosis is often a result of not finding a pulsatile abdominal mass on examination. In cases of frank rupture, patients may be cyanotic with mottled extremities, accompanied by severe hypotension, tachycardia, and altered mental status. Aortoduodenal fistulas may present as an upper gastrointestinal bleed followed by exsanguination and hemorrhagic shock.

Laboratory tests

Patients presenting with the signs and symptoms listed above should raise concern for symptomatic AAA or RAAA. The following tests should be requested: a complete blood count (CBC) to evaluate for blood loss; a complete metabolic panel (CMP) to assess acid/base balance as well as renal function and hepatic function; type and crossmatch to prepare for potential massive transfusion of packed red blood cells, platelets, and fresh frozen plasma; and a coagulation profile consisting of PT, aPTT, and INR for correction of coagulation factors as needed. If the patient is hemodynamically unstable with suspicion of RAAA, then he or she should be taken to the operating room immediately regardless of the availability of test results so that the

bleeding can be controlled directly. In this situation, type-specific or universal donor blood products can be transfused.

Imaging

Plain radiographs of the abdomen are now used less frequently than CT and ultrasound, but they can help clinicians identify the presence of AAA in areas where the other modalities are not readily available. Findings of RAAA include aortic wall calcification extending beyond expected location and loss of psoas shadowing from retroperitoneal hematoma. One or both findings were present in 90% of patients in a retrospective review.[19] These could be particularly useful findings when a CT scanner is not readily available.

Another bedside imaging modality that can be used is ultrasound, which is being used increasingly by emergency physicians in trauma settings to conduct a focused assessment with sonography for trauma (FAST). With this technology, fluid collections in dependent recesses of the peritoneal cavity can be identified, and the aortic diameter can be assessed in less than five minutes.[20–22] Ultrasound can identify an AAA in a patient with high sensitivity and specificity.[22] Ultrasound cannot, however, rule out the rupture of an AAA.

Computed tomography remains the most useful tool available for diagnosis of RAAA. A non-contrast CT scan can identify an AAA as well as fluid within the retroperitoneum, indicating rupture (Figure 9.2). A CT scan with contrast provides precise anatomic information about the RAAA and thus indicates its suitability for endovascular repair or the need for open repair. Furthermore, the surrounding intra-abdominal and pelvic structures and organs can be evaluated as potential causes of the symptoms. Studies have documented that about 13% of patients with RAAA die within two hours after admission, with a median time between admission and death of 11 hours.[23,24] Therefore, it should be feasible in most instances to obtain a CT scan, but all patients should be monitored continuously and any signs of hemodynamic instability should prompt immediate transfer to the operating room.

Emergency department management

Initial assessment

When the differential diagnosis includes a high suspicion for RAAA, it is important to focus on this disease

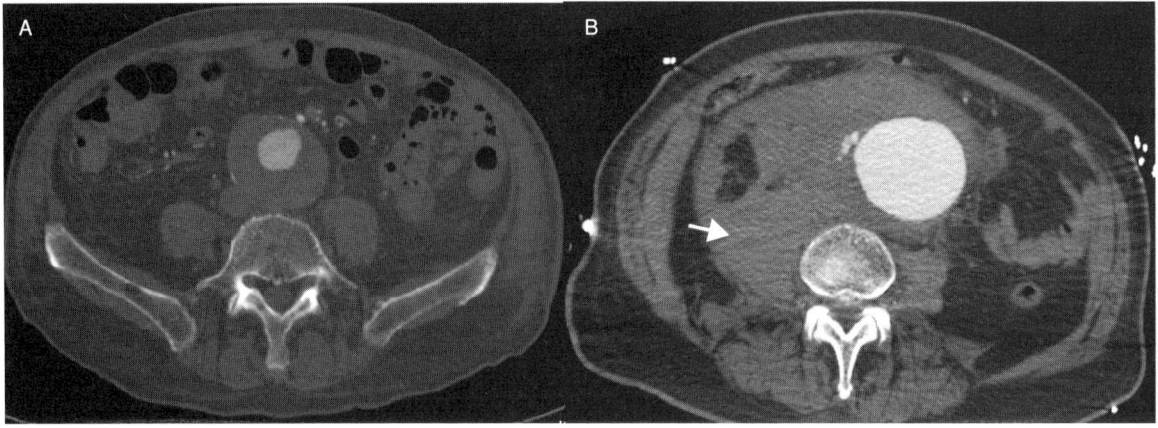

Figure 9.2 (A) AAA found on CT scan incidentally. (B) Ruptured AAA on CT scan with fluid/blood (arrow) in retroperitoneum.

process so as to confirm or exclude its presence. Immediate attention should be paid to the patient's hemodynamic status. Airway should be assessed, and two large-bore IV access lines should be placed for resuscitation. Appropriate laboratory tests and a specimen for crossmatch can be obtained at the time of placement of the IV lines. Prophylactic intubation should not be performed routinely in the emergency department, because the sedation needed for placement of an endotracheal tube can further decrease the blood pressure and exacerbate hemodynamic instability. Diagnostic imaging should be performed to exclude the presence of AAA. Ideally, bedside ultrasound would be followed with a CT scan. Thin-slice CT scan (1–3 mm cuts) with IV contrast is preferred because it can reveal the presence of retroperitoneal fluid or aneurysms of the splanchnic (splenic, hepatic, mesenteric vessels) or renal arteries. A RAAA can also be evaluated for appropriateness for endovascular repair, specifically assessing: the diameters of the aorta, iliac, and femoral arteries; the precise length and location of the aortic aneurysm; the presence of anatomic details such as accessory renal arteries; and superior mesenteric artery stenosis. If CT with contrast is not available, then a non-contrast CT scan can be performed, without the need for renal function tests, to evaluate the patient for an AAA and retroperitoneal fluid. If a CT scanner is not immediately available, a plain film can be obtained and used to identify a widened calcified aortic wall, as described above.

A quick physical assessment of the mental status for altered sensorium, of the abdomen for a pulsatile mass, and of the femoral and distal lower extremity for pulses and perfusion can increase or diminish suspicion of RAAA with ongoing internal hemorrhage. The lack of a pulsatile abdominal mass and the presence of femoral and distal lower extremity pulses do not reduce or eliminate the possibility of RAAA. Finally, a vascular surgeon should be consulted immediately to ascertain the need for operative repair. If the institution does not have the appropriate resources, arrangements should be made to transfer the patient to a regional center capable of handling a RAAA. Transfer increases the time to definitive repair, and a concomitant rise in the mortality rate is seen within the first 24 hours after transfer; however, for patients who survive after repair, the length of intensive care unit stay and hospitalization are similar regardless of the transfer time.[25]

In the emergency department, the resuscitative strategy should be to implement permissive hypotension. The goals of this strategy are to maintain the patient's mental status and consciousness, to avoid cardiac ST-segment depressions, and organ ischemia. These goals can typically be achieved at a systolic pressure of 50 to 70 mmHg.[26] The idea is that aggressive resuscitation to a blood pressure higher than 100 mmHg can lead to further hemorrhage by overcoming the tamponade that stabilized the initial hemorrhage.[26–28] There is no evidence that resuscitation is better with blood than with crystalloids. If blood is available, it can be given to maintain organ perfusion and consciousness until definitive surgical repair can be performed.

Definitive treatment

Definitive treatment for RAAA is prompt endovascular or surgical intervention. Endovascular repair requires a team of X-ray technologists, nurses, and operating room personnel and readily available fluoroscopic equipment and appropriately sized endovascular devices. If the CT scan shows common femoral arteries of adequate caliber, access is gained via surgical exposure of both common femoral arteries. The wires, catheters, and devices are introduced and deployed through the exposed vessels under fluoroscopic guidance. The access arteries are then repaired surgically. If the repair is successful, the patient can be moved to a monitored setting postoperatively. The initial results of RAAA treated with endovascular repair are favorable. Averaging results from several retrospective database reviews and meta-analysis shows that this approach has reduced the 30-day mortality rate from 44.6% to 27.7% in comparison with open repair.[6]

Traditional surgical repair is performed by bringing an awake patient to the operating room and then prepping and draping that patient after ensuring that all appropriate monitoring lines and catheters are in place. Once the operation is ready to begin, the patient is anesthetized and intubated just prior to incision. The reason for the delay in intubation is to prevent a decrease in blood pressure from the anesthetics. A midline laparotomy or retroperitoneal flank incision is made, with quick dissection to the aorta, controlling any free bleeding. Once the hemorrhage has been controlled, the rest of the structures can be dissected free, and the aneurysmal portion of the aorta can be replaced with prosthetic graft, most often a polyester woven graft that can go down as far as the common femoral arteries, if necessary. For postoperative recovery, the patient will be taken to the intensive care unit.

Inpatient care

The care of patients after endovascular repair of RAAA is less intense and has less morbidity compared to open surgical repair. Inpatient care is directed at managing complications from endovascular treatment, which include renal dysfunction requiring temporary and sometimes permanent hemodialysis, abdominal compartment syndrome from hematoma requiring drainage, embolization of thrombus to visceral organs or lower extremities causing ischemia, colonic ischemia, and wound infection.

Inpatient care after open surgical repair is more complex and requires a longer length of stay in the intensive care unit and the hospital. A myriad of complications can develop: myocardial infarction, arrhythmias, respiratory failure requiring tracheostomy, colonic ischemia, renal dysfunction, hepatic failure, postoperative bleeding, and multiorgan failure. Bown and colleagues calculated the incidence of multiorgan failure to be 3.8% after elective repair, 38% after urgent repair, and 64% after repair of a ruptured aneurysm.[29] In the same series, the mortality rate among patients with multisystem organ failure after open RAAA repair was as high as 69%, compared with a 0% mortality rate in patients without multisystem organ failure after open RAAA repair. Frequently, these patients require discharge to a rehabilitation center for long-term postoperative care.

Clinical approach when resources are limited

1. Identify acutely ill patients by examination, and establish large-bore intravenous access.
2. Perform a quick physical assessment, looking for pulsatile abdominal mass, lower extremity pulses, and ischemia.
3. Perform bedside abdominal ultrasound to assess the aortic diameter or request a plain film radiograph to look for a calcified aortic wall to confirm the diagnosis.
4. Obtain surgical consultation to assess the need for transfer to a regional medical center.
5. Begin a permissive hypotension resuscitation strategy.

Pearls and pitfalls

Pearls

1. If the patient has back or abdominal pain, a pulsatile abdominal mass, and hypotension, he or she has a RAAA until proven otherwise.
2. Perform bedside imaging (preferably ultrasound) to identify the presence of an AAA.
3. Obtain a CT scan with intravenous contrast as the gold standard, even if laboratory data are not yet available, as this is a life-and-death situation. Otherwise, perform non-contrast CT to assess for fluid in the retroperitoneum and the presence of AAA.

4. Obtain surgical consultation early.
5. Use a permissive hypotension resuscitation strategy to minimize the chances of further hemorrhage.

Pitfalls

1. Not recognizing the classic triad of findings of RAAA.
2. Considering other diagnoses before excluding RAAA in a hemodynamically unstable patient with back pain or abdominal pain.
3. Not obtaining surgical consultation early to assess the need to transfer the patient to a regional medical center.
4. Aggressive resuscitation to blood pressure greater than 100 mmHg.
5. Intubating a conscious patient who is maintaining his or her own airway, even if RAAA is suspected.

Critical actions

- Perform a quick physical examination to assess for abdominal pain, pulsatile mass, and hypotension
- Obtain bedside ultrasound imaging of the abdominal aorta
- Obtain thin-slice CT scans with contrast
- Use permissive hypotension resuscitation
- Obtain urgent vascular surgery consultation

References

1. Johnston KW, Rutherford RB, Tilson MD, *et al.* Suggested standards for reporting on arterial aneurysms. Subcommittee on Reporting Standards for Arterial Aneurysms, Ad Hoc Committee on Reporting Standards, Society for Vascular Surgery and North American Chapter, International Society for Cardiovascular Surgery. *J Vasc Surg* 1991; 13: 452–8.
2. Pearce WH, Slaughter MS, LeMaire S, *et al.* Aortic diameter as a function of age, gender, and body surface area. *Surgery* 1993; 114: 691–7.
3. Mureebe L, Egorova N, Giacovelli JK, *et al.* National trends in the repair of ruptured abdominal aortic aneurysms. *J Vasc Surg* 2008; 48: 1101–7.
4. Giles KA, Pomposelli F, Hamsdan A, *et al.* Decrease in total aneurysm related deaths in the era of endovascular aneurysm repair. *J Vasc Surg* 2009; 49: 543–50.
5. Bown MJ, Sutton AJ, Bell PR, Sayers RD. A meta-analysis of 50 years of ruptured abdominal aortic aneurysm repair. *Br J Surg* 2002; 89: 714–30.
6. Lindsay T. Abdominal aortic aneurysms: ruptured. In Cronenwett JL, Johnston KW, eds. *Rutherford's Vascular Surgery*, 7th edition. Philadelphia: Saunders Elsevier; 2010: 1994–2013.
7. Gloviczki P, Pairolero PC, Mucha P Jr, *et al.* Ruptured abdominal aortic aneurysms: repair should not be denied. *J Vasc Surg* 1992; 15: 851–9.
8. Brewster DC, Cronenwett JL, Hallett JW Jr, *et al.* Guidelines for the treatment of abdominal aortic aneurysms. Report of a subcommittee of the Joint Council of the American Association for Vascular Surgery and Society for Vascular Surgery. *J Vasc Surg* 2003; 37: 1106–17.
9. Powell JT, Brown LC, Forbes JF, *et al.* Final 12-year follow-up of surgery versus surveillance in the UK Small Aneurysm Trial. *Br J Surg* 2007; 94: 702–8.
10. Lederle FA, Johnson GR, Wilson SE, *et al.* Yield of repeated screening for abdominal aortic aneurysm after a 4-year interval. Aneurysm Detection and Management Veterans Affairs Cooperative Study Investigators. *Arch Intern Med* 2000; 160: 1117–21.
11. Lederle FA, Wilson SE, Johnson GR, *et al.* Immediate repair compared with surveillance of small abdominal aortic aneurysms. *N Engl J Med* 2002; 346: 1437–44.
12. Fillinger M. Abdominal aortic aneurysms: evaluation and decision making. In Cronenwett JL, Johnston KW, eds. *Rutherford's Vascular Surgery*, 7th edition. Philadelphia: Saunders Elsevier; 2010: 1928–48.
13. Lesperance K, Andersen C, Singh N, *et al.* Expanding use of emergency endovascular repair for ruptured abdominal aortic aneurysms: disparities in outcomes from a nationwide perspective. *J Vasc Surg* 2008; 47: 1165–70.
14. Harkin DW, Dillon M, Blair PH, *et al.* Endovascular ruptured abdominal aortic aneurysm repair (EVRAR): a systematic review. *Eur J Vasc Endovasc Surg* 2007; 34: 673–81.
15. Dillavou ED, Muluk SC, Makaroun MS. A decade of change in abdominal aortic aneurysm repair in the United States: have we improved outcomes equally between men and women? *J Vasc Surg* 2006; 43: 230–8.
16. McPhee JT, Hill JS, Eslami MH. The impact of gender on presentation, therapy, and mortality of abdominal aortic aneurysm in the United States, 2001–2004. *J Vasc Surg* 2007; 45: 891–9.
17. Akkersdijk GJ, van Bockel JH. Ruptured abdominal aortic aneurysm: initial misdiagnosis and the effect on treatment. *Eur J Surg* 1998; 164: 29–34.
18. Lederle FA, Walker JM, Reinke DB. Selective screening for abdominal aortic aneurysms with physical

examination and ultrasound. *Arch Intern Med* 1988; 148: 1753–6.

19. Tornwall ME, Virtamo J, Haukka JK, *et al*. Life-style factors and risk for abdominal aortic aneurysm in a cohort of Finnish male smokers. *Epidemiology* 2001; 12: 94–100.

20. Shuman WP, Hastrup WJ, Kohler TR, *et al*. Suspected leaking abdominal aortic aneurysm: use of sonography in the emergency room. *Radiology* 1988; 168: 117–19.

21. Knaut AL, Kendall JL, Patten R, Ray C. Ultrasonographic measurement of aortic diameter by emergency physicians approximates results obtained by computed tomography. *J Emerg Med* 2005; 28: 119–26.

22. Dent B, Kendall RJ, Boyle AA, Atkinson PR. Emergency ultrasound of the abdominal aorta by UK emergency physicians: a prospective cohort study. *Emerg Med J* 2007; 24: 547–9.

23. Lloyd GM, Bown MJ, Norwood MG, *et al*. Feasibility of preoperative computer tomography in patients with ruptured abdominal aortic aneurysm: a time-to-death study in patients without operation. *J Vasc Surg* 2004; 39: 788–91.

24. Boyle JR, Gibbs PJ, Kruger A, *et al*. Existing delays following the presentation of ruptured abdominal aortic aneurysm allow sufficient time to assess patients for endovascular repair. *Eur J Vasc Endovasc Surg* 2005; 29: 505–9.

25. Hames H, Forbes TL, Harris JR, *et al*. The effect of patient transfer on outcomes after rupture of an abdominal aortic aneurysm. *Can J Surg* 2007; 50: 43–7.

26. Crawford ES. Ruptured abdominal aortic aneurysm [editorial]. *J Vasc Surg* 1991; 13: 348–50.

27. Roberts K, Revell M, Youssef H, *et al*. Hypotensive resuscitation in patients with ruptured abdominal aortic aneurysm. *Eur J Vasc Endovasc Surg* 2006; 31: 339–44.

28. Alric P, Ryckwaert F, Picot MC, *et al*. Ruptured aneurysm of the infrarenal abdominal aorta: impact of age and postoperative complications on mortality. *Ann Vasc Surg* 2003; 17: 277–83.

29. Bown MJ, Nicholson ML, Bell PR, Sayers RD. The systemic inflammatory response syndrome, organ failure, and mortality after abdominal aortic aneurysm repair. *J Vasc Surg* 2003; 37: 600–6.

Chapter

10

Blunt aortic injury

David J. Skarupa and Jay Menaker

Blunt thoracic trauma is often associated with multiple injuries and has a high rate of morbidity and mortality. Injury to the great vessels is one of the most lethal blunt chest injuries, because of the risk of exsanguination, either acutely or in a delayed fashion. Vessels at risk of injury from blunt trauma are the thoracic aorta (most common), the innominate artery, the vena cava, and the pulmonary veins. The most common site of injury is at the isthmus of the proximal descending thoracic aorta.[1] Other segments of the thoracic aorta that are susceptible to blunt injury are the ascending aorta or transverse arch (3–23%), the mid or distal descending thoracic aorta (8–13%), and other sites (11–19%), including the abdominal aorta.[1–4] The most common cause of blunt aortic injury (BAI) is the motor vehicle crash (MVC), and many patients die at the scene. If BAI is untreated, approximately 30% of those who survive to the hospital will die within 24 hours.[2] High clinical suspicion, prompt medical management, expeditious diagnosis, and early surgical consultation are imperative.

Pathology and pathophysiology

The pathologic entities of BAI include dissection, transection, rupture, and pseudoaneurysm. Dissection is defined as an intimal tear that is worsened as blood flow cleaves the intimal and medial layers of the artery, creating a longitudinal separation of the arterial wall layers.[5] Transection refers to a full-thickness injury of the entire arterial circumference, whereas rupture is a partial-circumference, full-thickness arterial wall injury. If a person survives to the hospital with this injury, it is likely because the intact parietal pleura has contained the hematoma and prevented free rupture and immediate death.

Blunt aortic injury may also be partial thickness and evolve into a pseudoaneurysm (false aneurysm). A pseudoaneurysm forms when a hole in the artery wall allows extravasation of blood into a contained space outside the artery. The wall of the pseudoaneurysm is formed by periarterial hematoma or compressed surrounding tissue, not components of the injured arterial wall. Most patients with this type of injury are immediate survivors. The most common location of these pathologic entities is the isthmus/descending aorta (approximately 70%), which is anatomically defined as 1 cm distal to the left subclavian artery at the site of the ligamentum arteriosum.[1,3,4]

The landmark study of BAI was conducted in 1958 by Parmley and colleagues, from the Armed Forces Institute of Pathology and Walter Reed US Army Hospital.[2] In their autopsy series of 275 patients, they found that 86% had died at the scene, mostly from massive mediastinal and pleural hemorrhage. Aortic wall injury was defined along a spectrum from simple subintimal hemorrhage to complete laceration of the aorta. The lesions were classified into six stages: intimal hemorrhage, intimal hemorrhage with laceration, medial laceration, complete laceration of the aorta, false aneurysm formation, and periaortic hemorrhage. The progression from injury to rupture is unpredictable, especially if untreated. It is suggested that partial-thickness injuries (of the intima and media) occur first, followed by disruption of the external aortic layers, leading to rupture. Animal studies have shown that sufficient strength exists after an intima-media partial-thickness injury before complete rupture occurs.[6] These histopathologic findings support a window for diagnosis and initiation of treatment.

Originally it was thought the mechanism of BAI was strictly a deceleration vector force that "stretched"

Vascular Emergencies, ed. Robert L. Rogers, Thomas Scalea, Lee Wallis, and Heike Geduld. Published by Cambridge University Press. © Cambridge University Press 2013.

the aorta. The weakness of the isthmus, along with the relative mobility of the ascending aorta and aortic arch and the descending aorta, supported this theory. Other pathophysiologic variables have been proposed: a sudden elevation in intra-abdominal pressure, which may explain the association between blunt aortic injury and diaphragmatic injury;[7] sudden elevations in blood pressure against an occluded aorta, creating endovascular pressure waves (the "water-hammer" effect);[8] entrapment of the aorta between the anterior chest wall and vertebral column (the "osseous pinch");[9] a lower thoracic or upper abdominal impact that results in cranial displacement of the mediastinum and torsion at the isthmus (the "shoveling effect");[10] and compression.[11] Although certain combinations of these forces have been suggested as causing injury to certain parts of the aorta, the combination of all of these forces is the most likely pathogenesis of BAI.

Epidemiology

The first description of a death attributed to BAI, caused by an equestrian incident, can be traced to the 1500s. However, BAI is predominantly an injury of modern industrialized societies, often resulting from MVCs. In the United States, the national incidence of BAI among all trauma admissions is 0.3%. It is estimated that 20 to 30 persons per one million sustain BAI each year.[12] In blunt trauma patients, BAI is the second most common cause of death; the first is traumatic brain injury.[13] Teixeira *et al.*[1] studied 304 blunt trauma fatalities that had a full autopsy performed. MVC was the most common mechanism of injury, occurring in 50% (101) of the cases. Two-thirds of the patients were male, and overall mean age was 43 (±21) years. Blunt aortic injury was diagnosed in 34% (102) of the patients. These demographics are similar in other studies conducted at urban and rural level I trauma centers.[14,15]

Early studies of risk factors for BAI after MVC suggested that frontal impact was the predominant directional force leading to this injury[8,16,17] and that restraints were not a significant factor.[18] Further investigations showed that lateral impact MVCs can cause significant chest trauma and BAI.[10,18] In a prospective multi-institutional study of hospital admissions involving BAI, published in 1997, head-on-collision was the most common mechanism of injury (72%) followed by side impact (24%) and rear impact (4%).[13] Crash scene investigations by Horton

and associates in Miami determined that total velocity change (ΔV) ≥ 20 mph (32 km/h) and vehicle intrusion ≥ 15 inches (38 cm) were the two most significant risk factors for BAI in MVCs. No relationship was demonstrated between the use of restraints and the incidence of BAI.[14] An earlier study reported that ejection from the vehicle doubled the risk of BAI.[16] Other less common mechanisms include equestrian incidents, blast injuries, auto–pedestrian crashes, motorcycle crashes, crush injury, and falls from heights greater than 30 feet (9 m) (the impact is approximately equivalent to that of a 30 mph [48 km/h] crash).[19] Blunt thoracic aortic injury has been reported after crashes at slow speeds (10 mph [16 km/h]) with the deployment of airbags.[20]

Patients with BAI can be classified as follows:[21] dead at the scene from hemorrhage, unstable during transport and likely to die from multisystem organ injury, and stable but likely to die from central nervous system injury. Morbidity and mortality rates for those who survive to the hospital are high, secondary to the constellation of injuries that occur.[13] Associated injuries include head injury, rib fractures, pelvic and long-bone fractures, and abdominal injuries and the coinciding pain. Factors that predict worse outcome are advanced age, hypotension on admission, hypothermia on admission, major head injury, major abdominal injury, and Injury Severity Score ≥ 25.[22] In one study, aortic repair (either endovascular stent or interposition graft) was the only variable associated with improved survival.[22] Long-term functional status is impaired in these patients. Individuals with BAI who survive are two times more likely to suffer major disability in feeding, locomotion, and/or expression.[22] Based on a review of the National Trauma Databank, Arthurs and colleagues calculated that one-third of patients could walk independently at discharge, and one-fifth suffered major feeding and expression disability.[22] Survival statistics and long-term outcomes may improve as prehospital management continues to become more efficient and effective, the treatment paradigm continues to shift toward endovascular stenting, and postoperative critical care continues to advance.

Diagnosis

History and physical examination

Although the history and physical examination after blunt thoracic trauma are often unreliable, elements of them should raise the physician's concern. The history is often obtained from prehospital personnel but can be provided by the patient. Description of the scene, mechanism of injury, time from injury, vital signs, neurologic status, and any changes during transport are critical components of the history. Ejection from the vehicle, time from extrication, and the location and degree of vehicular compartment deformation are also useful in the assessment.

During the physical examination, certain key elements should alert the examiner to the presence of BAI. Some patients state that lying down causes severe back pain so they therefore prefer to be upright; others are pale and clammy. Interscapular or retrosternal discomfort may be caused by aortic injury, but it is an unreliable sign. External signs of injuries that suggest BAI are a steering wheel imprint on the chest, left flail chest, and palpable fracture of the sternum and/or thoracic spine. Fabian et al.[13] clearly described a multitude of injuries that are associated with BAI: closed-head injury; multiple rib fractures; flail chest; pulmonary contusion; myocardial contusion; diaphragm rupture; spleen, liver, small bowel, and other abdominal injuries; spinal cord injury, pelvis, femur, tibia, upper extremity, maxillofacial, cervical spine, thoracic spine, and lumbar spine fractures. Yet a good number of patients have no obvious external signs of thoracic injury.[2,23]

One of the specific physiologic findings of thoracic aortic injury is abnormal blood pressure – hypotension and/or hypertension – specifically in the upper extremities.[23,24] Upper extremity hypertension is caused by compression of the aortic lumen by a periaortic hematoma or disruption of blood pressure receptors located near the injured aortic isthmus. An "acute coarctation syndrome" or "pseudocoarctation syndrome" might also be present. This manifests as acute upper extremity hypertension and weak pulses or lower extremity hypotension. The pathology underlying this syndrome is an intimal flap causing a ball-valve effect, resulting in partial aortic obstruction. A systolic murmur might be auscultated secondary to turbulent flow across the flap. Complete obstruction manifests as anuria and/or paraplegia. Unequal upper extremity blood pressure should alert the clinician to the possibility of associated subclavian or innominate artery injury. Generalized hypotension is likely related to acute blood loss. Other less common findings are hoarseness without laryngeal injury and superior vena cava syndrome.

The results of the laboratory workup usually do not change the management of an unstable injured person. Standard trauma panels should be performed, but their acquisition should not impede diagnosis or management. Despite numerous clues to the diagnosis of BAI, the most important factor is a high degree of clinical suspicion. Once suspicion is elevated, medical therapy should be initiated and imaging should be employed to solidify the diagnosis.

Imaging

A standard, portable, supine anterior-posterior chest radiograph (CXR) should be obtained with some degree of urgency. Although some may argue against it for a patient without signs of chest trauma, our practice is to obtain one expeditiously. The utility of the CXR in diagnosing BAI has been well studied. Chest radiography findings suggestive of BAI are widened mediastinum, indistinct aortic knob, left pleural effusion, apical cap, first and/or second rib fracture, tracheal deviation, depressed left bronchus, nasogastric tube deviation, and a normal chest X-ray.[13] Although, historically, emphasis has been placed on a widened mediastinum, this finding results from venous bleeding (i.e., from tearing of the adjacent bridging veins or the vaso vasorum of the aorta), not from a direct tear in the aorta. Schwab et al., in an article published in 1984, supported upright over supine chest radiography for diagnosing BAI.[25] This conclusion was corroborated by Mirvis et al.,[26] who documented the strengths and limitations of chest radiography and determined that no single radiographic sign or combination of signs is sufficient to identify all cases of BAI. In essence, a "funny-looking" mediastinum should spark a high degree of clinical suspicion (Figures 10.1 and 10.2).

In the past, a normal upright CXR was believed to be sufficient to clear a mediastinum and rule out aortic injury; however, this idea may not be valid. Multiple studies have shown a "normal" CXR is not sufficient to rule out aortic injury in high-risk blunt trauma patients. Woodring et al. reported on their review of the records of 656 patients, all of whom had aortic or brachiocephalic injuries. The mediastinum was interpreted as normal on CXR in 7.3% of cases.[27] The first multi-institutional study of BAI, by the American Association for the Surgery of Trauma, reported a similar rate of normal CXR despite the presence of BAI. Other investigators revealed multiple missed thoracic injuries, including BAI.[28,29] Exadaktylos

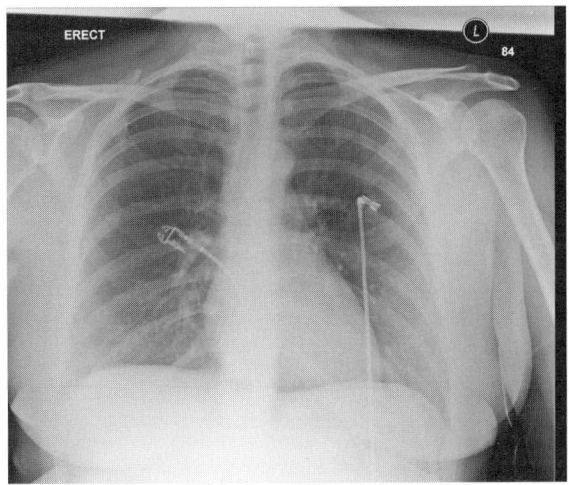

Figure 10.1 Normal chest radiograph.

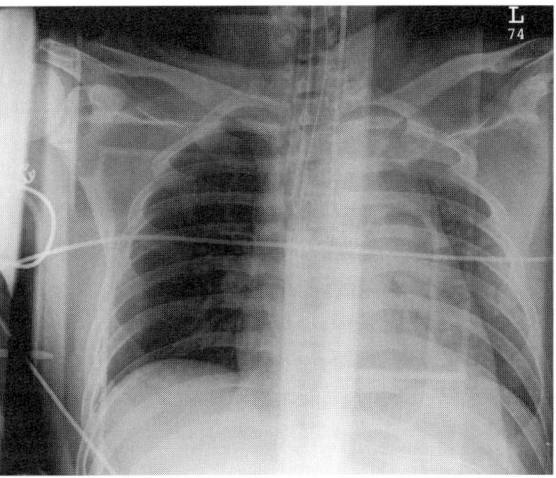

Figure 10.2 Abnormal mediastinum on chest radiograph.

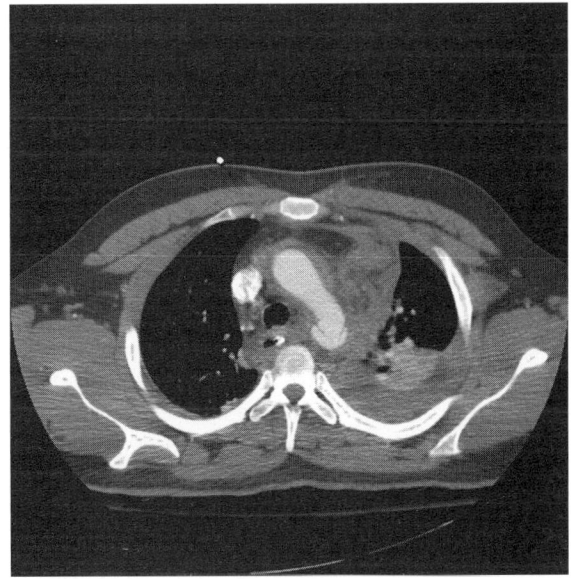

Figure 10.3 Axial CT corresponding to the chest radiograph with abnormal mediastinum from Figure 10.2.

and colleagues reported a 28% missed rate of BAI based on CXR readings. The authors suggested that all unrestrained drivers who crashed at speeds of 10 mph (16 km/h) or faster and all restrained drivers who crashed at speeds of 30 mph (48 km/h) or faster be evaluated for BAI with a contrast-enhanced CT scan of the chest. A study by Gammie and colleagues showed that BAI can be present despite a normal CXR and that the resulting delays in treatment can lead to significant morbidity.[30] Plurad *et al.* found that,

compared with CT scan, 13.9% of patients with BAI had a CXR that did not show any abnormality; all of these injuries required either thoracotomy or a stent graft for repair.[31] Given the high lethality of a missed and untreated BAI, we recommend that all patients with a high-risk mechanism undergo contrast-enhanced CT of the chest, regardless of the chest radiography findings.

Traditionally, biplanar aortography was the diagnostic test of choice. Today, this modality has been replaced nearly completely by CT scan. Mirvis *et al.* reported a sensitivity of 100%, a specificity of 99.7%, and an overall diagnostic accuracy of 99.7% for contrast-enhanced spiral CT in diagnosing BAI.[32] Direct CT findings of BAI include pseudoaneurysm, intimal flaps, aortic contour abnormalities, intraluminal thrombus, and pseudocoarctation (Figures 10.3 and 10.4). The newer modality of multidetector CT (MDCT) obtains higher-resolution images in less time than previous machines and provides 3D reconstructions (Figure 10.5). An MDCT of the chest with 3D reconstructions not only helps solidify the diagnosis, it also provides detailed information about anatomy, which is helpful in planning an endovascular repair if needed. A CT scan of the head should be performed simultaneously.

When the diagnosis is still uncertain, aortography is recommended (Figure 10.6). The disadvantage of this modality is transport of the trauma patient away from the resuscitation bay to the angiography suite for an indeterminate amount of time. If the angiogram confirms injury, the patient will need

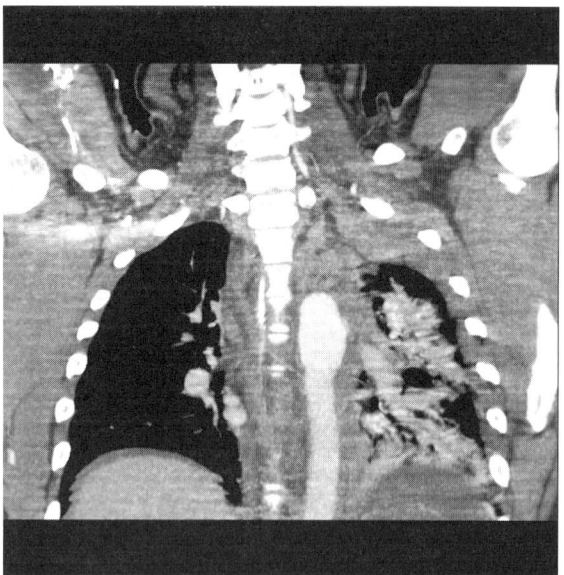

Figure 10.4 Coronal computed tomography scan of BAI.

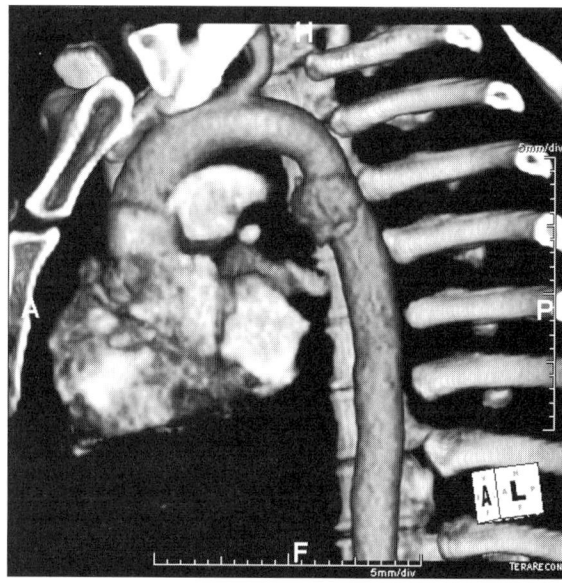

Figure 10.5 Computed tomography scan with 3D reconstruction of BAI.

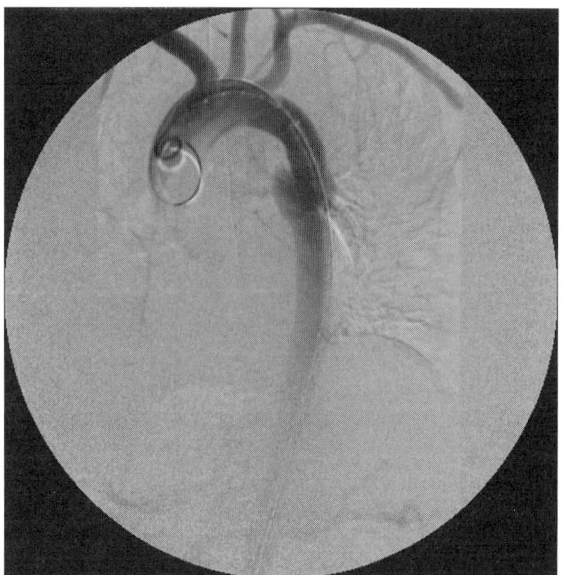

Figure 10.6 Angiography of patient with BAI. This patient was stented.

to remain in the cold angiography suite for stent deployment. The patient should be accompanied by an individual trained in critical care to ensure that proper monitoring and medical care are provided and to oversee resuscitation if it becomes necessary. The presence of the critical care provider will allow the interventionalist to focus on his/her task.

Recently, intravascular ultrasound (IVUS) has emerged as an important diagnostic modality for cases in which the diagnosis remains equivocal based on the CT findings. This technology can be added to the vascular surgeon's armamentarium if individuals credentialed in its use are readily available. Recent articles have documented its utility and have suggested it be used as the next step in diagnosing BAI when the contrast-enhanced CT is equivocal.[33,34] One study suggested it is superior to aortography, especially in diagnosing minimal aortic injury (defined as < 1 cm intimal flap with no or minimal periaortic hematoma).[33] Advantages of this technique are that it can be performed at the bedside, eliminating travel away from the resuscitation bay, and it can be used if high-resolution CT is not available.

Another alternative to CT scan is transesophageal echocardiography (TEE). This modality has been well studied for the evaluation of BAI and is an acceptable test.[34] It is especially valuable for the obese patient who does not fit in the CT scanner, for an unstable patient who cannot be transported to the CT scanner or angiography suite, and for intraoperative evaluation. TEE has several limitations: it is operator dependent, some patients cannot tolerate it, it cannot be performed secondary to some injuries, and it has "blind spots" (the ascending aorta and the aortic arch and its branches). The experienced echocardiographer might be able to manipulate the probe around the purported blind spots.

Magnetic resonance imaging (MRI) has also been employed, but it is best used as an ancillary modality. It is a time-consuming and expensive test that requires pretest screening. The previously mentioned modalities are superior and should be used first.

Pearls and pitfalls

- A high index of clinical suspicion for BAI is required.
- Adequate resuscitation and monitoring devices (central venous access, intra-arterial monitoring) are needed, especially for patients with prolonged prehospital transport times.
- Prompt medical therapy should be instituted prior to reaching a definitive diagnosis if the presence of BAI is highly suspected.
- Chest radiography is not an adequate screening test. All high-risk blunt trauma patients should have a contrast-enhanced CT scan of the chest, even if the initial CXR is "normal."
- If CT is not available and the patient is a high-risk blunt trauma patient, alternative diagnostic modalities should be employed – TEE, IVUS, or aortography.
- An abnormal mediastinum from periaortic hematoma or mediastinal hemorrhage is caused by tear of the adjacent bridging veins or the vaso vasorum of the aorta, not a direct tear in the aorta.
- Early discussion with surgical colleagues is recommended.
- Prompt disposition out of the emergency department is usually indicated, i.e., early transfer to definitive care or admission to an intensive care unit (ICU).

Clinical approach when resources are limited

- Maintain a high degree of clinical suspicion for the injury.
- Involve surgical colleagues early in the workup.
- Rely on physical examination findings.
- Obtain an erect/upright CXR if possible.
- Resuscitate the patient and institute anti-impulse therapy with central venous access and intra-arterial monitoring devices.

- Coordinate early transfer to a definitive care facility.

Emergency department management

During the first 15 minutes

Injury is a disease of time, and the clock is ticking. Information from the prehospital care providers helps with early triage (vital signs, signs of massive blood loss, paralysis, total body irradiation [TBI]). Mobilization of surgical specialists (e.g., trauma surgeon, vascular surgeons, and/or neurosurgeons) during transport can save valuable time once the patient arrives. Based on the information provided, a general assessment is made and resources are readied. After the patient arrives, another general assessment is performed. A primary survey is conducted following Advanced Trauma Life Support (ATLS) guidelines. The airway, breathing, and circulation are managed. Large-bore peripheral IV access is obtained. If central-line access is necessary, the subclavian or internal jugular vein opposite the side of suspected injury is preferred. The groin may need to be accessed for cardiac bypass or an endovascular approach. A general neurologic assessment is made. The patient is exposed and removed from the back board using standard spine precautions.

A portable, supine anterior-posterior CXR is obtained. Additional adjuncts to the primary survey such as FAST and pelvic radiography are performed as indicated. The secondary survey is performed expeditiously, and the patient is removed from the backboard using standard spine precautions.

The need for emergent operation is determined based on the patient's hemodynamic stability, physical examination findings, injury assessment, and chest radiography findings. Prompt surgical consultation is highly recommended. If a left hemothorax is identified, a left posterior-apical chest tube should be inserted and connected to an auto-transfuser. Aggressive resuscitation should ensue and further imaging obtained. MDCT with 3D reconstruction is the test of choice.[35] This will allow a more accurate diagnosis as well as the planning of endoluminal therapies. Alternatively, TEE or IVUS could be performed if personnel trained in these procedures are readily available.

Once the diagnosis of BAI is suspected, anti-impulse therapy should be initiated. The premise of this therapy lies in reducing aortic wall shearing

Table 10.1 Preferred medical management options

Drug	Mechanism	Onset	Duration of action	Dosage	Comment
Esmolol (Brevibloc)	β_1-Antagonist	60 seconds	Half-life: 4–16 min (mean, 9 min)	Infusion, 50–300 μg/kg·min	Full recovery from β-blockade 18–30 min
Labetalol (Trandate)	α- and β-Antagonist (1:7)	2–5 min; peak, 5–15 min	2–4 h	Infusion, 1–2 mg/min (up to 1–2 mg/kg)	
Nitroprusside (Nipride)	Arterial and venous dilator	Immediate	1–2 min	Infusion, 0.3–0.5 μg/kg·min (up to 10 μg/kg·min)	Cyanide toxicity; decreased cerebral blood flow; coronary steal
Nicardipine (Cardene IV)	Arteriolar dilator	1–2 min	40 min	Infusion, 5–15 mg/h	

force and lowering the ventricular ejection dynamic (*dp/dt*). This concept was originally described in 1965 by Wheat and colleagues, regarding the non-operative management of dissecting aortic aneurysms.[36] Based on the histopathologic similarities to aortic dissections, these physiologic principles have been extrapolated to BAI. Fabian *et al.* later recommended a target systolic blood pressure (SBP) below 100 mmHg (100 to 120 mmHg in older patients) or a mean arterial pressure (MAP) less than 80 mmHg and pulse less than 100 beats/minute and a mixed venous oxygen saturation of 65%. No patient with this medical management had an aortic rupture while waiting for repair.[37]

Medical management is imperative in these patients, and multiple options exist (Table 10.1). The priority in the management strategy is to reduce the heart rate. The preferred first-line agent is esmolol. A second-line agent is labetalol. It is imperative that heart rate is controlled first, as it reduces the shearing force against the aortic wall. If a vasodilator is used first, a reflexic tachycardic response will follow, increasing the shear force against the injured aorta. After the heart rate is controlled, a vasodilator such as nitroprusside can be added to reduce ventricular ejection dynamics. Caution should be used because it may be difficult to titrate in the under-resuscitated patient. An alternative and more modern drug is nicardipine. Nicardipine has a rapid onset of action but little or no negative inotropic effect. It has been observed not to produce coronary steal.

Our preference is to start anti-impulse therapy as soon as BAI is suspected and before imaging has verified the diagnosis. Other studies specifically looking at BAI and early β-blocker therapy have shown this approach to be safe.[37] In patients with concomitant traumatic brain injury, we aggressively reduce the heart rate and maintain the MAP within a tight range to ensure adequate cerebral perfusion pressure (CPP). If the patient has an intracranial monitoring device, this is slightly easier, but either way it is a balancing act between protecting the injured aorta and perfusing the brain. Care should be taken in titrating the heart rate in an under-resuscitated patient, since many of these individuals will be relatively hypovolemic and hypotensive secondary to their injuries. This is especially true in rural areas, where transport times are longer (i.e., > 60 min vs. min in urban areas); these patients may arrive significantly behind in their resuscitation. Tight pharmacologic management of heart rate and blood pressure is imperative. Once they are controlled, priorities for definitive management of the patient's injuries can be addressed (e.g., BAI, TBI, long-bone fixation).

First few hours

Medical management is paramount, as well as early surgical consultation. Tight blood pressure parameters should be maintained and medication titrated following intra-arterial blood pressure recordings. An upper extremity central venous catheter should be placed and utilized for resuscitation, administration of medications, and monitoring goals of resuscitation. The management plan should be discussed with the consulting surgeon(s) early and a plan set in motion for either expeditious transfer to a definitive care facility or admission to the ICU. These patients require high-level, dedicated critical care management. No reason exists for these injured patients to linger in any emergency department during the golden hour.

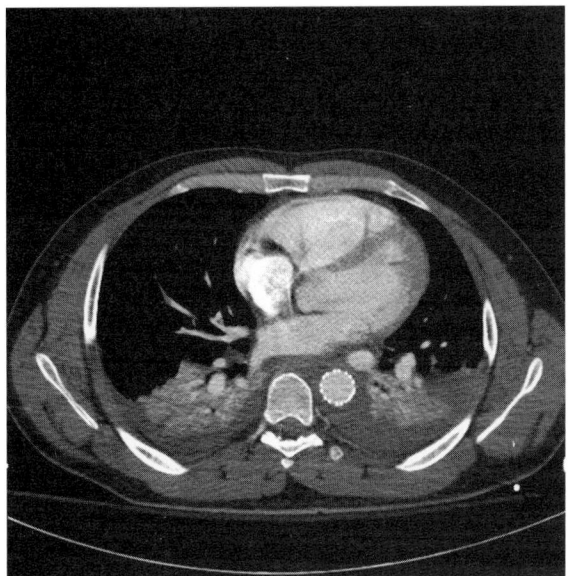

Figure 10.7 Axial computed tomography scan following endovascular stent deployment.

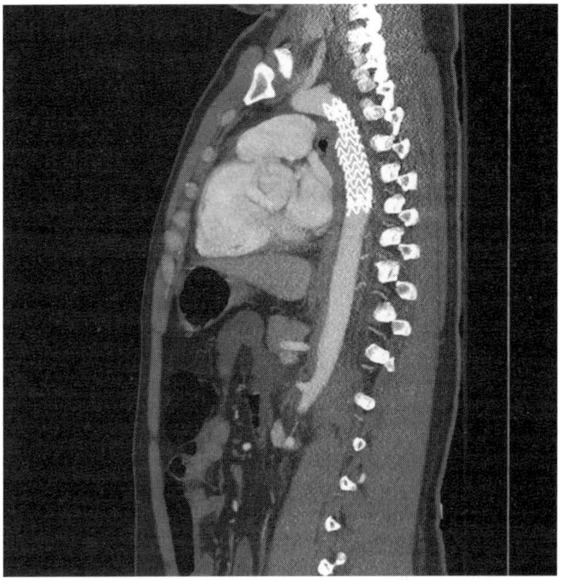

Figure 10.8 Sagittal computed tomography scan following endovascular stent deployment.

Definitive treatment (outside the ED)

Broadly speaking, patients with BAI are categorized into one of two treatment strategies: operative or non-operative. Anti-impulse therapy with β-blockers and vasodilators are the foundation of treatment. The stable patient can be admitted to the ICU with strict goals of heart rate, SBP or MAP, and definitive repair performed in a delayed fashion. Non-operative management or planned delayed repair should be aborted once ominous signs suggesting progression of BAI and impending rupture are identified. Such signs are a rapid increase in the size of a mediastinal hematoma or pleural effusion, anuria for more than six hours, limb ischemia, or free leak of contrast within the thorax.[23] Patients with any of these signs may require an emergent operation. Surgical consultation is wise early in the workup. If the facility does not have the necessary capabilities or is not a level I trauma center, the nearest definitive care facility should be contacted early and arrangements made for transfer. The treatment plan and goals during transfer should be discussed with the accepting surgeon. If imaging has been obtained, it should be transferred via telemedicine or at least via a modern universal medium for viewing by the receiving facility. At the definitive care facility/receiving facility, resources should be readied and a plan instituted once the patient arrives. Other in-juries should be assessed and prioritized (e.g., simultaneous craniotomy and need for heparinization). Imaging should be reviewed and the patient's candidacy for open versus endoluminal therapy evaluated.

Traditionally, BAI was treated with a left posterior lateral thoracotomy and either an interposition graft or a primary repair, with or without bypass. Its mortality and morbidity rates were high, most notably paraplegia. Paraplegic rates were associated with aortic cross-clamp times.[13] Bypass techniques allowed longer clamp times without increased rates of paraplegia. Advances in vascular imaging and endoluminal devices have provided the surgeon with the option of endovascular stenting (Figures 10.7 and 10.8). Endovascular stenting for this injury was originally reserved for high-risk polytrauma patients and the elderly. Today, it is the initial treatment of choice and has been shown to have lower rates of morbidity and mortality.[38] Enhanced imaging techniques and endovascular options have revolutionized the diagnosis and management of this injury.

Inpatient care

The characteristics of the injury and its relationship to the great vessels, especially the left subclavian artery, are important in the surgical repair of BAI. Based on anatomy, it is sometimes necessary to cover the left subclavian artery with an endovascular stent. The findings from a pulse examination of all four extremities should be recorded prior to repair and documented postoperatively. Mild ischemic changes of the left upper extremity can occur postoperatively with coverage of the left subclavian artery. This may manifest as a decreased pulse, which may improve over time to digital ischemia. After patients become more active, they might complain of upper extremity effort fatigue. These signs and symptoms should be addressed promptly. A subclavian-to-carotid bypass may be needed.

Vertebral artery flow may also be compromised, resulting in vertebrobasilar ischemia. Symptoms include vertigo, dizziness, drop attacks, diplopia, perioral numbness, alternating paresthesias, tinnitus, dysphasia, dysarthria, and ataxia. If two or more of these symptoms are present, a vascular surgeon should be notified for further workup.

The sites of vascular access should be monitored for signs of infection, bleeding, hematoma, pseudoaneurysm, and embolic phenomenon to the digits. If any of these are present, they should be addressed promptly. Postoperative CT should be performed to document stent placement and evaluate for stent complications, such as endoleak or stent migration. This evaluation should be coordinated with the trauma surgery team, vascular surgery team, and the intensive care team.

Intensive critical care is required for these patients not only for the BAI but also because many of them have polytrauma. Early involvement with physical therapy, occupational therapy, and cognitive therapy is wise. Once their injuries are repaired definitively, most of these patients require some sort of assistance and will be discharged to a rehabilitation facility.

References

1. Teixeira PG, Inaba K, Barmparas G, et al. Blunt thoracic aortic injuries: an autopsy study. *J Trauma* 2011; 70(1): 197–202.

2. Parmley LF, Mattingly TW, Manion WC, et al. Nonpenetrating traumatic injury of the aorta. *Circulation* 1958; 17(6): 1086–101.

3. Feczko JD, Lynch L, Pless JE, et al. An autopsy case review of 142 nonpenetrating (blunt) injuries of the aorta. *J Trauma* 1992; 33(6): 846–9.

4. Burkhart HM, Gomez GA, Jacobson LE, et al. Fatal blunt aortic injuries: a review of 242 autopsy cases. *J Trauma* 2001; 50(1): 113–15.

5. Rogers FB, Osler TM, Shackford SR. Aortic dissection after trauma: case report and review of the literature. *J Trauma* 1996; 41(5): 906–8.

6. Stemper BD, Yoganandan N, Pintar FA, et al. Multiple subfailures characterize blunt aortic injury. *J Trauma* 2007; 62(5): 1171–4.

7. Rizoli SB, Brenneman FD, Boulanger BR, et al. Blunt diaphragmatic and thoracic aortic rupture: an emerging injury complex. *Ann Thorac Surg* 1994; 58(5): 1404–8.

8. Lundevall J. Traumatic rupture of the aorta, with special reference to road accidents. *Acta Pathol Microbiol Scand* 1964; 62: 29–33.

9. Crass JR, Cohen AM, Motta AO, et al. A proposed new mechanism of traumatic aortic rupture: the osseous pinch. *Radiology* 1990; 176(3): 645–9.

10. Katyal D, McLellan BA, Brenneman FD, et al. Lateral impact motor vehicle collisions: significant cause of blunt traumatic rupture of the thoracic aorta. *J Trauma* 1997; 42(5): 769–72.

11. Richens D, Field M, Neale M, et al. The mechanism of injury in blunt traumatic rupture of the aorta. *Eur J Cardiothorac Surg* 2002; 21(2): 288–93.

12. Hill DA, Duflou J, Delaney LM. Blunt traumatic rupture of the thoracic aorta: an epidemiological perspective. *J R Coll Surg Edinb* 1996; 41(2): 84–7.

13. Fabian TC, Richardson JD, Croce MA, et al. Prospective study of blunt aortic injury: Multicenter Trial of the American Association for the Surgery of Trauma. *J Trauma* 1997; 42(3): 374–83.

14. Horton TG, Cohn SM, Heid MP, et al. Identification of trauma patients at risk of thoracic aortic tear by mechanism of injury. *J Trauma* 2000; 48(6): 1008–14.

15. Durham CA, McNally MM, Parker FM, et al. A contemporary rural trauma center experience in blunt

traumatic aortic injury. *J Vasc Surg* 2010; 52(4): 884–90.

16. Greendyke RM. Traumatic rupture of aorta; special reference to automobile accidents. *JAMA* 1966; 195(7): 527–30.

17. Sevitt S. Traumatic ruptures of the aorta: a clinico-pathological study. *Injury* 1977; 8(3): 159–73.

18. McLellan BA, Rizoli SB, Brenneman FD, *et al.* Injury pattern and severity in lateral motor vehicle collisions: a Canadian experience. *J Trauma* 1996; 41(4): 708–13.

19. Scalea T, Goldstein A, Phillips T, *et al.* An analysis of 161 falls from a height: the 'jumper syndrome'. *J Trauma* 1986; 26(8): 706–12.

20. Brinkman WT, Bavaria JE. Vascular trauma: thoracic. In Cronenwett JL, Johnston KW, eds. *Rutherford's Vascular Surgery*, 7th edition. Philadelphia: Saunders Elsevier; 2010: 2330.

21. Mattox KL, Wall MJ Jr, Lemaire S. Thoracic great vessel injury. In Feliciano DV, Mattox KL, Moore EE, eds. *Trauma*, 6th edition. New York: McGraw Hill Medical; 2008: 589.

22. Arthurs ZM, Starnes BW, Sohn VY, *et al.* Functional and survival outcomes in traumatic blunt thoracic aortic injuries: an analysis of the National Trauma Databank. *J Vasc Surg* 2009; 49(4): 988–94.

23. Symbas PN. Great vessels injury. *Am Heart J* 1977; 93(4): 518–22.

24. Symbas PN, Tyras DH, Ware RE, *et al.* Traumatic rupture of the aorta. *Ann Surg* 1973; 178(1): 6–12.

25. Schwab CW, Lawson RB, Lind JF, *et al.* Aortic injury: comparison of supine and upright portable chest films to evaluate the widened mediastinum. *Ann Emerg Med* 1984; 13(10): 896–9.

26. Mirvis SE, Bidwell JK, Buddemeyer EU, *et al.* Value of chest radiography in excluding traumatic aortic rupture. *Radiology* 1987; 163(2): 487–93.

27. Woodring JH. The normal mediastinum in blunt traumatic rupture of the thoracic aorta and brachiocephalic arteries. *J Emerg Med* 1990; 8(4): 467–76.

28. Exadaktylos AK, Sclabas G, Schmid SW, *et al.* Do we really need routine computed tomographic scanning in the primary evaluation of blunt chest trauma in patients with "normal" chest radiograph? *J Trauma* 2001; 51(6): 1173–6.

29. Demetriades D, Gomez H, Velmahos GC, *et al.* Routine helical computed tomographic evaluation of the mediastinum in high-risk blunt trauma patients. *Arch Surg* 1998; 133(10): 1084–8.

30. Gammie JS, Shah AS, Hattler BG, *et al.* Traumatic aortic rupture: diagnosis and management. *Ann Thorac Surg* 1998; 66(4): 1295–300.

31. Plurad D, Green D, Demetriades D, *et al.* The increasing use of chest computed tomography for trauma: is it being overutilized? *J Trauma* 2007; 62(3): 631–5.

32. Mirvis SE, Shanmuganathan K, Buell J, *et al.* Use of spiral computed tomography for the assessment of blunt trauma patients with potential aortic injury. *J Trauma* 1998; 45(5): 922–30.

33. Azizzadeh A, Valdes J, Miller CC 3rd, *et al.* The utility of intravascular ultrasound compared to angiography in the diagnosis of blunt traumatic aortic injury. *J Vasc Surg* 2011; 53(3): 608–14.

34. Patel NH, Hahn D, Comess KA. Blunt chest trauma victims: role of intravascular ultrasound and transesophageal echocardiography in cases of abnormal thoracic aortogram. *J Trauma* 2003; 55(2): 330–7.

35. Mirvis SE, Shanmuganathan K. Diagnosis of blunt traumatic aortic injury 2007: still a nemesis. *Eur J Radiol* 2007; 64(1): 27–40.

36. Wheat MW Jr, Palmer RF, Bartley TD, *et al.* Treatment of dissecting aneurysms of the aorta without surgery. *J Thorac Cardiovasc Surg* 1965; 50: 364–73.

37. Fabian TC, Davis KA, Gavant ML, *et al.* Prospective study of blunt aortic injury: helical CT is diagnostic and antihypertensive therapy reduces rupture. *Ann Surg* 1998; 227(5): 666–77.

38. Demetriades D, Velmahos GC, Scalea TM, *et al.* Operative repair or endovascular stent graft in blunt traumatic thoracic aortic injuries: results of an American Association for the Surgery of Trauma Multicenter Study. *J Trauma* 2008; 64(3): 561–71.

Thoracic aortic aneurysm

John A. Elefteriades

Thoracic aortic aneurysms are subdivided into those located in the ascending aorta and those in the aortic arch and descending thoracic aorta. They are treated differently, except in the setting of rupture. Following a brief review of pathophysiology and epidemiology, this chapter addresses these types of aneurysms in regard to their management by emergency physicians and other acute care providers.

Aortic aneurysm is defined clinically as an aorta measuring more than 3.5 to 4.0 cm in the ascending aorta or more than 4 cm in the aortic arch or descending aorta. A pseudoaneurysm is a focal dilation of the aorta, where the wall consists only of mediastinal tissues (i.e., a contained rupture, with the adventitia violated). Classification of aortic aneurysms is based on location, shape, and cause. The location of the aneurysm affects its clinical manifestations and reflects the natural history of the disease. Diagnostic and treatment options differ, depending on the location of the aneurysm.

The ascending aorta starts at the aortic annulus and extends to the take-off of the innominate artery and the end of the pericardial reflection onto the aorta (hence, cardiac tamponade can be an issue with rupture of this type of aneurysm). The ascending aorta is further subdivided into the aortic root and tubular portion of the ascending aorta. The aortic arch extends from the proximal orifice of the innominate artery to the distal orifice of the left subclavian artery. The descending thoracic aorta extends from the distal left subclavian orifice to the diaphragm. If the aneurysm crosses the diaphragm, it is called a thoracoabdominal aneurysm.

Aneurysms can be saccular or fusiform. Saccular aneurysms involve short portions of the aorta, with eccentric dilation connected to the aortic lumen by a neck. Fusiform aneurysms involve a longer segment of the aorta, with circumferential dilation of the aorta along the length of the aneurysm.

Ascending aortic aneurysms are typically fusiform and are divided into three categories depending on the involvement of the aortic root. The first category is the supracoronary type, in which the annulus of the valve and the aortic root are of normal size and the remainder of the ascending aorta is aneurysmal (Figure 11.1).[1] The second is annuloaortic ectasia or the Marfanoid type (according to whether the patient has Marfan's syndrome or not). In this type, the aortic annulus and the most proximal portion of the aorta are dilated (Figure 11.1).[1] The third type is tubular diffuse enlargement, in which the aortic annulus and proximal aorta are somewhat dilated, as is the remainder of the ascending aorta (giving it a tubular appearance) (Figure 11.1).[1] The type of ascending aortic aneurysm and patient's age largely determine the type of repair required (see below).

Pathophysiologic classification of thoracic aortic aneurysms is also useful because of its treatment implications. Descending thoracic aneurysms, as discussed below, are typically associated with atherosclerosis, are fusiform, and begin distal to the origin of the left subclavian artery.[2] If they cross the diaphragm, they are called thoracoabdominal aneurysms. Ascending aortic aneurysms, by comparison, are rarely atherosclerotic, being caused instead by inherited connective tissue disease (Figure 11.2).[1] Other rare causes include infection (mycotic aneurysms or syphilitic) and inflammation (Takayasu's arteritis, Behçet's disease, giant cell arteritis).

Pathophysiology/epidemiology

The wall of the aorta is composed of intima, media, and adventitia (Figure 11.3). The media is composed

---

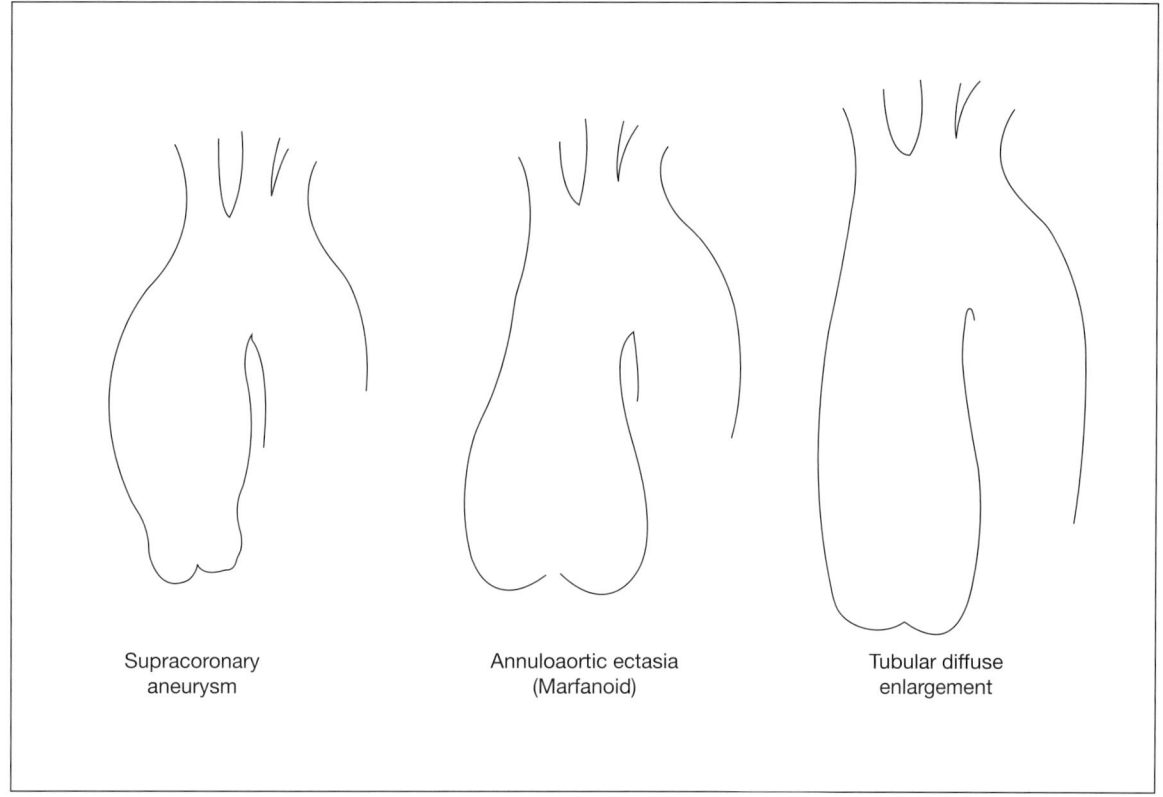

Supracoronary
aneurysm

Annuloaortic ectasia
(Marfanoid)

Tubular diffuse
enlargement

Figure 11.1 Three common patterns of ascending aortic aneurysm disease: supracoronary, annuloaortic ectasia, and tubular. (Reprinted from Elefteriades,[1] with permission from Elsevier.)

primarily of smooth muscle cells in a matrix of collagen, elastin, and other structural proteins, including but not limited to glycosaminoglycans, fibrillin, and fibronectin.[3] In general, the strength of the aortic wall is determined by the relative amounts of normal collagen (strength) and elastin (recoil). Defects in collagen or elastin can cause medial degeneration and aneurysmal disease of the aorta.

In idiopathic medial degeneration, degenerative changes within the media weaken the aortic wall, increasing wall tension and permitting aneurysmal dilatation to occur. The result can be aortic dissection, intramural hemorrhage, or rupture. Medial degeneration occurs normally with aging but is accelerated by hypertension.[4]

Marfan's syndrome is the most prevalent inherited connective tissue disorder, with a prevalence of 1 in 3000 to 5000. Various genetic defects result in defective fibrillin, which is a major component of elastin. Abnormal elastic properties result, and progressive aortic dilation occurs. Marfan's patients also get mitral valve prolapse and left ventricular dilation, but aortic root dilation is the most common cause of morbidity and mortality.[5]

Ehlers–Danlos syndrome is a rare connective tissue disorder. In patients with this condition, type III collagen is defective, resulting in a variety of vascular abnormalities, mostly in the thorax and abdomen.[6]

Loeys–Dietz is an autosomal dominant aortic aneurysm syndrome with systemic involvement. The phenotype overlaps considerably with Marfan's syndrome (aortic aneurysms, arachnodactyly, dural ectasia), with additional features including bifid uvula, cleft palate, generalized arterial tortuosity, and widely spaced eyes.[6]

Familial thoracic aortic aneurysms and dissections constitute an entity coming to be known in patients without Marfan's, Ehlers–Danlos, or Loeys–Dietz syndromes. The Yale database, containing clinical information from more than 1,600 patients, indicates that 21% of aneurysm patients have a first-order relative with a known or likely aneurysm.[7]

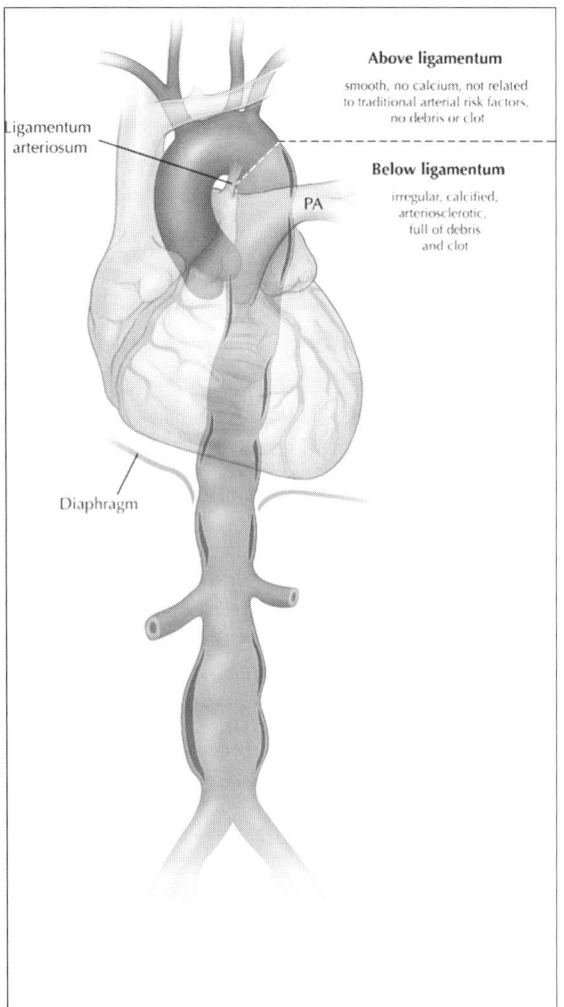

Above ligamentum
smooth, no calcium, not related to traditional arterial risk factors, no debris or clot

Below ligamentum
irregular, calcified, arteriosclerotic, full of debris and clot

Ligamentum arteriosum

PA

Diaphragm

Figure 11.2 Aortic aneurysm is really two diseases: ascending disease differs markedly from descending/abdominal disease. Note that thoracic aneurysm disease divides naturally into two patterns, separated at the ligamentum. Above the ligamentum, the aorta is thin, but not atherosclerotic; below the ligamentum, as with abdominal aortic aneurysms, heavy arteriosclerosis and calcification predominate. PA, pulmonary artery. See plate section for color version. (Figure illustration by Rob Flewell.)

Turner's and Noonan's syndromes are associated with aortic root dilation.

Bicuspid aortic valve disease occurs in 1 to 2% of the US population, and its presence is associated with a "bicuspid aortopathy." Because this congenital disorder is so common, it accounts for many more dissections than the better-known Marfan's disease.[8]

Chronic aortic dissections, Stanford Type A (ascending) or B (descending), tend to dilate over time. Patients with these conditions are prone to aneurysm formation. Poorly controlled hypertension makes them more likely to develop aneurysms.[9]

Diagnosis

History

Most thoracic aortic aneurysms are silent. The first signs and symptoms are secondary to rupture.[1] For most patients, the first symptom is death or a devastating complication that threatens to cause death. Only 5 to 10% of patients present with symptoms prior to rupture, thus permitting early detection and treatment in this small subset.[1] The most common symptom associated with thoracic aortic aneurysm is pain, ostensibly from stretching of aortic tissue or impingement of adjacent structures. The pain associated with ascending aortic aneurysms is usually felt retrosternally. In contrast, descending aneurysmal pain is felt in the interscapular location in the back (which, fortunately, is rarely a site for musculoskeletal pain). Lateral or posterior chest pain can also occur secondary to compression or erosion into ribs or vertebral bodies. Close attention must be paid to patients' reports, as they can usually distinguish deep visceral pain from musculoskeletal pain. Aneurysmal pain is also independent of patient position and movement, in contradistinction to musculoskeletal pain.

Rupture of the ascending aorta produces chest pain and possibly shock secondary to cardiac tamponade. Rupture of the descending aorta may produce hypovolemic shock and pain in location commensurate with the location of the rupture.

Other symptoms associated with thoracic aneurysms are less common but worth mentioning because an astute clinician can use them to complete the picture in certain cases. Ascending aneurysm can present as congestive heart failure, secondary to aortic insufficiency. If the aortic annulus is involved, then dilation of this portion of the aorta pulls the aortic valve leaflets apart, resulting in aortic regurgitation and subsequent heart failure. Ascending aneurysms can also obstruct or distort the trachea, causing respiratory symptoms. Compression of the superior vena cava may produce venous congestion of the head, neck, and upper extremities.

Descending or arch aneurysms can produce dysphagia (dysphagia lusoria) or hoarseness secondary to direct impingement of the esophagus or recurrent

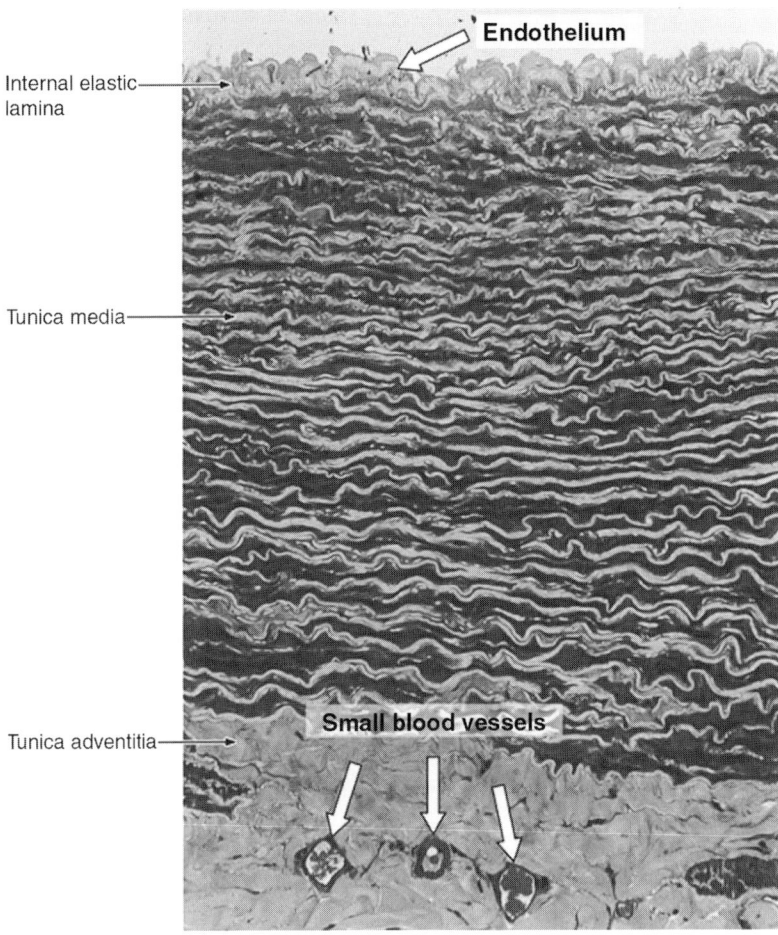

Internal elastic lamina

Tunica media

Tunica adventitia

Figure 11.3 Transverse section of the wall of a large elastic artery demonstrating the well-developed tunica media containing elastic lamellae (pararosaniline–toluidine blue stain; medium magnification). (Reproduced with permission from Junqueira and Carneiro.[3])

laryngeal nerve, respectively. Descending aneurysms can produce hemoptysis from erosion into the parenchyma of the lung or bronchi. Hematemesis can also result from erosion into the esophagus. Finally, descending aneurysms can present with distal embolic phenomena and associated symptoms because mural thrombi are quite common in these patients and often mobile.

As mentioned earlier, most thoracic aortic aneurysm cases are silent until rupture, so aneurysmal disease of the thoracic aorta is usually found incidentally on CT scans, echocardiograms, or MRI done for other reasons. For the purposes of this book, it is worth dividing the presentations of patients into: (1) those in whom you suspect acute rupture or dissection and (2) those who might harbor symptomatic thoracic aneurysms (without acute rupture or dissection). The immediate clinical implications for these two categories are drastically different.

Additional history important to obtain concerns potential family patterns of aneurysm disease. As mentioned earlier, a variety of heritable conditions (especially for the ascending aneurysm location) predispose individuals to aneurysms and to dissection and rupture. Specifically, the emergency physician must inquire whether anyone in the patient's family has ever been diagnosed with aneurysmal disease or if a young family member experienced a sudden unexplained death (Figure 11.4). Aneurysm rupture mimics death from myocardial infarction and is often misdiagnosed as such, so suspect a family pattern of aneurysm with a history of such events.[10]

Physical examination

Ascending aneurysms are generally not detectable on physical examination unless they produce aortic regurgitation (annuloaortic ectasia). In these patients,

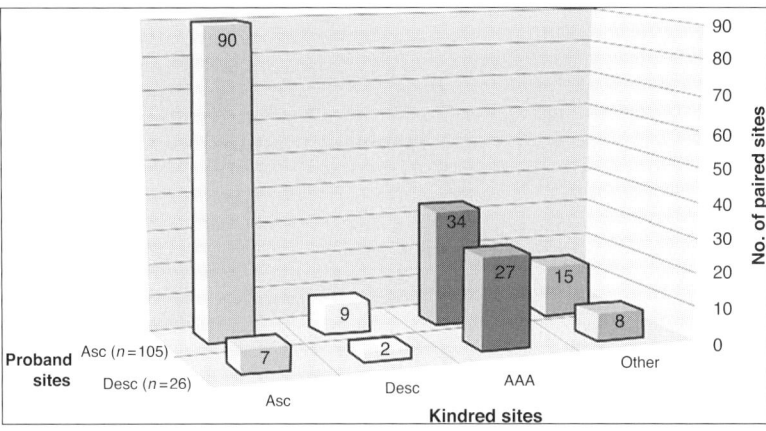

Figure 11.4 The location of the proband aneurysm influences the location of aneurysms in the family members. Probands with ascending aneurysms (Asc) have family members with ascending aneurysms, whereas probands with descending thoracic aneurysms (Desc) are more likely to have family members with abdominal aortic aneurysm (AAA).[10] (Figure provided by Rob Flewell.) (Reprinted from Albornoz et al., p. 1403,[11] with permission from Elsevier.)

a blowing diastolic murmur can be heard best at the right upper sternal border. Forced exhalation can bring the aorta closer to the sternum and accentuate this murmur, which often eludes detection. Rupture of an ascending aneurysm generally causes cardiac tamponade. Thus, physical examination findings may include muffled heart sounds, hypotension, distended neck veins, and pulsus paradoxus.

Descending aneurysms are also usually undetectable on physical examination, unless, on rare occasion, the patient has extreme aneurysmal dilation, which can be palpated through an attenuated chest wall. All patients in whom these diagnoses are being considered should have blood pressures taken in both upper extremities. A difference should alert the clinician to a possible dissection (discussed separately); of course, dissection not infrequently coincides with aneurysmal aortic disease.

Laboratory tests

A complete blood count, basic metabolic panel, and cardiac enzymes should be obtained on all patients with chest pain. Additionally, it is useful to request measurement of D-dimer because the absence of elevation in this value excludes two diagnoses in patients who present with chest pain: pulmonary embolism and aortic dissection.

Imaging

The major questions that need to be answered with imaging when aortic disease is suspected are as follows: Is the aorta aneurysmal (and how severely)? Is a

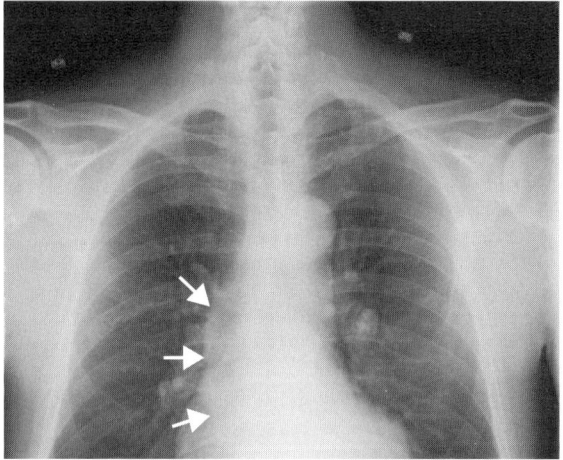

Figure 11.5 Chest film showing extension of the right upper mediastinal border (arrows), indicating an ascending aneurysm.

dissection present (where and how far)? Has the aorta ruptured?

An excellent initial screening test is the chest film. To the astute observer, chronic thoracic aneurysms will become apparent. An ascending aneurysm will show extension to the right of the upper mediastinal border. An arch aneurysm will show an exaggerated aortic knob.[12] Finally, a descending aneurysm will show up as a left deviated stripe of the descending aorta (Figures 11.5 and 11.6).[12] A chest film will also show a widened mediastinum after rupture or dissection of the ascending aorta.

Three types of 3D imaging will be helpful in evaluating patients with suspected thoracic aortic aneurysm or dissection. Most commonly used is the CT scan with IV contrast. A CT scan can give information about the

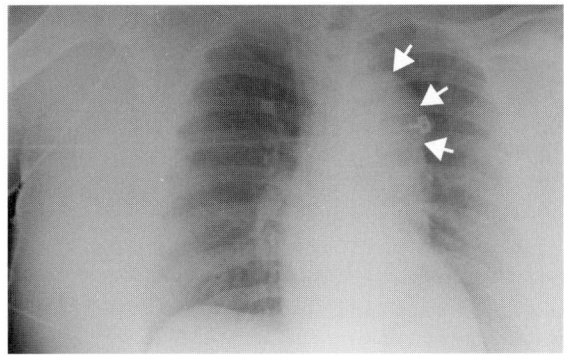

Figure 11.6 Exaggerated aortic knob and left deviated aortic stripe of the descending aorta, indicating an arch and descending aortic aneurysm.

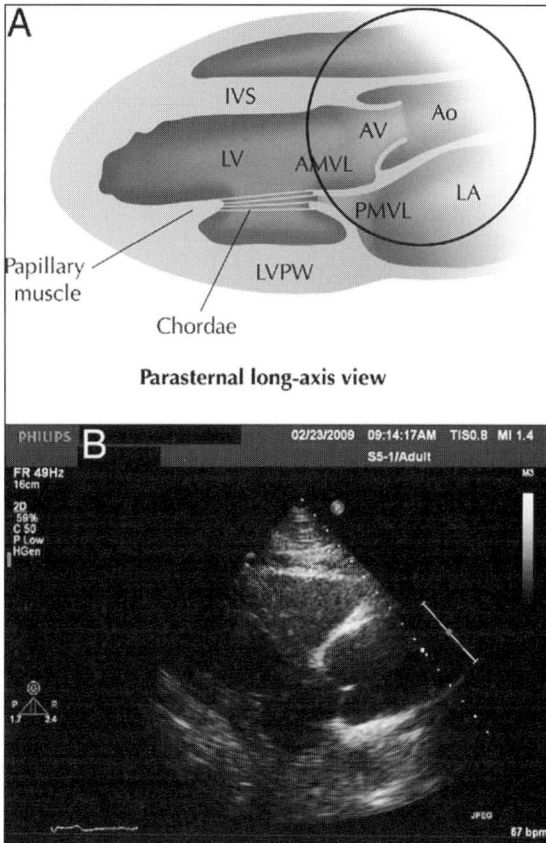

Figure 11.7 Schematic (A) and actual echocardiographic (B) images. Limited distance above the aortic valve (AV) for which the ascending aorta (Ao) can be seen on transthoracic echocardiography. AMVL, anterior mitral valve leaflet; IVS, interventricular septum; LA, left atrium; LV, left ventricle; LVPW, left ventricular posterior wall; PMVL, posterior mitral valve leaflet. (Panel A illustration by Rob Flewell.) (Reprinted from Elefteriades et al., [2] with permission from Elsevier.)

entire aorta within the chest/abdomen as well as information about the rest of the chest, including branches of the aorta.[13] Because CT is readily available, provides excellent images with ample information, and gives information that aortography cannot provide, without the risks associated with arterial puncture, it has become the gold standard for the assessment of aneurysmal disease in the aorta.[13] MRI gives much of the same information but is not as readily available in many emergency departments.

Transesophageal echocardiography (TEE) is also an excellent technique for evaluation of the thoracic aorta. One caveat is that there is a "blind spot" in the visualization of the aortic arch (which is obscured by the tracheal air column).[2] However, this procedure provides valuable information about potential pericardial/pleural effusions, cardiac tamponade, valve dysfunction, and left ventricular impairment. TEE can also diagnose ascending and descending thoracic aneurysms. The less invasive transthoracic echocardiography (TTE) examination can also provide most of this information, if the echo windows are good (e.g., patients without obesity or chronic obstructive pulmonary disease). The benefits and liabilities of TTE and TEE are illustrated in Figures 11.7 and 11.8.

The presence of a pericardial effusion on transthoracic echocardiogram without any other cause should raise suspicion for a ruptured ascending aneurysm. In this scenario, we recommend a CT scan to evaluate the aorta for aneurysmal dilation or dissection. Similarly, an unexplained pleural effusion can also represent a ruptured descending aneurysm. In this scenario, a CT scan is likely to be done for other reasons. We stress paying close attention to the aorta in these cases.

Emergency department management

Medical treatment of acute aortic syndromes

In the initial phase of management, blood pressure control is paramount in patients with a thoracic aortic aneurysm that has ruptured or in whom rupture is impending. Nitroglycerin and nitroprusside are used for this purpose because of their effectiveness in controlling blood pressure, rapid onset of action, and quick cessation of action upon discontinuation.[14] Typically, we aim for a systolic blood pressure of 90 to 100 mmHg, taking care not to cause oliguria or neurologic sequelae. With this in mind, in older patients with

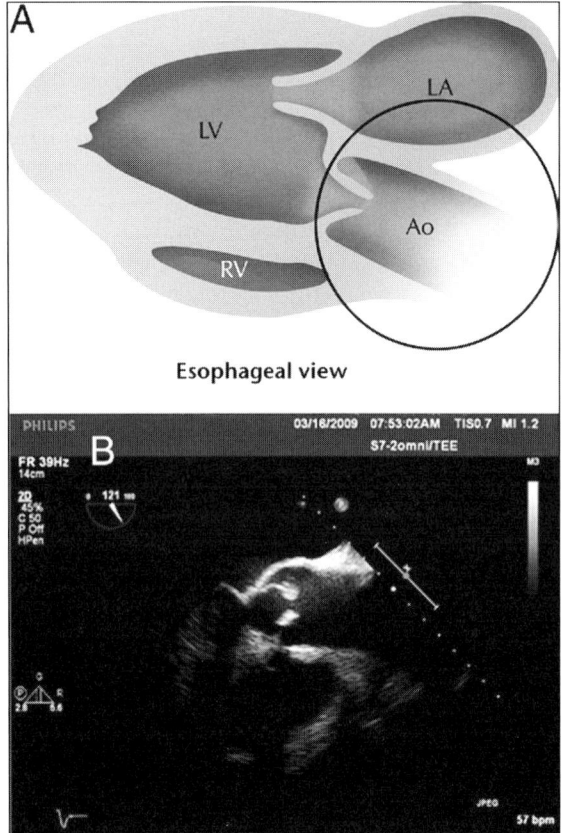

Figure 11.8 Schematic (A) and actual echocardiographic (B) images. Limited distance above the aortic valve for which the ascending aorta can be seen on transesophageal echocardiography. The tracheal air column interferes with visualization of the upper ascending aorta. RV, right ventricle; LV, left ventricle; Ao, ascending aorta; LA, left atrium. (Panel A illustration by Rob Flewell.) (Reprinted from Elefteriades *et al.*,[2] with permission from Elsevier.)

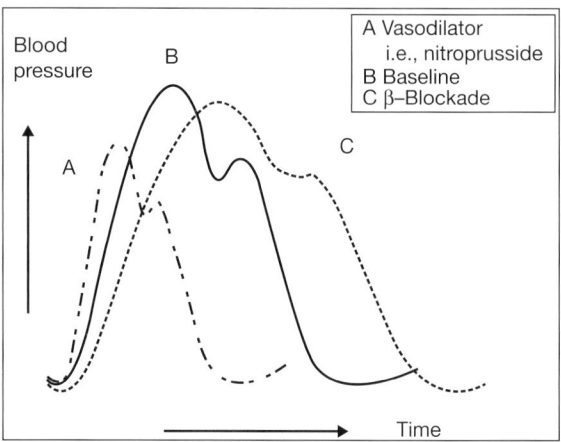

Figure 11.9 Pharmacologic anti-impulse therapy. Diagram of aortic pressure curves under various conditions. The continuous line (B) represents the baseline state. Administration of a vasodilator agent such as nitroprusside is represented by the dashed curve (A). There is significant decrease in pressure levels and acceleration in heart rate, but this is accompanied by the steepest slope of the ascending portion of the curve (increased *dp/dt* max). β-Blockade administration is represented by the dotted line (C). Although the degree of pressure lowering is usually smaller, the drug's negative inotropic and chronotropic effects result in decreased impulse and *dp/dt* max. (Reproduced with permission from Sanz *et al.* [14])

Differential diagnosis

The differential diagnosis for a presentation of aortic pathology is quite extensive. In addition, because aortic pathology presents in a variety of ways related to the organs involved, it has been termed the "great masquerader." For these reasons, a high index of suspicion is needed on the part of the clinician who first sees the patient. For instance, chest pain without an obvious cause requires that the thoracic aorta be imaged.

Acute coronary syndrome is commonly the initial diagnosis for patients in whom an aortic rupture/ dissection is eventually discovered. This is particularly important to recognize because administration of thrombolytics in the setting of aortic rupture or dissection can have obvious disastrous consequences. In one study, acute aortic syndromes were initially misdiagnosed 39% of the time and most commonly misdiagnosed as acute coronary syndrome.[15] For this reason, even if the leading diagnosis is acute coronary syndrome, at least a screening chest film should be done prior to coronary intervention (administration of a thrombolytic or performance of an angiographic intervention). In addition, a negative D-dimer rules out not only pulmonary embolism (on the differential) but also aortic dissection with near total accuracy.[16]

peripheral vascular disease, we may have to accept 120 to 130 mmHg as a target systolic blood pressure.

Dropping the afterload without decreasing the force of contraction, however, would actually increase the sheer stress on the aortic wall.[14] For this reason, we usually use a short-acting β-blocker (esmolol) in addition to afterload reduction. Afterload reduction and β-blockade are referred to as "anti-impulse" therapy (Figure 11.9).[14] To discourage rupture or propagation of a dissection, this therapy should be instituted regardless of whether the patient is going emergently to the operating room. Most often these therapies are instituted while the patient is being imaged to define the anatomic type of aneurysm/dissection. Definitive therapies then follow.

Caution should be exercised, however, since no cutoff value for D-dimer has been established.

The extensive list of diagnoses included in the differential diagnosis of thoracic aortic aneurysm includes musculoskeletal pain, pericarditis, pleural effusion, pneumothorax, pulmonary embolism, cholecystitis, ureteral colic, appendicitis, mesenteric ischemia, pyelonephritis, stroke, transient ischemic attack (TIA), and isolated limb ischemia.

Pearls and pitfalls

1. Have a high index of suspicion for aortic dissection or rupture.
2. Image freely.
   a. All patients with presumed acute coronary syndrome should have at least a screening chest film.
   b. The CT scan can be used to rule out/in three major diagnoses (triple rule-out CT)[13]:
      i. pulmonary embolism;
      ii. aortic aneurysm/dissection;
      iii. coronary artery disease.
3. A negative D-dimer rules out both pulmonary embolism and aortic dissection.[16] A clot within the false lumen of the dissection liberates D-dimer. The absolute magnitude of the D-dimer elevation correlates with the longitudinal extent of the dissection and the outcome. It should be stressed, however, that an appropriate cutoff level for D-dimer has not been established.
4. Look at the aorta even on CT scans done for other purposes. Aortic syndromes can present in a variety of ways.

Critical actions to take in the acute setting

In the acute setting, as outlined above, it is helpful to divide patients into two groups: (1) those with rupture or acute cardiorespiratory decompensation, who need instantaneous diagnosis and treatment, and (2) stable patients with a diagnosis picked up on imaging studies.

Those with rupture are likely to be unstable, in which case the airway needs to be controlled and managed in the same way as for a patient with cardiorespiratory embarrassment from other causes in the acute setting. If cardiac tamponade is suspected based on signs and symptoms, then a transthoracic echocardiogram should be obtained to assess for this possibility. If a pericardial effusion is seen, the patient should go directly to the operating room, where a transesophageal echocardiogram can be performed to confirm the diagnosis and visualize the aneurysm; definitive repair can be performed at that time. A patient with rupture of the descending aorta might present with instability and a large hemothorax. In this setting, a proper physical examination, supplemented by a chest film, can lead to the correct diagnosis. In the absence of trauma, a hemothorax on either side should alert the physician to the strong possibility of a ruptured descending thoracic aneurysm. Computed tomographic scan will confirm the diagnosis, and a trip to the operating room or to the hybrid suite (for operative or endovascular therapy) will follow.

For ambulatory patients, not distressed, presenting to the emergency department with symptoms possibly compatible with thoracic aortic aneurysm, aortic imaging is essential. In the ideal setting, the triple rule-out CT scan is the imaging study of choice (after a screening chest film). This is most ideal when a 64-slice CT scanner is available at the facility. If resources are limited (i.e., no CT scanner), and ascending aortic aneurysm is a possibility, then a transesophageal echocardiogram (TEE) can be done to evaluate the aorta, the aortic valve, the pericardial space, and the level of left ventricular function. If visualization is suboptimal, the TTE can be followed by a TEE. As mentioned earlier, the disadvantage of TEE is the blind spot in the aortic arch. On TEE, the descending thoracic aorta can be evaluated quite adequately, even if a CT scan is not feasible.

In the absence of rupture of the thoracic aorta or acute ascending dissection (see Chapter 7, Acute aortic dissection), where immediate operation is required, the patient with a thoracic aortic aneurysm needs blood pressure and heart rate control as the primary therapy. This is called "anti-impulse therapy" because decreasing the blood pressure and blunting the contractile strength of the heart (dp/dt) decrease the impact of each heartbeat on the vulnerable aortic wall.[14] Anti-impulse therapy is usually effected via IV nitroglycerin or nitroprusside. Blood pressure is monitored by arterial line in an intensive care unit. If the patient is effectively stabilized, a transition is made to oral therapy from IV afterload-reducing drugs and IV β-blockers (Figure 11.9). If β-blockers are contraindicated, then calcium channel blockers are an acceptable alternative.

Table 11.1 Algorithm for intervention for asymptomatic thoracic aortic aneurysms[17]

1. Rupture

2. Acute aortic dissection
   a. Ascending aorta requires urgent operation
   b. Descending aorta requires a "complication-specific approach"

3. Symptomatic states
   a. Pain consistent with rupture and unexplained by other causes
   b. Compression of adjacent organs, especially trachea, esophagus, or left main stem bronchus
   c. Significant aortic insufficiency in conjunction with ascending aortic aneurysm

4. Documented enlargement
   a. Growth ≥ 1 cm/yr or substantial growth and aneurysm is rapidly approaching absolute size criteria

5. Absolute size criteria (cm)

	Marfan's	**Non-Marfan's**
Ascending	5.0	5.5
Descending	6.0	6.5

The surgical intervention criteria for thoracic aortic aneurysms recommended by the Yale Center for Thoracic Aortic Disease are detailed in Table 11.1.[17] Rupture or acute ascending dissection requires immediate surgical intervention. A descending dissection requires a more complication-specific approach. Continued or persistent pain, compression of adjacent organs, and significant aortic insufficiency in conjunction with ascending aortic aneurysm also require urgent surgical therapy. Finally, size and growth criteria for surgical intervention are delineated. Documented enlargement of > 1 cm/yr or an absolute size of more than 5.5 cm for an ascending aneurysm (5.0 cm for Marfan's patients) or more than 6.5 cm for descending thoracic aneurysms (6.0 cm for Marfan's patients) are accepted criteria for intervention in asymptomatic patients. Symptomatic patients require surgical extirpation of the thoracic aneurysm regardless of size.

Definitive treatment (outside the ED)

Medical treatment of chronic aneurysms

Aggressive anti-impulse therapy is the main treatment for thoracic aneurysms that do not meet surgical criteria. The idea is to decrease the virulence of the impact of systole on the aortic wall. This treatment, although standard practice, is largely unproven in patients with thoracic aortic aneurysms. A study performed at Johns Hopkins with long-term follow-up has provided support in the Marfan's population, which has resulted in the standard practice for all patients.[18]

Habashi *et al.* recently demonstrated that angiotensin receptor blockers may prevent aneurysm growth in the Marfan's population. This action is thought to be due to down regulation of transforming growth factor beta (TGF-β).[19] Angiotensin-converting enzyme inhibitors may also have benefit, perhaps by decreasing the inflammatory milieu and vascular smooth muscle apoptosis.[20,21] In the abdominal aortic aneurysm population, statin therapy has also shown some potential benefit.[22–24] However, there are no data to support its use in patients with non-atherosclerotic or inherited thoracic aortic aneurysm syndromes.

Surgical therapy

The indications and urgency for surgical intervention are reviewed above. For ascending aneurysms, the type of operation depends largely on the involvement of the aortic root. If the aortic root is involved, then the aortic valve and root are replaced with a valve-conduit, with reimplantation of the coronary arteries (Figure 11.10). If the root is not involved, then replacement of the ascending aorta with a tube graft will suffice. For descending aneurysms, replacement with a tube graft spanning the length of the aneurysm is the operation of choice. Finally, if the patient has aneurysmal disease that involves the ascending aorta, the arch, and the descending aorta, then a two-stage "elephant trunk" procedure is required. At the first stage, usually the ascending and aortic arch are replaced with reimplantation of the innominate, left carotid, and left subclavian arteries (Figure 11.11). A "trunk" of graft is left within the lumen of the descending aorta for use at the second stage. During the second stage, the "trunk" is used after opening and resecting the aorta to sew distally on the descending aorta.

Summary

Thoracic aortic aneurysms represent a significant challenge for acute care providers and cardiovascular surgeons. A high index of suspicion is crucial to diagnosis and initiation of treatment of this disease; thus, a point of emphasis for us is to image freely and pay attention to the aorta on imaging tests done for other reasons. Medial degeneration is the leading cause of ascending

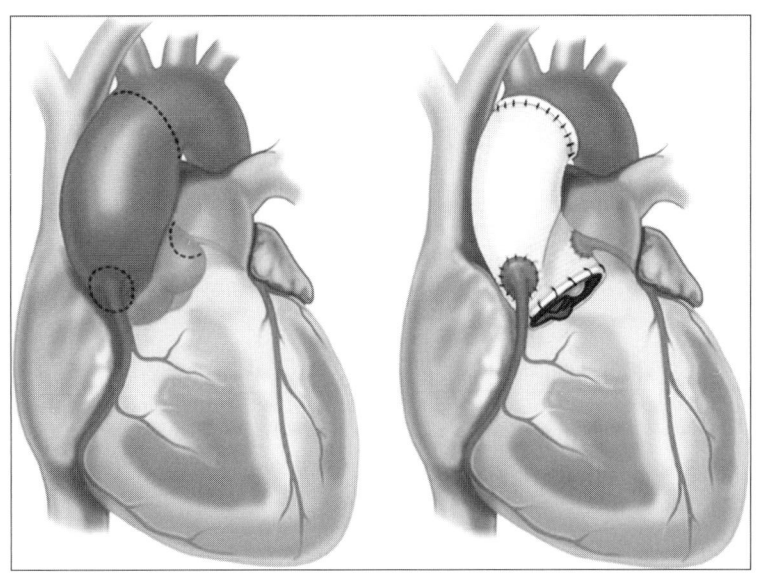

Figure 11.10 Composite graft replacement of ascending aorta and aortic valve, with reimplantation of coronary artery "buttons." See plate section for color version. (Reprinted from Isselbacher.[25] Used with permission ©Massachusetts General Hospital Thoracic Aortic Center.)

aneurysms, which can be idiopathic or accelerated by heritable conditions. Descending or arch aneurysms are caused by chronic dissection, hypertension, or atherosclerosis. These causes, along with the symptom complex, should guide the initial history, physical examination, and subsequent workup. Acute aortic syndromes (rupture/impending rupture) should be treated immediately with anti-impulse therapy while the workup is being completed and surgical treatment is being arranged. The mainstay of workup is a CT scan or an echocardiogram, but additional clues along the way can be gained from simple tests such as D-dimer and a chest film. An astute clinical team, evaluating the indications and arranging appropriate and timely treatment, can be life-saving for many patients with this disease.

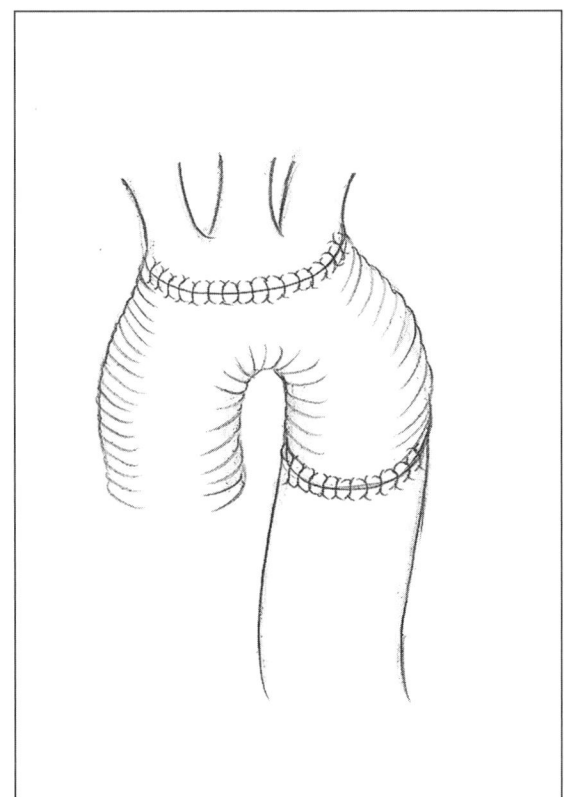

Figure 11.11 Methods of reimplantation of head vessels (with or without subclavian artery) using a Carrel patch of aortic tissue. When the subclavian artery is not included in the patch (to save time and improve exposure [preferred technique at Yale]), it is reimplanted separately after completion of the aortic arch reconstruction. (Reproduced with permission from Griepp and Elefteriades.[26])

References

1. Elefteriades JA. Thoracic aortic aneurysm: reading the enemy's playbook. *Curr Probl Cardiol* 2008; 33: 203–7.

2. Elefteriades JA, Farkas EA. Thoracic aortic aneurysm: clinically pertinent controversies and uncertainties. *J Am Coll Cardiol* 2010; 55: 841–57.

3. Junqueira LC, Carneiro J. The circulatory system. In Junqueira LC, Carneiro J. *Basic Histology: Text and Atlas*, 11th edition. New York: McGraw-Hill Access Medicine [electronic format]; 2005: 215–33.

4. Yun KI. Ascending aortic aneurysm and aortic root disease. *Coron Artery Dis* 2002; 13(2): 85–92.

5. Milewicz DM, Dietz HC, Miller DC. Treatment of aortic disease in patients with Marfan syndrome. *Circulation* 2005; 111(11): e150–7.

6. Germain DP, Herrera-Guzman Y. Vascular Ehlers-Danlos syndrome. *Ann Genet* 2004; 47(1): 1–9.

7. Coady MA, Davies RR, Roberts M, *et al.* Familial patterns of thoracic aortic aneurysms. *Arch Surg* 1999; 134(4): 361–7.

8. Edwards WD, Leaf DS, Edwards JE. Dissecting aortic aneurysm associated with congenital bicuspid aortic valve. *Circulation* 1978; 57(5): 1022–5.

9. DeBakey ME, McCollum CH, Crawford ES, *et al.* Dissection and dissecting aneurysms of the aorta: twenty year follow-up of five hundred twenty-seven patients treated surgically. *Surgery* 1982; 92(6): 1118–34.

10. Lorelli DR, Jean-Claude JM, Fox CJ, *et al.* Response of plasma matrix metalloproteinase-9 to conventional abdominal aortic aneurysm repair or endovascular exclusion: implications for endoleak. *J Vasc Surg* 2002; 35: 916–22.

11. Albornoz G, Coady MA, Roberts M, *et al.* Familial thoracic aortic aneurysms and dissections – incidence, modes of inheritance, and phenotypic patterns. *Ann Thorac Surg* 2006; 82: 1400–5.

12. Elefteriades JA, ed. *Acute Aortic Disease.* New York: Informa Healthcare; 2007.

13. Napoli A, Anzidei M, Francone M, *et al.* 64-MDCT imaging of the coronary arteries and systemic arterial vascular tree in a single examination: optimisation of the scan protocol and contrast-agent administration. *Radiol Med* 2008; 113: 799–816.

14. Sanz J, Einstein J, Fuster V. Acute aortic dissection: anti-impulse therapy. In Elefteriades JA, ed. *Acute Aortic Disease.* New York: Informa Healthcare; 2007: 229–50.

15. Hansen MS, Nogareda GJ, Hutchison SJ. Frequency of and inappropriate treatment of misdiagnosis of acute aortic dissection. *Am J Cardiol* 2007; 99(6): 852–6.

16. Elefteriades JA. Legal considerations in acute aortic diseases. In Elefteriades JA, ed. *Acute Aortic Disease.* New York: Informa Healthcare, 2007: 331–45.

17. Coady MA, Rizzo JA, Hammond GL, *et al.* What is the appropriate size criterion for resection of thoracic aortic aneurysms? *J Thorac Cardiovasc Surg* 1997; 113: 476–91.

18. Shores J, Berger KR, Murphy EA, *et al.* Progression of aortic dilatation and the benefit of long-term beta-adrenergic blockade in Marfan's syndrome. *N Engl J Med* 1994; 330(19): 1335–41.

19. Habashi JP, Judge DP, Holm TM, *et al.* Losartan, an AT1 antagonist, prevents aortic aneurysm in a mouse model of Marfan syndrome. *Science* 2006; 312: 117–21.

20. Ahimastos AA, Aggarwal A, D'Orsa KM, *et al.* Effect of perindopril on large artery stiffness and aortic root diameter in patients with Marfan syndrome: a randomized controlled trial. *JAMA* 2007; 298: 1539–47.

21. Yetman AT, Bornemeier RA, McCrindle BW. Usefulness of enalapril versus propranolol or atenolol for prevention of aortic dilation in patients with the Marfan syndrome. *Am J Cardiol* 2005; 95:1125–7.

22. Kertai MD, Boersma E, Westerhout CM, *et al.* Association between long-term statin use and mortality after successful abdominal aortic aneurysm surgery. *Am J Med* 2004; 116: 96–103.

23. Sukhija R, Aronow WS, Sandhu R, *et al.* Mortality and size of abdominal aortic aneurysm at long-term follow-up of patients not treated surgically and treated with and without statins. *Am J Cardiol* 2006; 97: 279–80.

24. Diehm N, Becker G, Katzen B, *et al.* Statins are associated with decreased mortality in abdominal, but not in thoracic aortic aneurysm patients undergoing endovascular repair: propensity score-adjusted analysis. *Vasa* 2008; 37: 241–9.

25. Isselbacher E. Contemporary reviews in cardiovascular medicine: thoracic and abdominal aneurysms. *Circulation* 2005; 111: 816–28.

26. Griepp R, Elefteriades JA. Surgical procedures: a primer. In Elefteriades JA, ed. *Acute Aortic Disease.* New York: Informa Healthcare; 2007: 251–68.

Acute upper limb ischemia

Kamil Vallabh

Acute ischemia of the upper limb is relatively less common than lower limb ischemia. Because of the rich proximal collateral circulation in the neck, shoulder girdle, and elbow and the relatively low metabolic requirement from the smaller muscle mass, amputation is seldomly performed for upper extremity ischemia/gangrene. Loss of an upper limb can have devastating occupational and functional implications, so every emergency physician must be able to identify and manage upper limb ischemia appropriately.[1,2]

Pathophysiology

More than 90% of cases of acute upper limb ischemia are caused by embolic occlusion, and two-thirds of these emboli are of cardiac origin.[1] The source of the embolus is usually the left atrium, in association with atrial fibrillation. Other sources of emboli include those from thrombus in a dilated left ventricle, prosthetic valves, and paradoxic emboli.[3] Emboli also originate from ulcerated atherosclerotic plaques in the aortic arch or proximal large vessels as well as from thrombosed aneurysms in these vessels.[1] The thrombotic causes of acute upper limb ischemia include complications from atherosclerosis in the larger proximal vessels or thrombosis of aneurysmal arteries.

Less common causes of upper limb ischemia are trauma (blunt, penetrating, or iatrogenic), external compression of an arterial lumen from aortic or vascular dissection, thoracic outlet syndrome, and compartment syndrome. Vasospastic causes include Raynaud's disease and vasculitic diseases such as Buerger's disease, temporal arteritis, and Takayasu's arteritis.[4] Hypercoagulable states can also cause acute upper limb ischemia.

Table 12.1 Signs and symptoms of acute ischemia: the "five Ps"

Pain

Pallor

Pulselessness

Paresthesia

Paralysis

Epidemiology

Patients with acute upper limb ischemia tend to be in an older age group, compared with those with lower limb ischemia, with a slight female predominance.[5,6]

Diagnosis

History

A thorough history is essential in establishing the diagnosis of upper limb ischemia and should include occupational, pharmacologic, and medical aspects.[2] The patient's hand dominance should always be documented. Ask the patient specifically about a history of atrial fibrillation, previous myocardial infarctions, and valvular heart disease. Concurrent back or chest pain could indicate aortic dissection. Inquire about a history of vasculitis, as a quarter of acute upper limb ischemia is caused by arteritis.[4]

The typical symptoms of acute ischemia are represented by the "five Ps" (Table 12.1). Important factors that need to be elucidated about pain include its location, quality, onset, and duration. Pain is usually localized to the area distal to the obstruction. The sudden onset of pain points to an embolic cause, whereas a subacute onset usually indicates a thrombotic source. Occlusion can lead to tissue loss in a

---

Vascular Emergencies, ed. Robert L. Rogers, Thomas Scalea, Lee Wallis, and Heike Geduld. Published by Cambridge University Press. © Cambridge University Press 2013.

significantly shorter time than the widespread belief of a four- to six-hour window for reversibility of limb ischemia. Beyond six hours, tissue loss and disability are inevitable.[7] Paresthesia and paralysis secondary to ischemic neuropathy and myonecrosis, respectively, represent late stages of acute limb ischemia and are harbingers of an unsalvageable limb.[4] The absence of one or more of these signs and symptoms does not exclude ischemia.[7]

The symptoms of chronic ischemia are varied and include forearm claudication, although this is uncommon because of the rich collateral circulation around the shoulder and the smaller muscle mass in the upper limb. Neurologic symptoms brought about by arm movements are associated with proximal subclavian artery occlusion in the subclavian steal syndrome. Raynaud's phenomenon and embolic phenomena ("painful blue finger") are indicative of digital ischemia.

Physical examination

The clinical evaluation should include comparison of the affected limb with the unaffected side. A systematic physical examination from the fingertips to the thoracic cavity should be performed.

Examination of the hand. Inspect the hand for signs of digital and palmar ischemia. Look for pallor, cyanosis, ulceration, gangrene, splinter hemorrhages, and digital embolic phenomena. Any evidence of signs of underlying connective tissue disease, e.g., rheumatoid arthritis and scleroderma, should be documented.

Examination of the pulses. Palpation for the presence or absence of all peripheral pulses – radial, ulnar, brachial, axillary, and supraclavicular subclavian – is vital. Consider atrial fibrillation if the pulses are irregularly irregular. These arteries also need to be palpated for the presence of aneurysms. Assess the radial pulse with the arm abducted and externally rotated if thoracic outlet compression is suspected.[8,9] The Allen test should also be performed. It is a useful test for detecting the presence and site of occlusion in small arteries beyond the wrist.[8,9]

Blood pressure. Measure the blood pressure in both arms. A difference of more than 20 mm Hg is significant and indicative of stenosis or occlusion of the subclavian or axillary artery.

Base of the neck/supraclavicular fossa. Palpate the base of the neck for the presence of a cervical rib. The subclavian artery is displaced upward by a cervical rib and will therefore be palpable above the clavicle. Compression or stenosis of this artery may reveal a bruit or thrill in the supraclavicular fossa.

Neurologic function. Sensory and motor function of the hand must be assessed in all patients.

Bedside tests

Obtain segmental blood pressure measurements in the upper limb at the brachial, forearm, and wrist level. Request an electrocardiogram to assess for atrial fibrillation.

Laboratory tests

During the emergency department assessment of a patient with upper limb ischemia, the following tests should be requested:

- hemoglobin and platelet count;
- type and screen – because of possible hemorrhagic risk with anticoagulation;
- creatinine – because of nephrotoxic risk of angiography contrast agents;
- PT/PTT – for heparinization treatment;
- creatinine kinase – if myonecrosis is suspected.

Additional tests that do not necessarily need to be performed urgently during the emergency department evaluation include those that assess for underlying hematologic and connective tissue diseases as well atherosclerotic risk.

Imaging

Plain films. Obtain a chest film in patients with suspected thoracic outlet syndrome to look for a cervical rib or first rib anomaly.

Duplex ultrasonography. Ultrasound with color flow and Doppler waveforms provides information regarding vascular flow and patency.[4,9–13] Useful in the assessment of patients with upper limb ischemia, duplex ultrasonography allows visualization of vessels from the aortic arch to the palmar arch.[8,14–16] This examination is operator dependent and time intensive, but it is neither invasive nor nephrotoxic. Consider duplex ultrasonography if there is a high risk for contrast-induced nephropathy, severe contrast allergy, or equivocal examination results for acute limb ischemia.

Digital subtraction angiography. This is the gold standard for imaging in patients with limb ischemia. It offers the advantage of allowing therapeutic intervention (intra-arterial lysis) during the imaging procedure. However, it is a relatively invasive test, with a risk of contrast nephropathy.[4,17] Angiography should be the first-choice imaging approach for acute limb ischemia, because of the benefit of being able to diagnose and treat an arterial occlusion at the same time.

Computed tomography angiography. CTA offers several advantages: it is non-invasive and provides a means of evaluating a patient for aortic dissection while looking at run-off vessels in the extremities. Its disadvantages are that it is a time-intensive procedure with the risk of nephrotoxicity. It has not been well studied in its application for acute limb ischemia.[4]

Magnetic resonance angiography. MRA does not risk nephrotoxicity and does not involve ionizing radiation. It is very time intensive and is unavailable after hours in most medical facilities. Currently, it has no role in the evaluation of acute limb ischemia.[4]

Treatment of patients with active limb ischemia should not be delayed by sending them for ultrasound, CT, or MRI.[4]

Emergency department management

First 15 minutes

Initial assessment. Assessment and management of the airway, breathing, and circulation should take priority. After obtaining a history, perform a focused physical examination, which should include evaluation of the limb as well as a cardiovascular examination. Palpation of pulses is often inaccurate, so all patients with suspected upper limb ischemia should have a Doppler assessment of all peripheral pulses to determine if a flow signal is present.

Emergency department treatment

Improve limb perfusion pressure by placing the extremity in a dependent position.

Aspirin. The administration of aspirin reduces the chances of a vascular event by 25%.[4,18–20]

Unfractionated heparin. Unfractionated heparin should be administered to reduce the propagation of thrombus. It decreases the morbidity and mortality rates associated with acute limb ischemia.[4,21] It is contraindicated in cases of ischemia caused by aortic dissection, compartment syndrome, and vascular trauma.

Analgesia. Administer intravenous opioids for pain relief.

Studies needed acutely

If there is evidence that the ischemia is complete, the patient must be taken directly to the operating room because angiography will introduce delay. If the ischemia is incomplete, preoperative angiography should be performed, since simple embolectomy or thrombectomy is unlikely to be successful. Thrombolysis can be instituted at the time of angiography in addition to giving a "roadmap" for distal bypass. Most patients with acute arm ischemia require urgent revascularization, but some selected cases can be managed successfully by an endovascular approach.[22] Consult a vascular specialist to determine the best therapeutic approach.

Definitive treatment

The most reliable method of establishing arterial inflow into a limb is surgical intervention. Up to a third of patients treated conservatively will have an unsatisfactory outcome, with an amputation rate of 6%.[23]

In most cases of acute upper limb ischemia, the cause is either thrombosis or embolism. A preoperative angiogram is not necessary in a clear-cut case of embolism; however, an angiogram may be useful in making the distinction between embolism and thrombosis and in planning an operative strategy. Embolectomy can be performed under local anesthesia through a transbrachial approach. Thrombolytic agents can be an effective method of removing thrombus from occluded vessels.[24]

Treatment of acute upper limb ischemia

An initial conservative approach may significantly reduce the operative rate and hence reduce potential operative complications in a generally elderly and comorbid population. Patients presenting with acute upper limb ischemia have a tendency to have a large number of systemic medical problems,[25–27] which makes them more susceptible to surgical complications. Those with embolism often have ischemic heart disease with atrial fibrillation, cardiac failure, or a recent myocardial infarction. Conservative management takes advantage of the anatomic difference of greater collateral arterial supply in the arm compared with the lower extremities.

Early diagnosis and treatment are essential in determining the outcome from upper limb ischemia. Before embolectomy became routine, conservative treatment was the only available treatment. This included heparin, re-hydration, bed rest, and treatment of contributing medical conditions such as cardiac failure or dysrhythmias.[6] An active approach to upper limb ischemia is safe and effective in reducing the likelihood of late complications.[13] Surgical embolectomy with a Fogarty catheter is the most frequent and successful surgical procedure performed for acute upper limb ischemia.[6,28]

Although peripheral thrombolysis is well established in the management of lower limb ischemia, there are very few reports explaining its role in upper limb ischemia.[29] Catheter-directed thrombolysis is based on the principle that activation of fibrin-bound plasminogen to the active enzyme plasmin is the most effective means of lysing pathologic thrombi. Thrombolytic agents have also been used successfully intraoperatively to improve the outcome of patients with upper limb ischemia.[30]

Successful thrombolysis should be followed by endovascular or open surgical revision of any lesion unmasked after dissolution of the thrombus. Endovascular modalities such as balloon angioplasty with or without stenting can be performed at the conclusion of thrombolysis, usually through the same access site used for the infusion. It may thus avoid the stress of emergency vascular reconstruction.[31]

Inpatient care

Unless the patient has medical contraindications, long-term anticoagulation should be provided after embolectomy,[6,32–34] particularly when the heart is the source, as there is a high risk of recurrent embolism.[6,35–37]

If there are any residual signs of reduced vascular supply, or no obvious embolic source, further workup may be beneficial. This includes echocardiography, angiography, or duplex Doppler evaluation of the upper limb blood vessels.

Complications

Reperfusion injury

The generation of highly reactive oxygen free radicals caused by the reintroduction of oxygenated blood after a period of ischemia causes more damage than the ischemia alone. The local effects of reperfusion injury include limb swelling due to increased capillary permeability, which can cause compartment syndrome; impaired muscle function secondary to ischemia; and subsequent muscle contracture if the muscle infarcts. General effects include acidosis and hyperkalemia due to leakage from the damaged cells. This can cause cardiac arrhythmias and myoglobinemia, which can be complicated by acute tubular necrosis. Acute respiratory distress syndrome may also develop.[38]

Compartment syndrome

Reperfusion causes increased capillary permeability and edema within the muscle compartment. Prevention of this devastating complication by expeditious revascularization and fasciotomy are the key steps in management.[38]

Chronic pain syndromes

Chronic pain syndromes result from peripheral nerve injury caused by the acute ischemia.[38]

Clinical approach when resources are limited

Arteriography is not always required in the emergency situation. In a typical case of embolic occlusion, the diagnosis can be made by physical examination alone, with confirmation by non-invasive testing.[2] If computerized tomography or angiography is unavailable, Doppler ultrasound can be used to assess flow and extent of the injury.

> ### Critical actions
>
> - Utilize Doppler ultrasonography to confirm the diagnosis of acute limb ischemia.
> - Commence anticoagulation therapy to limit the propagation of thrombus.
> - Provide analgesia.
> - Consult a vascular specialist.

Pearls and pitfalls

- The typical symptoms of acute ischemia are represented by the "five Ps."
- Most cases of acute upper limb ischemia are caused by embolic occlusion.
- Treatment of patients with active limb ischemia should not be delayed by sending them for ultrasound, CT, or MRI.
- Most patients need anticoagulation with heparin.
- Consult a vascular specialist early.

References

1. van Marle J. Upper limb ischaemia. Student Lecture, Netcare Unitas Hospital, Pretoria, South Africa. Available at http://vascucare.co.za/index_htm_files/Lectures/UpperLimbIschaemia-web.pdf. Accessed on April 12, 2012.

2. Yao JST, Flinn WR. Emergencies in upper extremity ischemia. In Bergan JJ, Yao JST, eds. *Vascular Surgical Emergencies*. Orlando, FL: Grune & Stratton; 1987: 469–85.

3. Tailor J. Acute limb ischaemia. *Student BMJ* [serial on the Internet] 2008; 16: 80–1. Available at: http://student.bmj.com/student/view-article.html?id=sbmj0802080. Accessed on April 11, 2012.

4. Lin M. Acute limb ischemia: what are the newest diagnostic treatment options? Boston, Massachusetts, Scientific Assembly, American College of Emergency Physicians, October 5–8, 2009.

5. Quraishy MS, Cawthorn SJ, Giddings AE. Central ischemia of the upper limb. *J R Soc Med* 1992; 85: 269–73.

6. Eyers P, Earnshaw JJ. Acute non-traumatic arm ischaemia. *Br J Surg* 1998; 85: 1340–6.

7. Chopra A. Thrombophlebitis and occlusive arterial disease. In Tintinalli JE, ed. *Emergency Medicine: A Comprehensive Study Guide*, 6th edition. New York: McGraw-Hill; 2004: 409–18.

8. Myers KA. Acute upper limb ischaemic states. In Chant ADB, Barron D'Sa, eds. *Emergency Vascular Practice*. London: Arnold; 1997: 38–54.

9. Longo GM, Pearce WH, Sumner DS. Evaluation of upper extremity ischemia. In Rutherford RB, ed. *Rutherford's Vascular Surgery*, 6th edition. Philadelphia: Elsevier Saunders; 2005: 1274–93.

10. Hutchinson DT. Color duplex imaging: applications to upper extremity and microvascular surgery. *Hand Clin* 1993; 9: 47–53.

11. Koman LA, Bond MG, Carter RE, *et al.* Evaluation of upper extremity vasculature with high-resolution ultrasound. *J Hand Surg* 1985;10: 249–55.

12. Payne KM, Blackburn DR, Peterson LK, *et al.* B-mode imaging of the arteries of the hand and upper extremity. *Bruit* 1986; 10: 168.

13. Trager S, Pignataro M, Anderson J, *et al.* Color flow Doppler: imaging the upper extremity. *J Hand Surg* 1993; 18: 621–5.

14. Baxter BT, Blackburn D, Payne K, *et al.* Noninvasive evaluation of the upper extremity. *Surg Clin North Am* 1990; 70: 87–97.

15. Harris J, Huang W, Tyrer P, *et al.* Clinical and photoplethysmographic assessment of thoracic outlet arterial compression. *J Vasc Technol* 1989; 13: 20–3.

16. Summer DS. Noninvasive assessment of upper extremity and hand ischemia. *J Vasc Surg* 1986; 3: 560–4.

17. Srodon P, Matson M, Ham R. Contrast nephropathy in lower limb angiography. *Ann R Coll Surg Engl* 2003; 85(3): 187–91.

18. Clagett GP, Sobel M, Jackson MR, *et al.* Antithrombotic therapy in peripheral arterial occlusive disease: the Seventh ACCP Conference on Antithrombotic and Thrombolytic Therapy. *Chest* 2004; 126(3 suppl): 609–26.

19. Braithwaite BD, Jones L, Yusuf SW, *et al.* Aspirin improves the outcome of intra-arterial thrombolysis with tissue plasminogen activator. *Br J Surg* 1995; 82: 1357–8.

20. Antiplatelet Trialists' Collaboration. Collaborative overview of randomised trials of antiplatelet treatment. Part I: Prevention of death, myocardial infarction, and stroke by prolonged antiplatelet therapy in various categories of patients. *BMJ* 1994; 308: 81–106.

21. Blaisdel FW, Steele M, Allen RE. Management of acute lower extremity ischemia due to embolism and thrombosis. *Surgery* 1978; 84: 822–34.

22. Whitbread T, Cleveland TJ. A combined approach to the treatment of proximal arterial occlusions of the upper limb with endovascular stents. *Eur J Vasc Endovas Surg* 1998; 15: 29–35.

23. Williams N, Bell PRF. Acute ischaemia of the upper limb. *Br J Hosp Med* 1993; 50: 579–82.

24. Baguneid M, Dodd D, Fulford P, *et al.* Management of acute nontraumatic upper limb ischaemia. *Angiology* 1999; 50: 715–20.

25. Jane E, Turner H, Loh A, *et al.* A conservative approach to acute upper limb ischemia. *Vasc Dis Manag* 2010; 7: 219–22.

26. Pedderson WC. Management of severe ischemia of the upper extremity. *Clin Plast Surg* 1997; 24: 107–20.

27. Perrault L, Lassonde J, Laurendeau F. Arterial surgery of the upper limb. *Ann Chir* 1991; 45: 765–9.

28. Hernandez-Richter T, Angele MK, Helmberger T, *et al.* Acute ischemia of the upper extremity: long term results following thrombembolectomy with the Fogarty catheter. *Langenbeck's Arch Surg* 2001; 386: 261–6.

29. Machleder HI. Disorders of major vessels. In Machleder HI, ed. *Vascular Disorders of the Upper Extremity*. New York: Future Publishing Company; 1989: 225–65.

30. Grover T, Gupta A, Agarwal S, *et al.* Upper limb ischaemia: a four year experience. *Indian J Surg* 2002; 64: 56–8.

31. Vinayagam K, Arumugam S, Rao UV, *et al.* Acute nontraumatic upper limb ischaemia: a protocol for management. *Indian J Surg* 2005; 67: 257–9.

32. Elliott JP Jr, Hageman JH, Szilagyi DE, *et al.* Arterial embolization: problems of source, multiplicity, recurrence, and delayed treatment. *Surgery* 1980; 88: 833–45.

33. Sachatello CR, Ernst CB, Griffen WO Jr. The acutely ischemic upper extremity: selective management. *Surgery* 1974; 76: 1002–9.

34. Davies MG, O'Malley K, Feeley M, *et al.* Upper limb embolus: a timely diagnosis. *Ann Vasc Surg* 1991; 5: 85–7.

35. Darling RC, Austen WG, Linton RR. Arterial embolism. *Surg Gynecol Obstet* 1967; 124: 106–14.

36. Green RM, DeWeese JA, Rob CG. Arterial embolectomy before and after the Fogarty catheter. *Surgery* 1975; 77: 24–33.

37. Ricotta JJ, Scudder PA, McAndrew JA, *et al.* Management of acute ischemia of the upper extremity. *Am J Surg* 1983; 145: 661–6.

38. Callum K, Bradbury A. ABC of arterial and venous disease: acute limb ischaemia. *BMJ* [serial on the Internet] 2000 March; 320(7237): 764–7. Available from www.biomedix.com/userfiles/file/Articles/ABCofArterialandVenousDisease.pdf. Accessed on September 20, 2012.

Chapter

13

Acute lower limb ischemia

Thomas S. Monahan

Ischemia, the absence of the flow of blood, is derived from the Greek words *ischo*, "to keep back," and *haima*, "blood."[1] *Acute limb ischemia* refers to the sudden cessation of the flow of blood to an extremity. The most common causes of acute limb ischemia are arterial embolism, thrombosis of an artery, trauma, and iatrogenic events (Figure 13.1).

Acute limb ischemia is a serious medical event associated with high morbidity and mortality rates. Few epidemiologic data are available to allow calculation of the incidence, but it is generally thought to approximate 140 per million persons per year.[2] Even patients who receive prompt care have amputation rates as high as 15% and a 30-day mortality rate as high as 25%.[3,4] Prompt recognition and treatment are essential for limb salvage in acute limb ischemia; delays in definitive treatment result in greater risk of limb loss.

A clear distinction must be made between *acute limb ischemia* and *critical limb ischemia*. Acute limb ischemia develops suddenly and represents a potentially imminent threat to life and limb. *Critical limb ischemia* is characterized by the presence of rest pain, tissue loss, or gangrene in an extremity that has been ischemic for more than two weeks.[2] This chapter focuses on the diagnosis and management of atraumatic acute limb ischemia.

Pathophysiology

Embolism

The most common cause of acute limb ischemia is arterial embolism. The widespread use of anticoagulation and advances in the care of patients with valvular disease have decreased the proportion of cases of acute limb ischemia stemming from arterial embolism. However, embolism still remains the most common cause of acute limb ischemia, accounting for more than half of the cases.[3–6] The word *embolism* is derived from the Greek word *embolisma*, meaning "something thrust in."[1] Emboli can lodge in any artery in the body, resulting in immediate ischemia. Emboli tend to lodge at points where arteries change caliber, typically immediately distal to a bifurcation, or at an area of anatomic compression, such as the superficial femoral artery as it passes through the adductor magnus hiatus (Hunter's canal). With an embolism lodged in an artery, thrombus then propagates proximally and distally in response to slow or absent flow. Propagation of the thrombus results in further ischemia as collateral blood vessels become occluded.

Emboli are considered either cardiac or non-cardiac. Cardiac emboli are associated with cardiac pathology. The most common source of cardiac embolization (accounting for half of all embolic events) is a thrombus in the left atrium associated with atrial fibrillation.[6] Embolization can also occur after myocardial infarction. Myocardial infarction that causes septal hypokinesis can give rise to intraventricular thrombi, which can then embolize.

Less common cardiac emboli are those originating through a patent foramen ovale (PFO) and from an atrial myxoma. A PFO results in a right-to-left intracardiac shunt due to the failure of the foramen ovale to close during postpartum development. Approximately 25% of people have a PFO, and they are usually asymptomatic. The presence of a right-to-left intracardiac shunt allows passage of venous thromboemboli to the systemic arterial circulation. Passage of thromboemboli most commonly presents as stroke; however, in 3%

Vascular Emergencies, ed. Robert L. Rogers, Thomas Scalea, Lee Wallis, and Heike Geduld. Published by Cambridge University Press. © Cambridge University Press 2013.

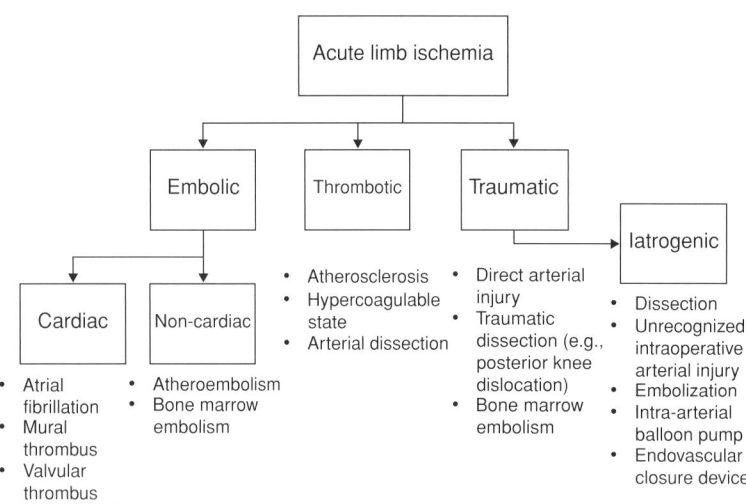

Figure 13.1 Etiology of acute limb ischemia.

of patients, the thrombus lodges in the lower extremity.[7] Atrial myxoma is a benign cardiac neoplasm composed of fibroblast-derived cells. These tumors are typically found in the left atrium. In more than a quarter of patients with atrial myxoma, the tumor fractures, resulting in embolization. Although most of these embolic events result in stroke, there are reports of atrial myxoma causing acute limb ischemia.[8,9]

Non-cardiac embolism refers to embolism arising from a source outside the heart. The most common source is a mural aortic thrombus. Patients with atherosclerosis are at higher risk of this type of embolization. Another common source of arterial embolism is a popliteal aneurysm. These aneurysms are often clinically silent until they embolize the final tibial vessel, resulting in acute limb ischemia. A myriad of other arterial emboli have been described in the literature, ranging from tumor emboli[10] to the nematode *Ascaris lumbricoides* [11] to a bullet.[12] However, these are rare occurrences, often confined to case reports in the literature.

Thrombosis

The prevalence of atherosclerosis, the formation of lipid-laden plaque in arteries, is rising in the United States and the rest of the world. Fifteen to twenty percent of persons over the age of 70 have clinically significant atherosclerosis.[13] Consequently, there has been an increase in the number of cases of acute limb ischemia related to *in situ* thrombosis

of atherosclerotic lesions. Acute coronary ischemia is generally thought to be caused by the rupture and subsequent thrombosis of an unstable coronary artery plaque. There are few data to suggest that this is the predominant mechanism of lower extremity acute ischemia. Another mechanism by which atherosclerosis can progress acutely to occlusion is a low-flow state. Decrease in flow across a lesion, in response to dehydration, sepsis, or cardiogenic shock, can lessen flow across a lesion, resulting in stagnation of blood and subsequent thrombosis of the affected vessel.

Another source of *in situ* thrombosis is thrombosed peripheral aneurysms, the most common being popliteal aneurysms.[14] Unlike aortic aneurysms, which cause morbidity and mortality by rupture, popliteal aneurysms result in morbidity through thrombosis and embolism of tibial vessels. Dissection is another cause of *in situ* thrombosis. In dissection (either *de novo* dissection of a native artery or traumatic dissection [iatrogenic or otherwise]), a tear develops in the arterial wall, creating a "true" and a "false lumen." As the false lumen propagates distally, the "true" lumen can become occluded, resulting in thrombosis and acute ischemia.

Although less common than in venous thromboembolism, acute arterial occlusion has been associated with hypercoagulable states, which can be either congenital (e.g., factor V Leiden, antithrombin III deficiency, prothrombin 20210a) or acquired (e.g., heparin-induced thrombocytopenia, malignancy).[15] Hypercoagulable states alone or in conjunction with other risk factors can lead to acute limb ischemia.

Trauma

Although the focus of this chapter is atraumatic acute limb ischemia, trauma is a significant enough cause of acute limb ischemia that its brief mention is warranted. Traumatic mechanisms of injury can disrupt the iliac artery, common femoral artery, superficial femoral artery, or popliteal artery. Additionally, ischemia can be the result of direct compression of one of these structures, as in patients with displaced femur fractures. Trauma can also result in arterial dissection at any level, resulting in acute limb ischemia as described above. Acute lower extremity ischemia is often associated with popliteal artery dissection resulting from an aortic dissection. Finally, trauma can result in embolism from a large number of sources, including bone marrow in patients with femur fracture.[16]

Iatrogenic injury is a subset of traumatic injury that can result in acute limb ischemia. Acute limb ischemia is often identified in the cardiothoracic intensive care unit (ICU). Acute limb ischemia has been well described in patients in cardiogenic shock requiring support from an intra-aortic balloon pump (IABP).[17] The dramatic increase in the number of endovascular procedures being performed has been accompanied by an increased number of iatrogenic complications. Inadvertent dissection of the common femoral artery can occur while obtaining arterial access. Plaque in the common femoral artery can be dislodged, causing distal embolization. Finally, devices designed to close arterial access sites have also been associated with acute limb ischemia from embolization.[18,19]

Morbidity and mortality

Even patients who receive prompt care for an acute arterial ischemia have amputation rates ranging up to 15% and a 30-day mortality rate as high as 25%.[3,4] Prompt recognition and treatment are essential for limb salvage; delays in definitive treatment result in greater risk of limb loss. The survival and amputation rates depend largely on the cause of the ischemia and patient-specific risk factors. Young age is a positive predictor of amputation-free survival, whereas heart disease, CNS disorders, and active malignancy are all predictive of decreased amputation-free survival.

The rate of survival without amputation is dependent on the appearance of skin changes and rest pain,[20] not on the duration of ischemia. Patients with advanced atherosclerotic disease typically have an extensively developed collateral circulation. Patients with increased collateralization can often tolerate acute limb ischemia better than patients with normal native arterial circulation and no collateralization.

Diagnosis

History

The diagnosis of acute limb ischemia is based primarily on the history and physical examination. The prime objective of the history is to establish the diagnosis. The history of the present illness is essential to establish the time of onset of symptoms. Patients describe the recent onset of rest pain or paresthesia. The duration of symptoms, as well as the presence of sensory or motor deficits, is important for establishing the severity of disease and the potential for limb salvage. Diminished motor or sensory function is an ominous finding that mandates prompt intervention for limb salvage.

Solicitation of the patient's medical and surgical history should be directed toward narrowing the differential diagnosis and identifying the cause of the occlusion. Pertinent elements in the history indicate the cause of ischemia. The patient's history of cardiac disease, including dysrhythmia, valvular disease, and myocardial infarction, should be documented. Risk factors for atherosclerosis and the presence of leg pain before the acute event raise suspicion of thrombosis of a native vessel secondary to atherosclerotic disease. Previous ischemic and thrombotic events should be noted. A history of deep vein thrombosis should lead the practitioner to consider a PFO or hypercoagulable state. Although it seems obvious, the patient should be questioned about recent trauma or medical procedures.

Physical examination

Acute limb ischemia is classically associated with the "five Ps" (see Table 12.1). Pain is often severe and exacerbated by movement or exertion. Pain with compression of the lower leg is associated with muscle necrosis and is an ominous sign, often indicative of a non-salvageable limb. Pulselessness refers to the

Table 13.1 Categories of acute limb ischemia

Category	Description/prognosis	Findings		Doppler signals	
		Sensory loss	Muscle weakness	Arterial	Venous
I Viable	Not immediately threatened	None	None	Audible	Audible
IIa Marginally threatened	Limb salvage if promptly treated	Minimal or none (toes only)	None	Inaudible	Audible
IIb Immediately threatened	Salvage with immediate revascularization	More than toes, rest pain	Mild to moderate	Inaudible	Audible
III Irreversible	Major tissue loss or permanent nerve damage inevitable	Profound, anesthetic	Profound, rigor	Inaudible	Inaudible

Adapted from Rutherford et al.[21]

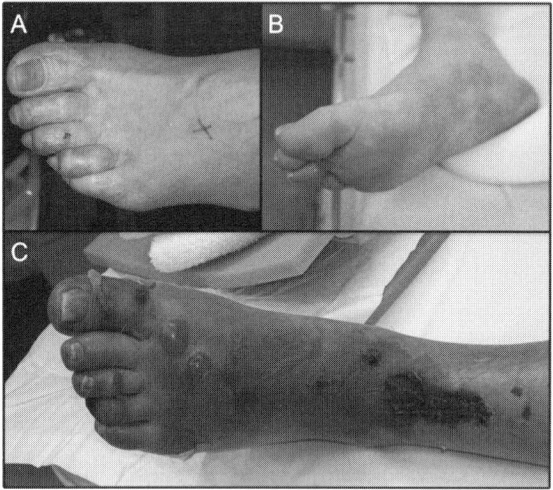

Figure 13.2 Appearance of acutely ischemic lower extremities. The limb in panel A, Rutherford IIa, is marginally threatened. Note the significant pallor. The limb in panel B, Rutherford IIb, is immediately threatened. The first signs of mottling are present. Note the areas of blanching over the forefoot. These areas represent significantly delayed capillary refill. The limb in panel C, Rutherford III, suffers from irreversible ischemia. This limb demonstrates fixed mottling. Also present is blistering and rigor (not apparent in the photograph). It is important to understand that the difference between marginally and immediately threatened limbs is not obvious based on appearance alone. See plate section for color version.

absence of pedal pulses. If these pulses are absent, Doppler signals should be obtained. The ankle brachial index should be calculated immediately to confirm or exclude the diagnosis of limb ischemia. Most acutely ischemic limbs appear pale (Figure 13.2) and are cool to touch. The change in temperature is often referred to as "poikilothermia," an alternate member of the "five Ps." Paresthesia, or diminished sensation, is associated with acute limb ischemia. Often the paresthesia is limited to the toes or forefoot. As the whole foot becomes involved and paresthesia progresses to anesthesia, the prognosis for limb salvage becomes quite poor. The final "P" is paralysis. Motor deficit, a late finding in acute limb ischemia, can range from modest weakness to profound paralysis and rigor. Paralysis and rigor are late findings and are indicative of a limb beyond salvage.

In addition to the "five Ps" of acute limb ischemia, a careful examination of the entire vascular system is important. The heart should be examined with an emphasis on the identification of irregular heart rate (atrial fibrillation) and murmur (valvular disease). Peripheral pulses over the upper and lower extremity must be assessed for quality and symmetry. The importance of these elements of the physical examination cannot be over-emphasized.

The differential diagnosis for acute limb ischemia includes aortic dissection and acute aortic occlusion. It is possible to diagnose both of these entities on physical examination. Asymmetric femoral or brachial pulses in a patient with back pain should raise concern for aortic dissection. Acute aortic dissection can also be associated with diminished motor function of one or both lower extremities. Paralysis affecting proximal muscles should also raise suspicion for aortic dissection. Aortic occlusion results in absent bilateral femoral pulses. The diagnostic algorithm of these pathologies differs significantly from that for acute limb ischemia. Prompt treatment is essential for favorable outcomes in all three conditions. Establishing a likely diagnosis on physical examination decreases the use of tests that are not useful and ultimately decreases the time to definitive treatment and improves the probability of limb salvage.

As for most clinical pathologies, a classification system has been developed to gauge the severity of acute limb ischemia. This system describes four categories (Table 13.1[21]):

I   viable
IIa   marginally threatened
IIb   immediately threatened
III   irreversible ischemia.

Most importantly, this classification system serves as a guide to identify limbs that have irreversible ischemia with no chance of salvage. In this scenario, patients should be directed to primary amputation. Limbs with category III ischemia have profound sensory loss and profound weakness that can progress to frank rigor. These limbs lack *both* arterial and venous signals. Fixed mottling and blistering (Figure 13.2) frequently accompany the aforementioned signs of irreversible ischemia. It is important to understand that the difference between marginally and immediately threatened limbs is not obvious based on appearance alone.

Laboratory studies to obtain in the emergency department

Time to definitive treatment is one of the most important factors in limb salvage. Acute limb ischemia is diagnosed on the findings from the history and physical examination. Laboratory studies are not essential in the diagnostic process, but their results will aid in management decisions.

The first intervention in the management of acute limb ischemia is anticoagulation; therefore, baseline measurements of prothrombin time (PT) and partial thromboplastin time (PTT) are useful. An operative intervention will likely be required for most patients; consequently, a type and screen should be obtained. The hemoglobin level is important to guide the possible need for blood transfusion. Finally, serum chemistry is important when planning for intervention. Because intravenous contrast is often used in imaging studies, it is important to know the patient's creatinine level. Finally, as a consequence of ischemia, the threatened limb will become acidotic and hyperkalemic. When the limb is reperfused, these byproducts of acidosis and ischemia enter the circulatory system and can have a profound physiologic impact.[22]

Imaging to obtain in the emergency department

Once a diagnosis is made, all efforts should focus on definitive treatment. Examination with a hand-held Doppler confirms the diagnosis and aids in assessing the prognosis for limb salvage (Table 13.1). Given the widespread availability of handheld Doppler machines, most practitioners consider this examination part of the physical examination. In general, formal vascular laboratory studies do not contribute significantly to the diagnosis and only increase time to definitive treatment. Similarly, CT angiogram generally provides limited additional information and also delays treatment. Additionally, CT angiogram, even with multidetector scanners and time-resolved protocols, mandates the use of intravenous contrast, [23] increasing the risk of contrast-induced nephropathy.[24]

An electrocardiogram can be useful in identifying the cause of ischemia (e.g., atrial fibrillation, acute myocardial infarction). This study is inexpensive, easy to obtain, and widely available. Patients suspected of having acute limb ischemia should have an electrocardiogram as part of their emergency department evaluation. An echocardiogram can demonstrate cardiac sources of embolism; however, this imaging is not necessary before definitive treatment and *should not delay care*. It is important, however, to obtain an echocardiogram prior to discharge from the hospital. The findings on echocardiography might influence postoperative management.

Emergency department management

The first 15 minutes

Identification of the category of limb ischemia (Table 13.1)[21] establishes the next steps in management (Figure 13.3). Class I and II ischemia should be considered for revascularization, and class III ischemia should be considered for primary amputation. When the decision is made to attempt revascularization, the urgency of repair is also dictated by the category of ischemia: class IIb ischemic limbs are immediately threatened and should be triaged to emergent revascularization. The classification of ischemia and decision to intervene should be made in consultation with a vascular specialist.

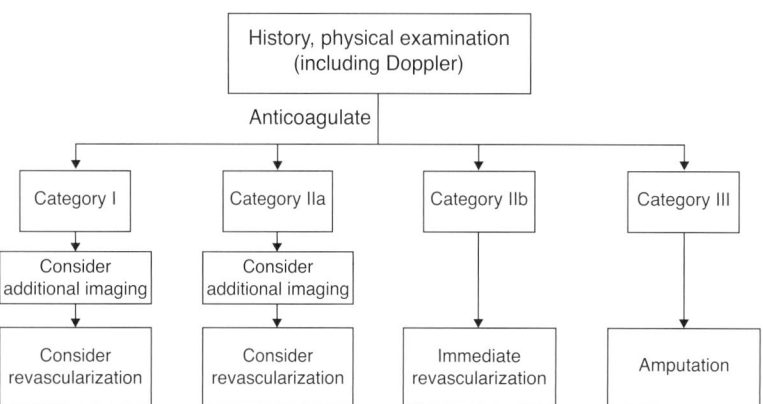

Figure 13.3 Management algorithm for acute limb ischemia. Adapted from Rutherford *et al.*[21]

Once the decision to attempt revascularization has been made, the patient should be anticoagulated promptly. Unfractionated heparin is commonly used for this purpose. The standard dosage is based on a weight-based nomogram; a bolus of 80 IU/kg is administered followed by a continuous infusion of 18 IU/kg, with a target PTT of 1.5 to 2.3 times the normal value.[25,26] As a weight-based therapeutic agent, heparin can be particularly difficult to use in morbidly obese patients. Morbidly obese patients tend to be given lower doses of heparin per unit of body weight than non-obese patients, owing to practitioners' reluctance to administer the large doses indicated by the nomogram. In addition, morbidly obese patients take a significantly longer time to achieve therapeutic levels of heparin than their non-obese counterparts.[27] A solution to this problem lies in adjusting the nomogram for the morbidly obese. Myzienski and colleagues proposed the following formula to calculate a dosing weight:[28]

$$IBW + 0.3(ABW - IBW)$$

where IBW is ideal body weight and ABW is actual body weight.

The first few hours

All efforts associated with the care of patients with acute limb ischemia should be directed toward definitive treatment. This point is particularly important for class IIb ischemia and less important for class I and III ischemia. The practice of vascular surgery has changed significantly over the past 20 years. Vascular surgeons now have many available tools for the treatment of acute limb ischemia. These measures include endovascular methods (pharmacomechanical

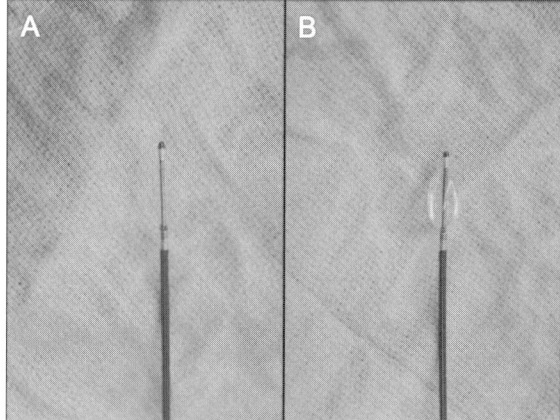

Figure 13.4 The Fogarty catheter. A Fogarty embolectomy catheter consists of a catheter-mounted balloon. The catheter is passed through the embolism in its deflated state (A), it is inflated (B), and the embolism is then swept out of the affected artery.

thrombolysis catheters, infusion catheters) and open surgical methods (Fogarty catheter, bypass surgery). Even in facilities where endovascular resources are not available, patients with limb ischemia can be treated successfully. These patients are better served by performing an urgent intervention than by delaying care for transport to a facility with advanced endovascular capacity.

Fogarty invented his embolectomy catheter and demonstrated its successful use in humans in 1963. This catheter revolutionized the field of vascular surgery and remains a powerful tool in the vascular surgeon's armamentarium for treatment of thromboembolism (Figure 13.4).[29] If a vascular surgeon is available and able to perform an embolectomy or bypass, the care of a patient with limb ischemia should not be delayed by a transfer to a higher level of care for angiography.

Patients with acute limb ischemia should be admitted to a unit with telemetry monitoring. This type of monitoring is important for several reasons. First, the cause of the ischemia could be a dysrhythmia (atrial fibrillation) or the sequela of a recent myocardial infarction. Acute ischemia causes a sudden change from aerobic to anaerobic metabolism in the affected skeletal muscle and a concomitant rise in the serum lactate concentration. These processes stimulate an increase in inflammatory mediators and produce systemic signs and sequelae of inflammation.[22] The systemic effects of these derangements are generally not observed until the limb is reperfused; however, the patient should be monitored closely for a potentially fatal dysrhythmia.

Clinical approach when resources are limited

The most essential element in the treatment of acute limb ischemia is early diagnosis and revascularization without delay; time to revascularization is an important predictor of limb salvage. When resources are limited, a vascular specialist might not be available. In this situation, the patient should be systemically heparinized (80 IU/kg). Often general surgeons have the training and ability to perform an embolectomy – a definitive treatment. If there is no provider with the training to perform an embolectomy, systemic heparinization should be continued while efforts are made to transfer to a facility with the needed resources. Often heparin alone is sufficient to at least lower the level of amputation that will be required in the future. If revascularization is not performed, signs of myonecrosis (acidemia, hyperkalemia, increasing serum myoglobin) should be monitored. If there is evidence of myonecrosis, early amputation will be necessary.

Definitive treatment

Catheter embolectomy

The cornerstone of definitive treatment for acute limb ischemia is removal of the embolism and restoration of distal flow. In patients with suspected embolism, knowledge of anatomy, typical patterns of embolism, and a careful physical examination will direct the

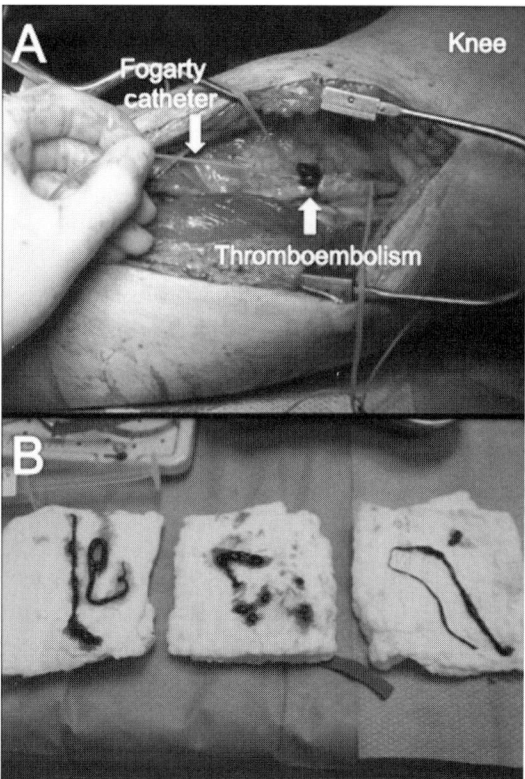

Figure 13.5 Surgical embolectomy. To perform an open embolectomy, exposure of the affected vessel is obtained. The vessel is controlled and a transverse arteriotomy is made. A Fogarty catheter is directed toward the embolism, inflated and swept toward the arteriotomy (A). The Fogarty catheter is repeatedly inserted until no more thromboembolism is retrieved. Thrombus will form in a vessel after an embolism occurs. Panel B depicts acute thrombus associated with an embolic event. See plate section for color version.

therapeutic approach. Embolisms typically lodge at areas where the caliber of an artery decreases. In the lower extremity, common locations include the bifurcation of the common iliac artery, the distal superficial femoral artery where it crosses the abductor magnus hiatus (Hunter's canal), the tibial peroneal trunk, and each of the tibial arteries. An absent femoral pulse suggests an iliac embolism; an absent popliteal pulse with a femoral pulse suggests occlusion at Hunter's canal. A palpable popliteal pulse suggests tibial involvement. Each of these scenarios dictates a different surgical approach.

Other therapeutic options

Occasionally, an embolectomy is not technically possible. In this setting, a surgical bypass is required to re-establish flow distal to the obstruction. Considerations for a surgical bypass include the identification of an appropriate distal target, selection of an inflow vessel, and choice of conduit. These considerations and their technical details are beyond the scope of the present discussion.

An alternative to open surgical embolectomy or bypass is catheter-directed thrombolysis. In this procedure, a catheter is directed into the area of thromboembolism and thrombolytics are infused for several hours. In reporting their initial experience with catheter-directed thrombolysis, Ouriel and associates documented six-month and one-year amputation-free survival rates comparable to those achieved with open embolectomy.[30] In this series, the thrombolysis group demonstrated a significant increase in bleeding complications compared with the open surgery group. The risk of bleeding was associated with the use of therapeutic heparin. When this treatment was eliminated, the risk of bleeding was decreased.

Some authors advocate centralizing the treatment of acute limb ischemia at centers with advanced endovascular facilities.[31] However, others contend that acute limb ischemia can be treated successfully without angiography.[32] Having access to an array of endovascular tools might be advantageous, but the time required to transport the patient to such a facility – especially a patient with an immediately threatened limb (Rutherford IIb) – might convert a limb from potentially salvageable to not salvageable.

Fasciotomy

Acute limb ischemia induces an inflammatory response[22] that causes swelling and edema. Edema becomes more pronounced after revascularization. Muscles, especially in the lower leg, are bound in firm, non-compliant fascial compartments. As swelling increases, tissue pressure increases and ultimately can rise above venous pressure, preventing venous outflow. This series of events is referred to as compartment syndrome. With the onset of compartment syndrome, nerves become compressed, causing motor weakness and altered sensation. The most sensitive, early sign of compartment syndrome is pain on passive motion. Motor weakness is a more ominous sign of advanced compartment syndrome. The loss of pulses is a late sign.

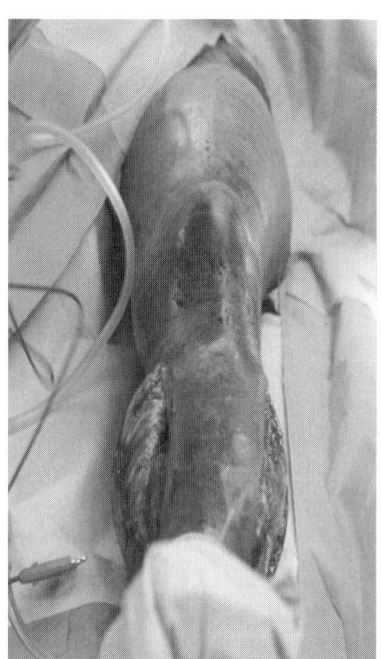

Figure 13.6
Fasciotomy. Fasciotomy should be considered for all patients with acute limb ischemia. Compartment syndrome occurs most commonly in the lower leg. The figure depicts a four-compartment fasciotomy performed with a two-incision approach. The anterior and lateral compartments can be released through a lateral incision, and the superficial and deep compartments are released through a medial incision.

In patients with acute limb ischemia, compartment syndrome usually does not develop until after revascularization. Its signs are not evident in the operating room. Prophylactic fasciotomy should be considered, with the goal of preventing potentially debilitating complications or the need to bring the patient back to the operating room.

Compartment syndrome occurs most frequently in the lower leg, but it can also involve the buttock, thigh, lower leg, and foot (Figure 13.6). In a complete lower-leg fasciotomy, four compartments of the lower leg are released: the anterior, lateral, superficial posterior, and deep posterior compartments.[33] Single-incision and two-incision approaches have been described.[33,34] Our approach is a two-incision lower-leg fasciotomy. The anterior and lateral compartments can be released through a lateral incision, and the superficial and deep compartments are released through a medial incision. Although this approach requires a second incision, it allows easy confirmation that all four compartments are adequately released. Some authors advocate a subcutaneous technique; however, this approach often results in incomplete fasciotomy and leads to a return to the operating room.[35]

Gluteal compartment syndrome, a rare complication of acute limb ischemia, should be suspected in patients with an unexplained rise in the serum myoglobin level. Iatrogenic gluteal compartment syndrome is often associated with prolonged periods of immobilization on the operating table in the lithotomy position.[36] The thigh and gluteal compartments can be released through a lateral incision. In the thigh, the posterior and medial compartments must be released. The anterior compartment rarely requires decompression. In gluteal compartment syndrome, care must be taken to ensure that the gluteus maximus, gluteus minimus, and gluteus medius are adequately released.

Inpatient care

Restoring blood flow to the affected limb does not end the evaluation and management of acute limb ischemia. A thorough investigation needs to be performed to identify and treat the underlying cause of ischemia. This evaluation should be deferred until after ischemia is reversed and should not delay definitive treatment. An echocardiogram is mandatory for all patients. It can reveal thrombus in the left atrium, mural thrombus, and a patent foramen ovale. An evaluation for hypercoagulable states is also mandatory. An evaluation should test for activated protein C resistance/factor V Leiden, prothrombin G20210A, deficiencies of protein C, protein S or antithrombin, and antiphospholipid antibodies.[37] Most patients being treated for acute limb ischemia should be maintained on antiplatelet therapy. Surgical and endovascular therapies damage the endothelium and place the patient at higher risk for rethrombosis of the treated vessel. Anticoagulation with a vitamin-K antagonist (warfarin) is administered, depending on the cause of the ischemia.

Summary

- Acute limb ischemia is a vascular emergency associated with a risk of death and amputation.
- Amputation-free survival depends on prompt diagnosis and definitive care.
- Treatment of acute limb ischemia does not require advanced endovascular equipment or techniques; care should not be delayed for transport to a facility with advanced endovascular capabilities.

Critical actions

- Prompt recognition of acute limb ischemia.
- Immediate anticoagulation with unfractionated heparin; this action will preserve flow in threatened collateral vessels.
- Early consultation with a vascular specialist.
- Revascularization without undue delay.

Pearls and pitfalls

- The "five Ps" – pain, pulselessness, pallor, paresthesia, and paralysis are excellent predictors of acute limb ischemia.
- Rigor, fixed mottling, blistering, and absence of arterial and venous Doppler signals strongly suggest a limb beyond salvage.
- The diagnosis of acute limb ischemia can be subtle – especially in patients with atherosclerosis and peripheral arterial disease. Acute limb ischemia should be on the differential diagnosis for any patient with peripheral arterial disease and lower extremity symptoms.
- Delay in diagnosis and treatment results in poor prognosis for limb salvage, and frequently amputation.

References

1. Stedman TL. *Stedman's Medical Dictionary*, 28th edition. Philadelphia: Lippincott Williams & Wilkins; 2006.

2. Norgren L, Hiatt WR, Dormandy JA, *et al*. Inter-society consensus for the management of peripheral arterial disease (TASC II). *J Vasc Surg* 2007; 45(suppl): S5–67.

3. Abbott WM, Maloney RD, McCabe CC, *et al*. Arterial embolism: a 44 year perspective. *Am J Surg* 1982; 143: 460–4.

4. Ender Topal A, Nesimi Eren M, Celik Y. Management of non-traumatic acute limb ischemia and predictors of outcome in 270 thromboembolectomy cases. *Int Angiol* 2011; 30: 172–80.

5. Tawes RL Jr, Harris EJ, Brown WH, *et al*. Arterial thromboembolism. A 20-year perspective. *Arch Surg* 1985; 120: 595–9.

6. Fagundes C, Fuchs FD, Fagundes A, *et al*. Prognostic factors for amputation or death in patients submitted to vascular surgery for acute limb ischemia. *Vasc Health Risk Manag* 2005; 1: 345–9.

7. Dao CN, Tobis JM. PFO and paradoxical embolism producing events other than stroke. *Catheter Cardiovasc Interv* 2011; 77: 903–9.

8. Coley C, Lee KR, Steiner M, Thompson CS. Complete embolization of a left atrial myxoma resulting in acute lower extremity ischemia. *Tex Heart Inst J* 2005; 32: 238–40.

9. Val-Bernal JF, Acebo E, Gómez-Román JJ, Garijo MF. Anticipated diagnosis of left atrial myxoma following histological investigation of limb embolectomy specimens: a report of two cases. *Pathol Int* 2003; 53: 489–94.

10. Xiromeritis N, Klonaris C, Papas S, Valsamis M, Bastounis E. Recurrent peripheral arterial embolism from pulmonary cancer. Case report and review of the literature. *Int Angiol* 2000; 19: 79–83.

11. Ashraf HZ, Ahangar AG, Dar FA, *et al.* Popliteal artery embolism by *Ascaris lumbricoides*: a case report. *Ulus Travma Acil Cerrahi Derg* 2009; 15: 619–20.

12. Pavy C, Lebreton G, Sanchez B, Roques F. Aortic bullet embolization revealed by peripheral ischemia after a thoracic gunshot wound. *Interact Cardiovasc Thorac Surg* 2011; 12: 520–2.

13. Selvin E, Erlinger TP. Prevalence of and risk factors for peripheral arterial disease in the United States: results from the National Health and Nutrition Examination Survey, 1999–2000. *Circulation* 2004; 110: 738–43.

14. Kropman RH, Schriver AM, Kelder JC, Moll FL, de Vries JP. Clinical outcome of acute leg ischaemia due to thrombosed popliteal artery aneurysm: systematic review of 895 cases. *Eur J Vasc Endovasc Surg* 2010; 39: 452–7.

15. Dorweiler B, Neufang A, Kasper-Koenig W, *et al.* Arterial embolism to the upper extremity in a patient with factor V Leiden mutation (APC resistance) – a case report and review of the literature. *Angiology* 2003; 54: 125–30.

16. Johnson MJ, Lucas GL. Fat embolism syndrome. *Orthopedics* 1996; 19: 41–9.

17. Busch T, Sîrbu H, Zenker D, Dalichau H. Vascular complications related to intraaortic balloon counterpulsation: an analysis of ten years experience. *Thorac Cardiovasc Surg* 1997; 45: 55–9.

18. Teso D, Karmy-Jones R. Distal embolism of percutaneous arterial closure device resulting in critical limb ischemia. *J Vasc Interv Radiol* 2010; 21: 1487–8.

19. Aerden D, Creeten E, Van den Brande P. Two cases of an embolized femoral closure device in the popliteal artery causing ischaemia. *Acta Chir Belg* 2010; 110: 357–60.

20. Ouriel K, Veith FJ. Acute lower limb ischemia: determinants of outcome. *Surgery* 1998; 124: 336–42.

21. Rutherford RB, Baker JD, Ernst C, *et al.* Recommended standards for reports dealing with lower extremity ischemia: revised version. *J Vasc Surg* 1997; 26: 517–38.

22. Blaisdell FW. The pathophysiology of skeletal muscle ischemia and the reperfusion syndrome: a review. *Cardiovasc Surg* 2002; 10: 620–30.

23. Sommer WH, Helck A, Bamberg F, *et al.* Diagnostic value of time-resolved CT angiography for the lower leg. *Eur Radiol* 2010; 20: 2876–81.

24. Liu Y, Tan N, Zhou YL, *et al.* The contrast medium volume to estimated glomerular filtration rate ratio as a predictor of contrast-induced nephropathy after primary percutaneous coronary intervention. *Int Urol Nephrol* 2012; 44: 221–9.

25. Raschke RA, Reilly BM, Guidry JR, Fontana JR, Srinivas S. The weight-based heparin dosing nomogram compared with a "standard care" nomogram: a randomized controlled trial. *Ann Intern Med* 1993; 119: 874–81.

26. Clagett GP, Sobel M, Jackson MR, *et al.* Antithrombotic therapy in peripheral arterial occlusive disease: the Seventh ACCP Conference on Antithrombotic and Thrombolytic Therapy. *Chest* 2004; 126(3 suppl): 609S–26S.

27. Riney JN, Hollands JM, Smith JR, Deal EN. Identifying optimal initial infusion rates for unfractionated heparin in morbidly obese patients. *Ann Pharmacother* 2010; 44: 1141–51.

28. Myzienski AE, Lutz MF, Smythe MA. Unfractionated heparin dosing for venous thromboembolism in morbidly obese patients: case report and review of the literature. *Pharmacotherapy* 2010; 30: 324.

29. Meyers M, O'Leary JP. Fogarty and his catheter. *Am Surg* 1998; 64: 478–9.

30. Ouriel K, Veith FJ, Sasahara AA. A comparison of recombinant urokinase with vascular surgery as initial treatment for acute arterial occlusion of the legs. Thrombolysis or Peripheral Arterial Surgery (TOPAS) Investigators. *N Engl J Med* 1998; 338: 1105–11.

31. Clason AE, Stonebridge PA, Duncan AJ, *et al.* Acute ischaemia of the lower limb: the effect of centralizing vascular surgical services on morbidity and mortality. *Br J Surg* 1989; 76: 592–3.

32. Zaraca F, Stringari C, Ebner JA, Ebner H. Routine versus selective use of intraoperative angiography during thromboembolectomy for acute lower limb ischemia: analysis of outcomes. *Ann Vasc Surg* 2010; 24: 621–7.

33. Mubarak SJ, Owen CA. Double-incision fasciotomy of the leg for decompression in compartment syndromes. *J Bone Joint Surg Am* 1977; 59: 184–7.

34. Cooper GG. A method of single-incision, four compartment fasciotomy of the leg. *Eur J Vasc Surg* 1992; 6: 659–61.

35. Jensen SL, Sandermann J. Compartment syndrome and fasciotomy in vascular surgery: a review of 57 cases. *Eur J Vasc Endovasc Surg* 1997; 13: 48–53.

36. Henson JT, Roberts CS, Giannoudis PV. Gluteal compartment syndrome. *Acta Orthop Belg* 2009; 75: 147–52.

37. Khor B, Van Cott EM. Laboratory evaluation of hypercoagulability. *Clin Lab Med* 2009; 29: 339–66.

Chapter

14

Extremity aneurysms

Kristian A. Ulloa

Introduction

Extremity aneurysms are not as common as aortic aneurysms. When discovered, the majority of these peripheral aneurysms are located in the lower extremity. These aneurysms can be classified as either true aneurysms or pseudoaneurysms. True aneurysms involve degeneration of the entire arterial wall. Pseudoaneurysms, or false aneurysms, are simply a hole in the arterial wall or a disruption in an anastomosis, with continuous blood flowing between the hematoma and injured artery. Pseudoaneurysms are by far the more common type.

Another important way in which to classify extremity aneurysms is whether they are symptomatic or asymptomatic. Extremity aneurysms rarely present with rupture. More commonly, the presentation involves pain, compression of local structures such as nerves or veins, or distal embolization. Although not as dramatic as the presentation of a ruptured infrarenal aortic aneurysm, complications of extremity aneurysms can lead to severe debilitation.

Pseudoaneurysms of the femoral artery are the most common extremity aneurysm. These aneurysms are the result of injury to the artery, either iatrogenic or from trauma. Diagnostic and interventional procedures involving a transfemoral catheter are the most common cause of pseudoaneurysms overall. Among patients undergoing transfemoral catheterizations, a pseudoaneurysm develops in 1.2%.[1] The incidence of iatrogenic injury is even higher if an intervention such as angioplasty or stenting is performed. A pseudoaneurysm develops in up to 8% of patients after a transfemoral percutaneous intervention.[2] The higher incidence is likely due to the larger sheath size usually needed to perform an intervention, as well as the use of systemic anticoagulation.

Evaluation

Given the causes of iatrogenic pseudoaneurysms, the history is essential when evaluating a patient with a suspected arterial injury. The procedure may have been performed weeks prior to presentation, with symptoms developing indolently or abruptly. Typical complaints include groin pain, neuralgia, and distal ischemia. If the arterial injury was proximal or in proximity to the inguinal ligament, a concomitant pelvic hematoma may be present, which can cause back or flank pain, flank ecchymosis, and psoas irritation. Signs and symptoms of anemia related to blood loss may also be present, such as light-headedness, fatigue, tachycardia, and hypotension. Comparison of a pre-procedure hemoglobin level with a current level would be useful.

Physical examination of the groin, with particular attention to the puncture site, is critical. A prominent pulsatile mass, often tender to palpation, is often present. This prominence might not be easily noted in obese patients. Ecchymosis and induration are often more telling in this subset of patients. A bruit may be auscultated over the groin. Careful evaluation of the pulses distal to the suspected aneurysm is also essential, as extremity aneurysms, especially true aneurysms, are more likely to present with distal embolization of atheroma from the aneurysm sac than with rupture.

To definitively determine the presence of a pseudoaneurysm, duplex ultrasonography is indispensable. Portable ultrasound devices with color flow Doppler are universally available, and physicians can quickly develop the skill set needed to interrogate peripheral arteries for the presence of pseudoaneurysms. For extremity vessels, a 5- to 7-MHz probe is ideal because of the superficial nature of the femoral and brachial

Vascular Emergencies, ed. Robert L. Rogers, Thomas Scalea, Lee Wallis, and Heike Geduld. Published by Cambridge University Press. © Cambridge University Press 2013.

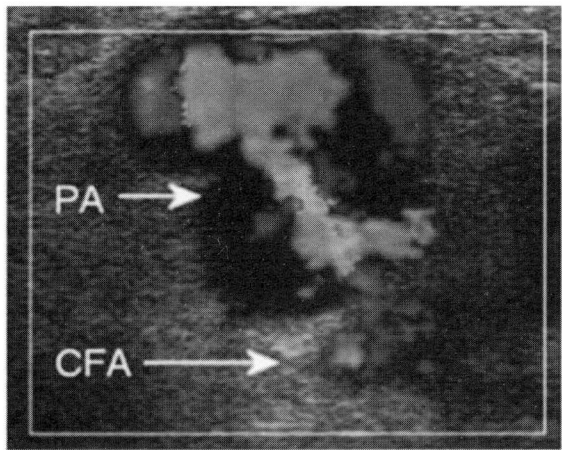

Figure 14.1 Peripheral pseudoaneurysm with characteristic to and fro Doppler flow pattern. PA, pseudoaneurysm; CFA, common femoral artery. See plate section for color version.

arteries, which are the most commonly injured arteries given their use for percutaneous access. The blood vessel should be identified initially in transverse orientation, and gentle compression will help distinguish the artery from the vein. The veins, as long as they are free of chronic venous disease or acute deep venous thrombosis, will compress. The arteries will demonstrate a thicker wall and appear pulsatile. Once these vessels are identified, the probe should be oriented in a longitudinal manner, which will allow visualization of a greater length of the vessel. Once the longitudinal view is obtained, color flow Doppler should be utilized, with visualization centered on the middle of the vessel at a 60° angle. Color Doppler velocity waveforms and spectra will appear pulsatile in the artery, with biphasic or triphasic waveforms, whereas continuous or phasic waveforms will be noted in the vein. Furthermore, venous Doppler waveforms will augment with compression of the extremity distal to the probe.

With the artery and vein in view, a thorough search should be performed for extraluminal color Doppler spectra. The presence of "to and fro" flow, or a yin-yang appearance, is classic for a pseudoaneurysm (Figure 14.1). On grayscale imaging, a heterogeneous periphery is often noted, which consists of varying degrees of thrombus. The neck of the pseudoaneurysm, which is the actual communication between the artery and the hematoma rind containing the extraluminal blood flow, must be identified clearly. The length and width of the neck are key determinants of the therapeutic

options. A wide-based, short neck usually dictates operative intervention, as these pseudoaneurysms are unlikely to thrombose spontaneously. Typically, a neck wider than 0.5 cm and shorter than 1.0 cm should be approached with caution, since thrombin injection of these pseudoaneurysms is fraught with the complication of distal embolization, given the width of the neck of the aneurysm. Narrow, long necks are the most favorable, since the high resistance in these necks makes spontaneous thrombosis of the pseudoaneurysm most likely.

Management

A few factors must be considered when determining the management of a pseudoaneurysm. Size, the presence or absence of anticoagulation, symptoms, and the potential for follow-up are important. First, the size of the flow-containing pseudoaneurysm sac must be determined. Pseudoaneurysms under 3 cm in maximal diameter typically can be managed with observation and repeat imaging, whereas larger ones usually require intervention. Eighty-nine percent of pseudoaneurysms under 3 cm in diameter will close spontaneously.[2] For the patient to safely undergo observation, however, duplex ultrasound should be repeated at two-week intervals until closure is demonstrated. This follow-up is why assessing the reliability of the patient is critical. Patients taking anticoagulants and those who complain of significant pain or compressive symptoms should have the pseudoaneurysm addressed.

Various options exist for the treatment of extremity pseudoaneurysms. These options include blind manual compression, ultrasound-guided compression, percutaneous ultrasound-guided thrombin injection, and operative repair. Compression therapy is a reasonable choice for initial management, as it is non-invasive. Reports about the efficacy of this therapy vary; the presence of anticoagulation appears to be the most important determinant of success. The results of only one randomized trial comparing manual compression versus ultrasound-guided compression have been published, and there was no significant difference in closure rates after 60 minutes of compression. However, the 90% closure rate and lack of data on pseudoaneurysm size in this trial require critical evaluation.[3] Most studies on manual and ultrasound-guided compression demonstrate closure rates under 60%.

For hemodynamically stable patients with favorable pseudoaneurysm neck anatomy, ultrasound-guided thrombin injection is an excellent choice, as it is minimally invasive and has a high success rate for closure. In a large, prospective registry, 89% of pseudoaneurysms ranging in size from 0.5 to 16.0 cm closed after one session of thrombin injection, and 99% closed after three sessions.[4] A prospective, randomized trial compared thrombin injection with ultrasound-guided compression. Although a very small sample size was used, there was a 100% closure rate with thrombin injection, while a 13% success was noted in the ultrasound-guided compression arm.[5]

Patients with wide, short-necked pseudoaneurysms typically require surgical intervention. Hemodynamically unstable patients should also be treated aggressively in the operating room, with exploration of the vessel and repair. Depending on the extent of injury, surgical repair may entail primary suture repair, patch angioplasty, or bypass. In extreme cases, ligation of the vessel may be necessary to obtain control of the bleeding, with arterial reconstruction at a later date when the patient is more stable. Preoperative management should include resuscitation with blood products and permissive hypotension, as aggressive augmentation of blood pressure may lead to rupture of the pseudoaneurysm sac and worsening hemorrhagic shock.

Some patients present with compressive symptoms. These include venous compression with concomitant deep venous thrombosis, neuralgia from nerve irritation, or compression and compromise of the skin from massive hematomas. These patients also benefit from operative repair, as evacuation of the hematoma is essential to resolution of their symptoms. Prevention of skin necrosis from a pressure ischemia due to a massive hematoma is also essential. Rarely, a thigh compartment syndrome can develop, requiring hematoma evacuation as well.

Mycotic pseudoaneurysms should also be treated surgically. One should suspect such an aneurysm in intravenous drug abusers who present with a pulsatile mass, hematoma, or pain in the groin or antecubital fossa. Ultrasound findings will demonstrate the classic "to and fro" color Doppler spectra; however, the pseudoaneurysm wall is often more irregular in appearance. Systemic signs of sepsis, such as fever and leukocytosis, may also be present. Blood cultures should be obtained. *Staphylococcus aureus* is present about 90% of the time.[6] Furthermore, plain radiographs should be taken of the area in question to rule out the presence of a foreign object, such as a needle. These patients should be treated with antibiotics and operative repair. The repair typically involves ligation of the injured artery, drainage of the pseudoaneurysm sac, and extra-anatomic bypass. For femoral artery mycotic pseudoaneurysms, an obturator bypass is often necessary. Percutaneous treatment does not lead to adequate source control, as the pseudoaneurysm should be treated like an abscess, and the residual hematoma within the sac must be completely drained with open surgery.

Other pathologic conditions affecting the extremity arteries

Another consideration when evaluating arterial injuries is arteriovenous fistula (AVF). During percutaneous procedures, the proximity of the artery and vein often leads to venous injury. When interrogating the vein, pulsatile color Doppler spectra will be noted in the outflow, proximal on the extremity to the AVF. On the arterial evaluation, proximal to the AVF, there may be low-resistance flow and loss of the typical triphasic waveform. The fistulous communication will have continuous, turbulent flow patterns. These fistulas should be surgically ligated if high-output heart failure develops.

True aneurysms of the extremity are far less common than pseudoaneurysms. Those involving the popliteal artery represent the majority. Unlike aortic and visceral aneurysms, popliteal artery aneurysms present with limb ischemia due to thromboembolic complications rather than rupture. Occasionally, compressive symptoms may result in the neuralgia of deep venous thrombosis. These patients are almost universally male. Chronic limb ischemia, manifested by claudication, rest pain, and absent pedal pulses, is found in 40% of patients. Acute, limb-threatening ischemia is the presentation in another 21%, with 40% of patients being asymptomatic.[7] Physical examination is very unreliable for the diagnosis of popliteal artery aneurysms. The initial test of choice is duplex ultrasonography. This test offers information on size and mural thrombus. For surgical planning, a thin-slice CT angiogram is often all that is necessary, although, traditionally, angiography has been employed as well.

It is essential to examine the contralateral popliteal artery as well as obtain imaging to rule out an abdominal aortic aneurysm. In fact, 50% of patients have a contralateral popliteal artery aneurysm, and about 33% of patients have a concomitant abdominal aortic aneurysm.[8]

The decision for treatment depends on the presentation. Patients with acute limb ischemia require prompt operative management, which begins with catheter-directed thrombolysis in order to obtain patency of an outflow vessel for arterial reconstruction with a bypass. Patients with more chronic symptoms and no immediate limb threat should undergo angiography for operative planning. A controversial subset of patients is the asymptomatic group. There is ongoing debate regarding repair of asymptomatic patients. Some argue that all popliteal aneurysms should be repaired because of the risk of acute limb ischemia. Others use aneurysm size, typically larger than 2.5 to 3.0 cm, as the cutoff for repair. No multicenter prospective trials have addressed this question.

Of course, an individualized approach is warranted. In patients who are good surgical candidates with minimal comorbidities and a relatively active lifestyle, repair seems justified to prevent ischemic complications. More frail, debilitated patients may best be observed until ischemic complications develop. Another point of contention is the choice of operation. In recent years, endovascular repair has shown much promise and is less invasive than open options. Although the patient samples are small and no randomized data exist, the patency rate associated with endovascular, covered stent repair of popliteal artery aneurysms is similar to that of open repair. After a mean follow-up of 54 months, Jung *et al.* demonstrated primary patency rates of nearly 85% in patients treated with endovascular popliteal artery aneurysm repair.[9]

Clinical approach when resources are limited

The history and physical examination are of great value in the clinical diagnosis of extremity aneurysms, especially regarding pseudoaneurysms. Information on recent trauma or percutaneous intervention is, essential to elicit during the patient interview. Also, a history of bypass surgery in the affected limb may raise suspicion for an anastomotic disruption leading to a pseudoaneurysm. Pain, ecchymosis, swelling, and a bruit over the affected area are also suggestive of

a pseudoaneurysm. When imaging modalities, such as ultrasound and CT scan, are limited, then a low threshold for operative intervention is warranted.

Exploration of the artery, with repair as indicated, can be both diagnostic as well as therapeutic. In the absence of resources for operative intervention, direct manual pressure may be held over the artery with the suspected pseudoaneurysm. A pulsatile mass can be palpated, and pressure should be directed over this area for 20 to 30 minutes. Prior to holding pressure, a detailed pulse examination and ankle-brachial index (ABI) should be obtained and repeated after pressure is withheld, in order to rule out thrombosis of, or embolization to, the native arteries.

When a true aneurysm is diagnosed or suspected, then transfer to a facility with imaging capabilities should be arranged. If there is evidence of distal embolization or thrombosis, then systemic anticoagulation should be initiated. Immediate transfer to a facility with the resources to provide operative intervention should not be delayed, as limb salvage requires restoration of perfusion within six to eight hours.

Extremity aneurysms may be seen in a broad spectrum of patients. Patients can be young intravenous drug abusers, elderly patients with coronary artery disease who have recently undergone catheterization, or relatively active men in their 60s. A high index of suspicion must be maintained and a detailed history and physical examination performed. Duplex ultrasonography is indispensable. Early consultation with a vascular surgeon is paramount to the timely treatment of these patients.

Critical actions

- Have a low threshold for obtaining diagnostic imaging when a pseudoaneurysm is suspected.
- Always examine the contralateral extremity when true peripheral aneurysms are suspected or confirmed, as bilaterality is common.
- All peripheral extremity aneurysms are associated with an increased incidence of abdominal aortic aneurysms, and the latter should always be ruled out.
- Follow-up duplex ultrasound is imperative after percutaneous treatment of pseudoaneurysms, in order to confirm therapeutic thrombosis of the pseudoaneurysm sac.

Pearls and pitfalls

- Always examine the contralateral extremity.
- Determine the degree of distal perfusion with a pulse examination and ankle-brachial index.

- When injection of a pseudoaneurysm is performed with thrombin, slow injection of the thrombin at the apex of the sac should be performed. Only when the position of the needle tip is confirmed should the thrombin be injected.
- Do not attempt percutaneous treatment when a mycotic aneurysm is suspected.
- Avoid delay of anticoagulation when ischemia is present. Obtain immediate vascular surgery consultation for limb ischemia and, if unavailable, arrange immediate transfer to a facility with the resources to obtain rapid revascularization.

References

1. Ohlow MA, Secknus MA, von Korn H, *et al.* Incidence and outcome of femoral vascular complications among 18,165 patients undergoing cardiac catheterisation. *Int J Cardiol* 2009; 135: 66–71.

2. Etemad-Rezai R, Peck DJ. Ultrasound-guided thrombin injection of femoral artery pseudoaneurysms. *Can Assoc Radiol J* 2003; 54: 118–20.

3. Paschalidis M, Theiss W, Kölling K, *et al.* Randomised comparison of manual compression repair versus ultrasound guided compression repair of postcatheterisation femoral pseudoaneurysms. *Heart* 2006; 92: 251–2.

4. Hofmann I, Wunderlich N, Robertson G, *et al.* Percutaneous injection of thrombin for the treatment of pseudoaneurysms: the German multicentre registry. *EuroIntervention* 2007; 3: 321–6.

5. Lönn L, Olmarker A, Geterud K, *et al.* Treatment of femoral pseudoaneurysms: percutaneous US-guided thrombin injection versus US-guided compression. *Acta Radiol* 2002; 43: 396–400.

6. Tan KK, Chen K, Chia KH, *et al.* Surgical management of infected pseudoaneurysms in intravenous drug abusers: single institution experience and a proposed algorithm. *World J Surg* 2009; 33: 1830–5.

7. Huang Y, Gloviczki P, Noel AA, *et al.* Early complications and long-term outcome after open surgical treatment of popliteal artery aneurysms: is exclusion with saphenous vein bypass still the gold standard? *J Vasc Surg* 2007; 45: 706–13.

8. Dawson I, Sie RB, van Bockel JH. Atherosclerotic popliteal aneurysm. *Br J Surg* 1997; 84: 293–9.

9. Jung E, Jim J, Rubin BG, *et al.* Long-term outcome of endovascular popliteal artery aneurysm repair. *Ann Vasc Surg* 2010; 24: 871–5.

Evaluation and management of thrombosed/occluded bypass grafts

Jonathan Kittredge and Kapil Gopal

Revascularization is performed to maintain the function and viability of lower extremities affected by decreased arterial perfusion, ranging from claudication to critical limb ischemia (rest pain, gangrene, or non-healing wounds). Revascularization can be approached with endovascular procedures such as balloon angioplasty and, as needed, the placement of stents or the creation of a surgical bypass of occluded arteries. The life expectancy of a bypass graft depends on a number of variables, including its location, the quality of the inflow and outflow vessels, the material with which the graft is constructed (vein, cadaveric vein or arterial grafts, or prosthetic material), the state of the patient's coagulation system, and the patient's habits (e.g., smoking).[1–3] This chapter will focus on how to manage patients who present with threatened vascular graft occlusion.

The reasons for graft occlusion or thrombosis are related to progression of atherosclerotic arterial occlusive disease that compromises the inflow or outflow of blood from the graft. This progression is often seen in tobacco users, diabetics, and renal failure patients. Flow-limiting stenosis can also develop within a venous or prosthetic graft. Patients with a history of thrombophilia or arrhythmias could experience a thrombotic or embolic event, especially if anticoagulation is part of the history. A graft can become occluded within days or years after the original surgery.

When a patient presents with sensorimotor symptoms and absent distal Doppler signals, strong consideration should be given to empiric anticoagulation to maximize the chance of salvaging the bypass graft or even the limb. For patients with compromised perfusion, the magnitude of limb threat is quantified by the Rutherford classification (see Table 13.1).[4] This classification hinges on the results of a neurologic examination and the presence of Doppler signals. Patients with some sensory loss but baseline motor function are commonly managed with an endovascular approach; those with more profound symptoms may require immediate operative intervention. Patients with limbs considered not salvageable require amputation.

Diagnosis

History

When a patient arrives with a new complaint of sudden change of feeling and function in a surgically revascularized limb, the status of the bypass must be assessed. Symptoms could include: pain; paresthesia, defined as new numbness, tingling, or weakness; and even paralysis. Because of the acute nature of graft thrombosis, these symptoms tend to have a relatively acute onset, frequently developing over minutes to an hour. Most patients can tell you exactly when and where they were when the thrombosis occurred. This is critical information for the vascular surgeon, and the timeline should be investigated in all cases. The differential diagnosis of acute limb ischemia includes acute and chronic neurologic injury and deep venous thrombosis of the contralateral limb.

Typically, a patient with a lower extremity bypass is very familiar with the symptoms of ischemia. The chief complaint will frequently be that the leg feels cool, numb, or painful. Symptoms of claudication are pain with a predictable amount of exertion, and its reversal upon resting. They classically occur in the calf or forefoot. Rest pain is caused by the inability of the vascular system to meet the metabolic needs of the

Vascular Emergencies, ed. Robert L. Rogers, Thomas Scalea, Lee Wallis, and Heike Geduld. Published by Cambridge University Press. © Cambridge University Press 2013.

limb at rest. To fulfill the diagnostic criteria, this pain must have been present and required opiate analgesia for two weeks. Patients commonly relate that symptoms of claudication or rest pain that were present before their bypass have recently recurred, and frequently they are worse than before their operation. In some cases, patients have not even had a classic bypass. They may have had long-segment stenting of their native arterial system. If a covered stent was used, the patient is viewed as having had a "percutaneous bypass," which behaves in much the same way as an open bypass graft when thrombosis occurs.

Neurologic injury associated with a thrombosed or occluded graft can manifest as a peripheral condition, as in spinal disease; a peripheral neuropathy, as in diabetes; or an acute injury, as in trauma. Spinal disease and traumatic injury are typically limited to the specific peripheral nerves or dermatomes involved and tend not to affect a limb as a whole. Similarly, central injury such as transient ischemic attack (TIA) or stroke will involve the processes handled in the affected portion of brain; therefore, symptoms will not be limited to sensory and motor involvement of an entire extremity. Other elements of the patient's medical history include the detection of arrhythmias, the presence of a hypercoagulable state, and the use of anticoagulants. Some patients are placed on empiric long-term anticoagulation after receiving a bypass graft, even without a history of a hypercoagulable state or arrhythmias.

Physical examination

The physical examination is critical in assessing the degree of ischemia. Pulses are rarely palpable in these patients, so the subjectivity of "palpable" pulses makes this measure unreliable. The demonstration of signals from a handheld Doppler transducer is more objective and reproducible. The presence of an arterial Doppler signal reliably confirms perfusion to the distal limb. A signal over the bypass graft itself is reassuring but can be misleading if the Doppler signal is proximal to the occlusion and has a characteristic "water hammer" quality. A "water hammer" Doppler signal has an abrupt end and no diastolic flow. The presence of pedal Doppler signals (anterior tibial, dorsalis pedis, and posterior tibial) suggests the limb has distal perfusion and therefore is not immediately threatened.

Ischemic limbs without Doppler signals might be viable because chronically ischemic limbs have multiple collateral vessels. Also, the location of a patient's bypass graft might be difficult to interpret from scars: it could be deep in an anatomic plane or subcutaneously in an extra-anatomic plane. Thus, a perfectly functioning subcutaneously tunneled bypass could be missed on examination by a practitioner who is unfamiliar with the course of the tunnel for the graft.

More important than the demonstration of distal signals is the functionality of the limb. A good neurologic and sensory examination is much more helpful in defining the immediate threat. Since nerves are far more dependent on blood flow than muscle or skin, the first change that will occur in an ischemic limb is loss of sensory function, followed by loss of motor function. Longstanding neuropathy must be considered in these (frequently diabetic) patients, and it is important to discuss with the patient if the foot feels different from the typical state or is moving less than normal. A foot that feels numb or "asleep" might still have sensation to light touch; making the distinction between a foot with light touch sensation and paresthesias is important in determining the severity of ischemia.

The appearance of the skin can be suggestive of ischemia, but this assessment can be challenging in patients with darker complexions. The presence of capillary refill is indicative of venous reflux, not of arterial supply. As such, these factors are suggestive but not diagnostic.

Laboratory tests

Important blood work includes complete blood count, basic metabolic panel, and coagulation profile. Metabolic derangements such as hyperkalemia and low bicarbonate levels can indicate active muscle ischemia and death. The coagulation profile will allow identification of the patient's anticoagulation status, indicate if the patient is taking oral vitamin-K antagonists, and elucidate any hypocoagulable state that would make it advisable to not begin pharmacologic anticoagulation therapy. Finally, a complete blood count will alert the physician to any occult anemia or bleeding, infections, or thrombocytopenia. A baseline platelet count will allow monitoring for heparin-induced thrombocytopenia; this patient cohort most likely has had previous exposure to heparin. Finally, a 12-lead electrocardiogram (ECG) should be obtained to assess for underlying arrhythmias or myocardial infarction, which may identify the cause of the occlusion or a condition that limits the treatment options available to the patient.

Imaging

Duplex ultrasonography can be very helpful in delineating the anatomy and status of the lower extremity's native arterial system and bypasses. The quality of the examination depends on the skills of the sonographer. Many hospitals have a non-invasive vascular laboratory that offers multilevel ankle-brachial index (ABI) and continuous Doppler waveform analysis as well as duplex of the lower extremities. The vascular lab staff tend to work closely with vascular surgeons and are familiar with the techniques used by these surgeons as well as the information they need to make management decisions. If the patient has Doppler signals, waveform analysis can be helpful in quantifying the degree of ischemia.

If a sonographer who is trained to perform these studies is not available, a single ABI can be calculated with measurements from an ordinary blood-pressure cuff. A ratio can be derived from the systolic blood pressure in the upper extremity and the ankle pressure of each leg. Ankle pressures are determined by placing the blood-pressure cuff above the ankle, inflating it until the Doppler pedal signal becomes absent, and then slowly releasing the inflation and recording the pressure at which the Doppler signal reappears. Many emergency departments have bedside ultrasound machines that can be used to locate a bypass graft and determine if color flow is present in the bypass. This information can help in the assessment of bypass graft occlusion.

Computed tomography angiography (CTA) of the affected limb can also be used to identify flow in the graft as well as the distal anatomy. In some settings, when a sonographer is not available but a CT scanner is, CTA can confirm the diagnosis. It is important to make sure the CTA includes the inflow and outflow vessels for the bypass to ensure complete visualization of the graft. Unfortunately, these studies require time, intravenous contrast, and a cooperative patient. Time should not be spent on this modality if the patient's limb appears to be threatened (decreased motor function, weakness, or paralysis). Urgent consultation with a vascular surgeon should be obtained. The vascular surgeon might elect to perform an angiogram of the ischemic extremity, as it can be both diagnostic and therapeutic.

In most cases, imaging modalities before intervention will not be available or helpful in the management of an occluded graft that is threatening a limb.

Because the immediate treatment is not likely to be altered by imaging studies, we do not believe they are needed to make a diagnosis or determine the urgency of intervention. The urgency of the intervention hinges on the results of sensory and motor examinations. At no time should an imaging modality delay the initiation of anticoagulation or a surgical intervention to re-establish perfusion.

Emergency department management

Initial assessment

Initial management of an ischemic limb is systemic anticoagulation. Typically, this is accomplished with a bolus of unfractionated intravenous heparin followed by continuous infusion. Although the administration of a therapeutic dose of low-molecular-weight heparin (e.g., enoxaparin) gives a more predictable effect, the duration of action of unfractionated heparin (~90 min) gives the option of stopping the administration and possible reversal with protamine if unexpected catastrophic hemorrhage occurs. Because the response to anticoagulation may be inadequate or the patient may develop a complication from it, the authors favor acute management with unfractionated heparin. If the patient has a history of heparin-induced thrombocytopenia, alternatives such as direct thrombin inhibitors should be used.

Patients who do not have a specific contraindication should be taking an antiplatelet agent to reduce cardiac risk; if the agent is aspirin or clopidogrel (Plavix) alone, it can be safely continued. If the patient is not on antiplatelet therapy, 325 mg of aspirin is adequate initial therapy.[5] If the patient is on dual antiplatlet therapy (aspirin and Plavix), then the risk of perioperative bleeding is slightly increased, but, due to the urgent nature of intervention, both of these agents can be continued.[6] Many patients are taking a systemic anticoagulant, typically warfarin, with or without an antiplatelet agent, and others are on systemic anticoagulation and dual antiplatelet therapy. The presence of a therapeutic INR or antiplatelet therapy does not obviate the need to initiate systemic anticoagulation with heparin or a direct thrombin inhibitor. Heparin has pleomorphic effects beyond simple anticoagulation, and rates of graft thrombosis are improved only modestly with therapeutic warfarin therapy.[7,8] Nonetheless, patients on both aspirin and warfarin therapy tend to have less severe ischemia after occlusion of their bypass.[3] Vascular surgery consultation should be obtained to determine the degree of ischemia and the therapeutic options available to the patient at the institution. If the necessary resources are not available, the patient may require transfer to a regional medical center.

Patients should be optimized as much as possible for an emergent surgical intervention. This includes fasting, initiation of intravenous hydration, obtaining the laboratory data mentioned earlier, as well as a type and screen for possible transfusion, and an ECG. Oral N-acetylcysteine can be initiated and intravenous sodium-bicarbonate hydration can be considered as adjuncts for possible endovascular procedures. The benefit of sodium bicarbonate and N-acetylcysteine over simple hydration in reducing the incidence of dye-induced nephropathy is being studied. In the absence of these agents, simple hydration with normal saline is indicated.[9–11]

The need for urgent operative intervention depends on the severity of ischemia and the response to anticoagulation. Contrary to historical teachings, there is no strict timetable for re-establishing flow to save an extremity; rather, therapy should be guided by the examination results and the patient's symptoms. Prosthetic bypass grafts can be salvaged up to 14 days after suspected onset of thrombosis or occlusion; whereas, although not well defined, the chances of salvaging an autogenous vein graft decrease significantly after 24 to 48 hours of suspected occlusion.

Severity of ischemia, both before and after initiation of anticoagulation, is an important factor in the need for urgent/emergent intervention. As outlined earlier, the motor and sensory examinations are more important than the palpability or presence of a pulse or Doppler signal. Limbs that until recently were sensate and had intact motor function are the most urgent cases, because these are limbs that are acutely threatened. Limbs that have profound sensory deficits with paralysis are likely unsalvageable.

Definitive treatment and inpatient care

Definitive management of acute thrombosis of bypass grafts depends on many factors. These include the type and location of the bypass and the graft, the status of the inflow and outflow vessels, the degree of ischemia in the limb, the age of the bypass, and the amount of time that has passed since the bypass occluded. In general, salvage of a bypass is preferred to performing a new bypass or amputation. The possibility of successful salvage is best in bypass grafts that have been occluded for less than 14 days and have good inflow and outflow vessels, in patients with a residual ABI of at least 0.33, and in clinical scenarios in which the occlusive thrombus can be traversed with a wire.[12,13] Limbs that have lost sensory or motor function need emergent revascularization for reperfusion. Depending on the degree of ischemia, the patient may require fasciotomy of the lower limb in response to swelling of the muscles upon reperfusion.

A bypass graft that has acute thrombosis can be salvaged with either surgical or endovascular techniques. Classically, open exploration of the bypass is performed with balloon embolectomy, with revision if there is an anatomic reason for bypass failure. After flow through the bypass is re-established, an angiogram needs to be performed to identify any anatomic reasons for graft failure. Anatomic reasons for thrombosis are related to time: occurrence within 30 days after the original surgery is caused by technical factors at time of surgery; occurrences within 30 days to 2 years are from stenosis induced by neointimal hyperplasia at the distal anastomosis or within an autogenous conduit; and occurrences more than two years after surgery are most likely from progression of atherosclerotic disease compromising the outflow vessels. Compromised flow is ultimately responsible for thrombosis, and the anatomic lesion can be treated by endovascular or surgical methods. If treatment or revision is not possible or is unsuccessful, a new bypass needs to be performed.

Over the past 20 years, an increasing amount of vascular intervention has been performed with endovascular techniques.[14] This shift has been driven by a noted benefit in limb salvage, perioperative morbidity, and shorter hospital stay.[12,13,15] Currently, this modality is reserved for limbs in which sensory loss is minimal (i.e., toes only) and motor function is largely preserved. Surgical thrombectomy with or without fasciotomy and/or graft revision is used in patients with a greater severity of ischemia, typically with significant motor involvement. Irrespective of the continuing evolution of this modality in both technique and application, after catheter-directed thrombolysis, the patient should be monitored in an intensive care bed for bleeding complications associated with the procedure.

Following successful revascularization, the patient will likely be on systemic anticoagulation. Depending on the cause of the thrombosis and the quality of the bypass procedure, patients may require long-term anticoagulation with an oral vitamin-K antagonist or low-molecular-weight heparin. Once a patient has had a bypass, regular ultrasonographic assessments can identify a failing bypass prior to its complete thrombosis. The long-term patency of bypasses is improved by intervening on a bypass prior to thrombosis (assisted primary patency), rather than attempting to salvage a thrombosed bypass graft (secondary patency).[8,16,17] Finally, regular follow-up will allow the vascular surgeon to stress the importance of risk factor modification (i.e., smoking cessation) and optimal medical management.

Clinical approach when resources are limited

1. Suspect acute thrombosis of a graft based on the history and physical examination.
2. Obtain a thorough history regarding the patient's present illness, previous medical conditions, and family history.
3. Perform a physical examination and a bedside Doppler examination and calculate the ABI to assess perfusion of the limb.
4. For patients with salvageable limbs, initiate systemic anticoagulation with unfractionated heparin.
5. Obtain vascular surgery consultation for further treatment or possible transfer.

Pearls and pitfalls

Pearls

1. Maintain high suspicion based on history and physical examination.
2. Initiate anticoagulation therapy in patients with salvageable limbs.
3. Obtain surgical consultation early.

Pitfalls

1. Awaiting confirmatory imaging in a patient with suspected graft thrombosis before initiating anticoagulation in a salvageable bypass graft and limb.

2. Not initiating anticoagulation in patients already on a vitamin-K antagonist.

Critical actions

- Determine the acuteness of symptoms.
- Perform a physical examination to assess motor and sensory function of the distal limb.
- Perform a handheld Doppler examination of the distal pedal vessels.
- Confirm the diagnosis with duplex ultrasonography or bedside ultrasound if available.
- Obtain vascular surgical evaluation.
- Initiate heparin anticoagulation.

References

1. Willigendael EM, Teijink JA, Bartelink ML, et al. Smoking and the patency of lower extremity bypass grafts: a meta-analysis. *J Vasc Surg* 2005; 42: 67–74.

2. Owens C, Ridker PM, Belkin M, et al. Elevated C-reactive protein levels are associated with postoperative events in pateints undergoing lower extremity vein bypass surgery. *J Vasc Surg* 2007; 45: 2–9.

3. Jackson MR, Johnson WC, Williford WO, et al. The effect of anticoagulation therapy and graft selection on the ischemic consequences of femoropopliteal bypass graft occlusion: results from a multicenter randomized clinical trial. *J Vasc Surg* 2002; 35: 292–8.

4. Rutherford RB, Baker JD, Ernst C, et al. Recommended standards for reports dealing with lower extremity ischemia: revised version. *J Vasc Surg* 1997; 26: 517–38.

5. Braithwaite BD, Jones L, Yusuf SW, et al. Aspirin improves the outcome of intra-arterial thrombolysis with tissue plasminogen activator. *Br J Surg* 1995; 82: 1357–8.

6. Korte W, Cattaneo M, Chassot PG, et al. Peri-operative management of antiplatelet therapy in patients with coronary artery disease. *Thromb Haemost* 2011; 105: 743–9.

7. Lever R, Smailbegovic A, Page CP. Locally available heparin modulates inflammatory cell recruitment in a manner independent of anticoagulant activity. *Eur J Pharmacol* 2010; 630: 137–44.

8. Brumberg RS, Back MR, Armstrong PA, et al. The relative importance of graft surveillance and warfarin therapy in infrainguinal prosthetic bypass failure. *J Vasc Surg* 2007; 46: 1160–6.

9. Katzberg RW, Lamba R. Contrast-induced nephropathy after intravenous administration: fact or fiction? *Radiol Clin North Am* 2009; 47: 789–800.

10. Tepel M, van der Geit M, Schwarzfeld C, *et al.* Prevention of radiographic-contrast-agent-induced reductions in renal function by acetylcystiene. *N Engl J Med* 2000; 343: 180–4.

11. Gonzales DA, Norsworthy KJ, Kern SJ, *et al.* A meta-analysis of N-acetylcystiene in contrast-induced nephrotoxicity: unsupervised clustering to resolve heterogeneity. *BMC Med* 2007; 5: 32–44.

12. Comerota AJ, Weaver FA, Hosking JD, *et al.* Results of a prospective, randomized trial of surgery versus thrombolysis for occluded lower extremity bypass grafts. *Am J Surg* 1996; 172: 105–12.

13. Jaffery Z, Thornton SN, White CJ. Acute limb ischemia. *Am J Med Sci* 2011; 342: 226–34.

14. Schrijver AM, de Borst GJ, Vos JA, *et al.* PS110. Catheter-directed thrombolysis as first line treatment of acute nontraumatic upper extremity ischemia. *J Vasc Surg* 2011; 53(6 suppl): 58S.

15. Limtungturakul S, Wongpraparut N, Pornatanarangsri S, *et al.* Early experience of catheter directed thrombolysis for acute limb ischemia of native vessels and bypass graft thrombosis in Thai patients. *J Med Assoc Thai* 2011; 94(suppl 1): S11–18.

16. Mattos MA, van Bemmelen PS, Hodgson KJ, *et al.* Does correction of stenoses identified with color duplex scanning improve infrainguinal graft patency? *J Vasc Surg* 1993; 17: 54–66.

17. Hobbs SD, Pinkney T, Sykes TC, *et al.* Patency of infra-inguinal vein grafts – effect of intraoperative Doppler assessment and a graft surveillance program. *J Vasc Surg* 2009; 49: 1452–8.

Penetrating extremity trauma – vascular aspects

Timothy Craig Hardcastle, Christopher Venter, and Daan den Hollander

The limbs are vital for mobility, dexterity, and daily activity; therefore injuries affecting the limb vasculature often lead to loss of economic productivity, morbidity, and even death.[1,2] Penetrating trauma is a common mechanism by which the limb vessels are injured. Gunshot wounds (Figures 16.1 and 16.2), stabbings, domestic incidents (e.g., contact with broken glass), and penetrating injuries with an underlying blunt mechanism (e.g., impalement during a motor vehicle collision) all risk injuring the vessels and nearby nerves.

Approximately 25 to 35% of penetrating limb injuries involve a vascular injury.[3] When an orthopedic injury is also present, the therapeutic decision-making process becomes more challenging.[3,4]

Epidemiologically, looking at the world from a trauma perspective, South Africa has the highest rate of penetrating interpersonal violence of any country not at war, and the highest rate of non-natural death.[5] It has thus been possible to build a respectable experience in the field of vascular trauma of the limbs in this country. Many ground-breaking articles published over the past few years originated in South Africa.[6–16] Elsewhere in the world, the conflicts in Afghanistan and Iraq have provided some unique insights into the challenges of military trauma care.[17–21] The presence of war always increases knowledge about the care of military and civilian trauma victims.

The following statistics, presented as a brief epidemiologic introduction, were extracted from the trauma database at Tygerberg Hospital in Cape Town (1998–2005). Limb trauma accounted for 53% of vascular injuries, not all of which were induced by a penetrating mechanism. In the 392 cases recorded, brachial arterial injury was the most common vascular

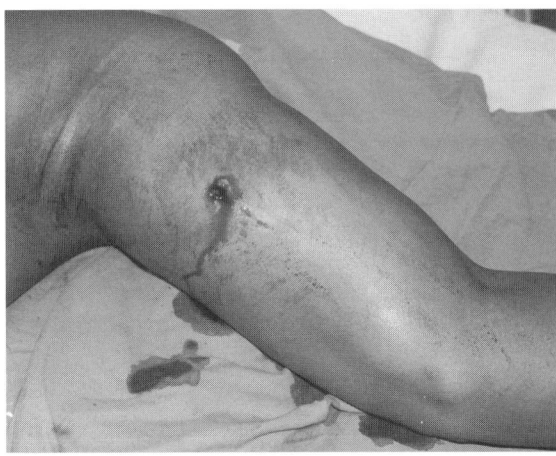

Figure 16.1 Medial arm gunshot wound of a patient with mid-brachial arterial injury.

injury,[14] followed by femoral artery injury,[22] and popliteal artery injury and injury to other below-knee vessels. Forearm vessel injuries were not documented in this database.

Prehospital care: assessment and management of limb trauma

Penetrating limb trauma may be a single injury or part of a complex penetrating injury profile. It is generally easy to visualize and identify on initial assessment. These injuries may be disabling but are rarely life-threatening. The prehospital injury spectrum includes open wounds, lacerations with or without active bleeding, open/compound fractures, amputations with vascular end-bleeding, and impaled objects (foreign bodies) plugging a vascular injury. The initial focus is assessment of other life-threatening injuries and initiation of resuscitation.

Vascular Emergencies, ed. Robert L. Rogers, Thomas Scalea, Lee Wallis, and Heike Geduld. Published by Cambridge University Press. © Cambridge University Press 2013.

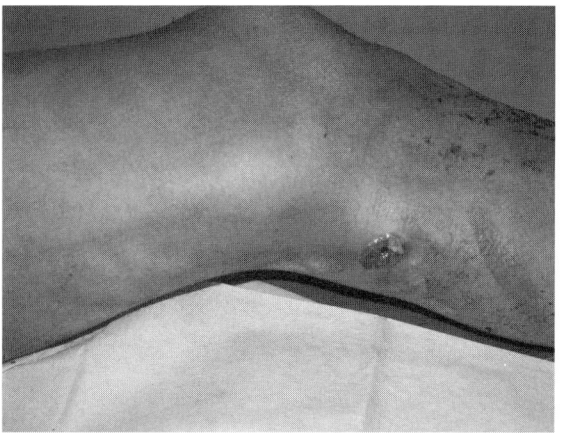

Figure 16.2 Gunshot exit wound below the popliteal fossa. The patient had distal femoral artery transection.

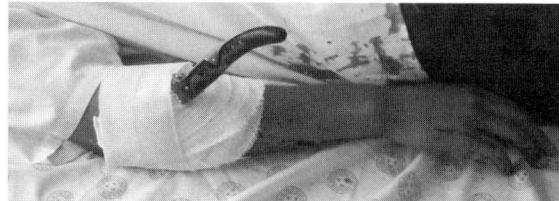

Figure 16.3 Foreign body impalement appropriately treated by prehospital paramedics.

The wounds need to be assessed by the medical care provider on scene and are treated according to the patient's status. If the penetrating limb trauma is a critical factor, the prehospital care provider needs to report this to the receiving facility so that the surgical team can intervene as soon as the patient arrives. Early hemorrhage control and rapid transfer to definitive care reduce the risk of loss of blood and limb. [23–25]

Bleeding wounds should be compressed and covered with sterile gauze, and a firm crepe compression bandage should be applied. The use of procoagulant wound-care products such as Celox or Chitosan may be considered if allowed by local protocol.[26–28] There is renewed interest in the temporary prehospital use of tourniquets of specific design to control massive arterial hemorrhage.[21,29]

Amputations are disabling and sometimes life threatening. They have the potential for massive blood loss, but the bleeding is self-controlled in many cases by vessel spasm or application of pressure to the stump. Tourniquets can be used if the blood loss from an amputation is uncontrollable in the prehospital environment.[28,29]

Impaled objects (foreign bodies) are injurious objects that enter the body and remain protruding out of the skin. The most important point is not to remove the object in the prehospital environment. With the skin as the pivot-point, any motion outside the body is reflected within the tissues, where the end of the object may further lacerate or harm sensitive structures and plugged vessels may be disturbed, causing rebleeding. The wound should be irrigated around the impaled object and dressed accordingly. The protruding object must be stabilized before transport (Figure 16.3).

Hospital care

Initial assessment

As for all trauma patients, those with penetrating trauma of the extremities should be transported rapidly to the nearest appropriate definitive care facility, ideally a regionally accredited trauma center with a trauma team. The composition of the trauma team may be determined by local policy or other circumstances; however, there is little evidence that bigger is better.[30]

The early assessment of the patient should follow the tried and tested systematic approach espoused by the Advanced Trauma Life Support (ATLS) philosophy.[31] In this approach, control of the airway, breathing, and circulation take precedence over assessment of limb injuries, with the notable exception of early control of massive bleeding. The risk of death associated with exsanguinating hemorrhage from a vascular injury cannot be overstated.

The early determination of whether there is severe physiological compromise is essential. This determination is best undertaken with the use of arterial blood gases, examining for lactic acidosis (arterial lactate > 5 mmol/L) or an elevated base excess (greater than 4), the degree of acidosis (pH < 7.25), and the core temperature on arrival at the emergency department (under 36.5 °C is associated with worse outcomes). These factors mandate the need for "damage control" philosophies, both during the initial phase of treatment (damage control resuscitation) and during surgery (damage control surgery).

When resuscitating a patient who has active ongoing bleeding, the early activation of a massive hemorrhage protocol must be considered. Such a protocol

Table 16.1 Clinical signs of vascular injury

Hard signs	Soft signs
Active arterial bleeding	History of significant bleeding
Absent distal pulse	Evidence of venous bleeding
Pulsatile or expanding hematoma	Non-expanding hematoma
Audible bruit	Diminished, but palpable, pulse
Distal ischemia (five Ps)*	Proximity to vessels
	Peripheral nerve injury

*See Table 12.1.

should be instituted at all hospitals that receive major trauma patients before such patients arrive. Essential topics to be addressed in the protocol are damage control resuscitation and limiting the amount of crystalloid fluid that can be transfused by the early use of natural colloid (blood and blood products).[32–34] The performance of a thromb-elastogram can be useful in providing early evidence of a coagulopathy and for guiding transfusion therapy.

Once the primary survey has been completed, all limbs should be examined in detail as part of the secondary survey. In particular, the clinician should assess the patient's distal pulses, neurologic function, and the presence of raised compartment pressures.

"Hard signs" are indicative of arterial injury, while "soft signs" may predict the presence of an injury, which may be venous or arterial (Table 16.1). Soft signs can also be present in patients who have no vascular injury; however, they may be caused by associated injuries rather than a direct injury to a blood vessel.

Twenty-five to thirty-five percent of patients with penetrating limb trauma have a vascular injury. The risk of vascular injury is based on the presumption that injuries to nearby structures increase the risk of injury to the associated vessels, which has not proved to be true in one well-publicized study.[35] The one exception to this general rule is shotgun injuries. Birdshot pellets can injure vessels as well as undergo distal embolization after they have come to rest in the tissues and enter the vasculature.

The classic picture of a cold, pale, pulseless, insensate, immobile limb (five Ps; see Table 12.1) is less common than the presence of one sign or a combination of a few of them. The presence of any of these signs in a firm, swollen limb with decreased hand or foot movement must raise the suspicion of compartment syndrome, which may develop even in the absence of an arterial injury. The consequence of missing compartment syndrome and an arterial injury is the same: avoidable loss of limb.

Bedside assessment with the use of a handheld audio-Doppler device is useful if there is any doubt about the presence of a vascular injury. Comparison of the Doppler signal and, most importantly, the occlusion pressure of the injured side with the contralateral uninjured side is useful in screening for an arterial injury. To test occlusion pressure, compress the injured limb vessel distal to the penetration with a blood-pressure cuff, observe the Doppler signal, and then repeat the technique on the uninjured side. A difference of more than 10 mmHg or a difference of more than 0.1 in the ankle-brachial index (ABI) suggests an injury, with a sensitivity of more than 90% but a specificity of only 60%.[36] The ABI is determined by dividing the systolic occlusion pressure of the lower limb by that of the upper limb, with a value above 0.9 accepted as normal.[37]

Pathology of penetrating vascular injury

Vascular injury can lead to the following spectrum of injuries:

- Vessel penetration with either uncontained bleeding or contained pseudoaneurysm.
- Vessel transection with active bleeding.
- Vessel transection with vasospasm (of the transected ends), clot formation, and occlusion, often with surprisingly little bleeding.
- Percussion injuries (found commonly with bullet wounds) cause intimal injury with early or sometimes late occlusion, often with diminished pulses or Doppler difference as the only early finding.
- Distal ischemia following occlusion.
- Non-occlusive injuries or pseudoaneurysms can be a source of distal embolization.
- Arteriovenous fistulas can be created, more commonly with knife injuries.
- Combination injuries are possible.

Civilian versus military

Penetrating injuries in civilians are most often caused by low-energy mechanisms such as knives, broken bottles, and small-caliber handguns, while penetrating trauma in military personnel is usually caused by high-energy forces such as explosive devices. The degree of destruction of the surrounding tissue is likely to be much greater with military wounds than with civilian wounds, so much more debridement will be required. The need for "damage control" techniques, such as vascular shunting, in the field is also more likely, since a soldier who is extricated under active fire conditions is likely to be more physiologically deranged than the civilian penetrating-trauma patient with short prehospital times and rapid extrication to well-staffed trauma units.

The use of improvised explosive devices (IEDs) has increased the amount of limb trauma in modern warfare, particularly in light of the improvements in body armor. Proximal bilateral traumatic amputations are now commonly treated by military medical services.[17–21]

Imaging: who, when, and how?

Blunt trauma tends to create complex vessel transection or extensive intimal injury and subsequent occlusion. In contrast, penetrating mechanisms often cause injury near the site of the skin wound, making clinical judgment and basic assessment tools adequate in many cases. Routine angiographic assessment is therefore much less commonly indicated than with blunt mechanisms of injury.

No patient with a penetrating injury and suspected vascular damage should be sent to the angiogram suite prior to discussion of the case with a suitably credentialed vascular or trauma surgeon. The surgeon may elect to explore the vessels empirically rather than undertake imaging that would delay definitive repair. Another option is on-table imaging.

In general, for patients with a single-level penetrating injury, with (hard) signs of vascular damage clinically apparent, imaging should be waived in favor of early surgical intervention. However, for hemodynamically stable patients with multiple-level injuries (e.g., above and below the knee) or with combined limb and trunk penetration, and with hard clinical signs, imaging is indicated. Wounds in a hemodynamically unstable patient should be explored operatively and on-table imaging undertaken if the injury is not readily apparent. The same may apply when multiple end-vessels have been disrupted and might be amenable to endovascular embolization therapy (e.g.,

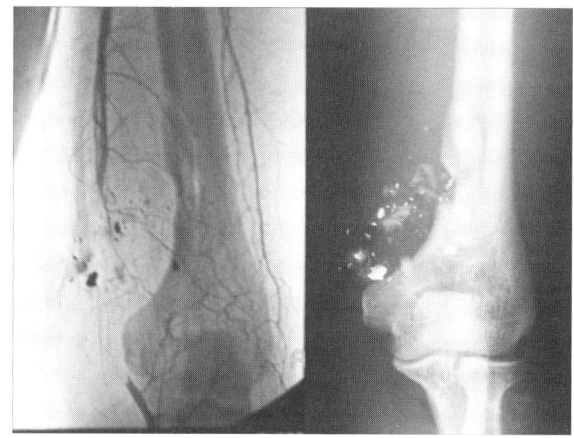

Figure 16.4 Brachial artery injury after gunshot to lower aspect of humerus identified on angiogram (the patient has other wounds of the forearm).

in the forearm or involving the below-knee vascular trifurcation).

In general, with penetrating trauma, the best imaging modality remains the conventional catheter-directed angiogram. This procedure can be performed in the emergency department with a simple direct proximal vessel puncture and prograde injection of intra-arterial contrast, using either an image intensifier or a plain film X-ray cartridge with suitable timing of the image (about three seconds after injection) (Figures 16.4 and 16.5).[38] The same technique can be carried out with the Lodox low-dose X-ray imaging device, currently in use in a number of major trauma units across the globe.[39,40] These techniques are more likely to identify minor, yet significant, injuries, which may be missed even with high-resolution computed tomography (CT) angiograms, commonly employed for whole-body trauma screening. Computed tomography angiography (CTA) is commonly used as a screening tool for vascular injury and may be more accurate in the neck than the limbs. CTA does have a higher miss-rate than that associated with conventional angiography.[41–43]

For hemodynamically stable patients, however, the use of formal digital subtraction angiography allows the detection and potential treatment of penetrating vascular injuries, particularly in positions that are difficult to access. This method gives the best quality imaging and is still the gold standard of vascular imaging.

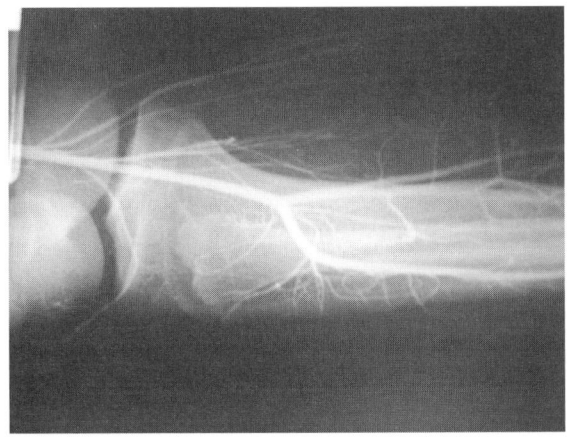

Figure 16.5 Normal on-table angiogram after gunshot through the calf.

Another option is duplex Doppler ultrasound technology, which is more useful over long straight vessels than around joints. This resource is not available after hours in many centers. It is somewhat user dependent and thus has lower sensitivity and specificity compared to angiography.[44]

What about the child?

Penetrating trauma is not uncommon as a cause of vascular injuries in children. In a series from Durban, 11 (28%) of 40 children under the age of 12 with vascular trauma were injured by a penetrating mechanism. In other series involving adolescents, the percentage is 55 to 92%.[45–49] Common mechanisms of injury among younger children are broken glass and lawnmowers, whereas adolescents are more commonly injured by gunshot and stab wounds.

Small children differ from adults in that their vasomotor responses to hypovolemia and local injury to a vessel are far more active. Because of this vasospasm response, it is difficult to provide an opinion on a possible vascular injury unless the child is well resuscitated and in a warm environment. Imaging may be necessary and non-invasive options should be considered as first line; however, it is important to remember that puncturing the small-diameter vessel of a young child is associated with a relatively high risk of complications, so catheter-directed angiography should be avoided unless the diagnosis of vascular injury is equivocal (i.e., decreased pulse, with ABI < 0.9).[49] Penetrating trauma victims with hard signs of vascular injury (arterial bleeding, peripheral ischemia) should be explored surgically without first undergoing angiography.

Operative techniques for children are similar to those for adults, but the vasospasm may make the procedure technically more difficult. Papaverine application may be necessary to reverse the spasm. Limb shortening may occur in all growing children after vascular injuries, whether they are treated conservatively or operatively, so they should be followed through their active growth stages. Although the management is controversial, current recommendations are to offer corrective surgery for children with limb discrepancies and a decreased ABI.[49]

Initial management: orthopedic and damage control aspects

The goal of the initial operative intervention should be to gain vascular control proximal and, preferably, distal to the suspected injury. The decision regarding definitive repair or implementation of damage control procedures can then be made in the context of the patient's physiologic condition combined with the presence of associated injuries, such as fractures.

If the limb is threatened, early revascularization with shunts and distal fasciotomy is preferred over complex immediate reconstruction (Figure 16.6). Orthopedic stabilization with an external fixation device or simple traction may be undertaken.[50] If the patient is stable, the limb is viable, and not much time has passed since the injury, then orthopedic fixation is best done initially, followed by definitive vascular repair. A decision regarding the need for fasciotomy can be delayed until the end of the procedure. Fasciotomy should be used liberally to prevent the dire consequences of compartment syndrome.[3,51]

Early consequences of penetrating vascular injury

The early consequences of penetrating vascular injury include blood loss, tissue hematoma, peripheral nerve injury (at the time of initial trauma or during rushed emergency surgery), muscle ischemia, and systemic complications (e.g., renal dysfunction and coagulopathy). The important aspects of limb viability and eventual patient survival should be balanced early in the decision-making process. It may be better to

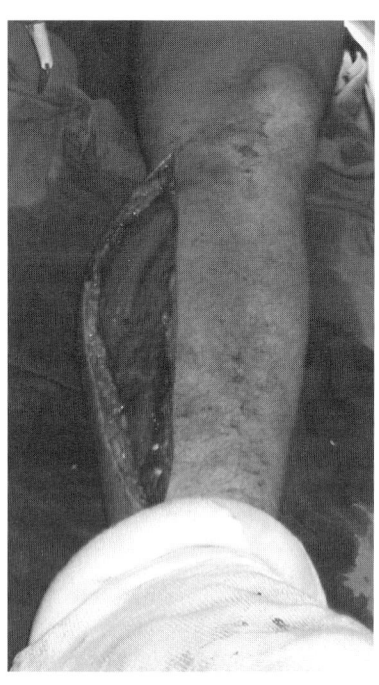

Figure 16.6 Medial aspect of lower limb fasciotomy after shotgun blast injury.

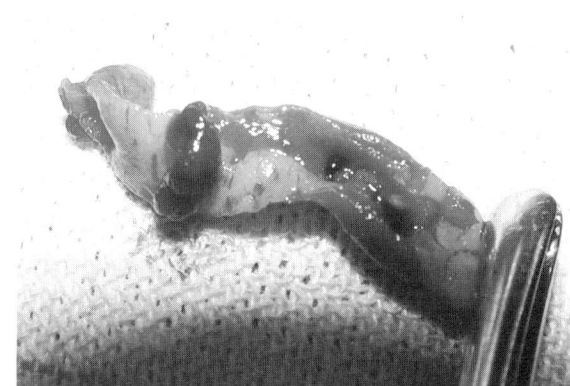

Figure 16.7 Intimal injury in arterial wall resection after percussion injury.

perform early amputation for a delayed presentation of a cold, swollen, insensate limb than to try to revascularize a dead limb, leading to systemic sequelae and the need for late amputation. This situation poses the medicolegal choices of life over limb, which must be made with the best interest of the patient in mind.[52] It may be better to have a good early amputation (followed by early rehabilitation) than a non-usable, yet viable "flail" limb resulting from neurologic damage.

Management of individual vessel injuries

Artery versus vein

As a general rule, arteries that are not end-vessels should be repaired, whereas most veins, including the popliteal and deep femoral veins, can be ligated without significant threat of loss of limb, provided liberal fasciotomy is performed. The popliteal and deep femoral veins should be repaired if simple end-to-end suture or lateral repair will suffice. If the vein is to be ligated and there is a concomitant arterial injury, consider harvesting the vein for the arterial repair from the vein to be ligated, particularly for injuries in the upper limb. Tradition, however, dictates that the harvested vein should come from an uninjured limb, without good evidence to support this contention.[3,50,51]

Technical aspects for definitive repair

Prophylactic antibiotic coverage with a first-generation cephalosporin is usually adequate, although current recommendations suggest doubling the usual dose (e.g., cefazolin, 2 g) and giving broader cover only if the wound is severely contaminated (additional Gram-negative coverage, e.g., amoxicillin-clavulanate or its equivalent).[53]

Proximal and distal control should be obtained away from the injury site, looping the vessels for easy control. The Rumel tourniquet is a useful device in this setting.[54] It eliminates the difficulty of gaining access through distorted tissue planes and hematoma. Once this control is achieved, then the injury can be exposed and assessed. Spasm does not generally occur in cases of penetrating trauma (except in small children), so a vessel that looks "in spasm" must be opened and the intimal layer inspected.[3] This is especially true with the percussion effect from gunshot and shotgun injuries.

After the vessel is opened, the next step is to clear any stasis clot from the vessel in both directions with the use of a Fogarty embolectomy catheter and then flush the open vessel with heparinized saline (1000 IU). Then the repair can be planned (see the section on Options for repair, below). After vessel continuity is re-established, a completion on-table angiogram should confirm vessel patency and good distal run-off (Figure 16.7).

Options for repair

Options for vascular repair are listed below:

- Simple lateral or transverse suturing.

- Debridement and primary end-to-end repair if the ends can be joined without tension.[51]
- Resection to healthy vessel ends and interposition of a vascular conduit: either a reversed autologous vein (especially for smaller vessels) or polytetrafluoroethylene (PTFE), which is associated with fewer septic complications than the more traditional Dacron grafts used in elective vascular surgery.[55]
- End arteries that have adequate collateral flow can be ligated.
- Endovascular repairs with covered stent grafts have been used for thoracic outlet and proximal limb vessels (subclavian and axillary) with access difficulties, mostly in stable patients, but are associated with complications and concerns about long-term patency. These procedures should be considered experimental at this stage.[19,56–59]

Repairs should always be covered with at least one layer of tissue other than skin and fascia to reduce the risk of infection and breakdown of the anastomosis. A closed suction drain is commonly left in the vicinity of the repair to drain lymphatic fluid seepage caused by dissection of tissue planes to access the vessels.[3,51]

Conservative management

With notable exceptions, such as minor intimal flaps from blunt injury, conservative management of penetrating arterial injury is uncommon. Suspected venous injury, however, can be managed expectantly, provided the skin wound is closed, no ongoing blood loss is evident, and the hematoma is not enlarging. Most venous injuries will coagulate and then recanalize over time.[60]

Upper limb

Most axillary brachial injuries should be repaired. One of the three vessels in the forearm below the elbow and branches in the hand can be ligated because of the extensive network of collaterals in those regions. The Allen test may support clinical decision-making regarding the need to revascularize the hand or forearm vessels, with non-perfusion of the distal limb indicating inadequate collateral blood supply. Below the axilla, the use of autologous vein is recommended because of the small size of the vessels.

Lower limb

The complex ileo-femoral junction and the common and superficial femoral arteries should be repaired with either autologous vein or PTFE. The femoral profunda branches into the thigh have significant collaterals and may be ligated. The troublesome vessel in the lower limb, with a high related amputation rate, is the popliteal artery, which is more commonly injured by blunt trauma (knee dislocation) than with penetrating injury. However, a number of these arteries were injured by penetrating trauma during the civil unrest in Ireland in the late 1980s, when collaborators were shot through the kneecaps! (D. Trunkey, personal communication, *James IVth Travelling Fellowship Report*, 1984.) This vessel is best repaired with autologous vein to ensure good distal run-off.[6]

The trifurcation vessels and foot vessels are often injured singly. They can be ligated, provided there is good clinical evidence of adequate collateral blood flow. Another option is endovascular embolization during catheter-directed angiography, provided the patient is stable enough to undergo such a procedure.

Postoperative complications

As with any surgical procedure or traumatic injury, wound sepsis, lymphatic leaks, and contaminated wounds require appropriate debridement. The open fasciotomy wound may initially require negative-pressure vacuum therapy and, eventually, flaps or skin grafts. Wounds that traverse the abdomen and limbs and high-velocity ballistic injuries are at high risk for necrotizing fasciitis, which should be sought vigilantly in all such cases. The management of these complications and the need for re-look operations are undertaken in line with standard surgical principles.

Of more importance are the specific consequences of the vascular injury and its repair; namely, reperfusion injury with resultant local sequelae (compartment syndrome) and systemic effects (myonephropathic or crush syndrome) (Figure 16.8). Ischemia/reperfusion injury is common after repair of vascular trauma. The traditional period of risk (> 6 hours of ischemia) is definitely not a fixed value. Significant muscle ischemia and cell death can occur within a much shorter time after injury. This pathophysiologic process manifests as swelling and tenderness in the compartments, caused by cellular edema, which is induced by loss of Na-K-ATPase cellular junctional function and the resulting efflux of myoglobin and potassium along with influx

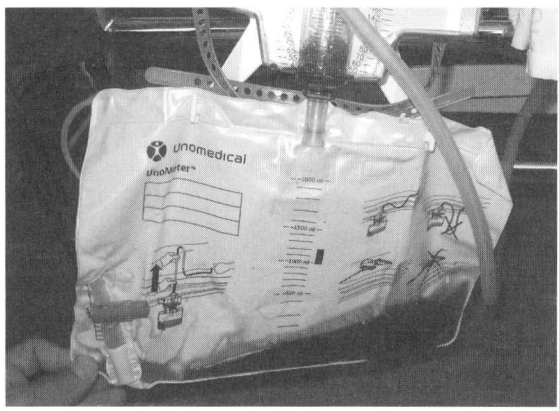

Figure 16.8 Myoglobinuria noted after reperfusion of ischemic muscle compartment in a patient with multiple penetrating wounds to the limb and abdomen (crush syndrome).

of sodium; cellular swelling occurs when water follows the sodium. Within the tight enclosure of a myofascial compartment, this leads to further compression ischemia and progression to neurovascular compromise. The situation is further complicated when the compartment contains a large primary hematoma. The important aspect of treatment is recognition and early fasciotomy.

Systemically, the more severe consequences occur after reperfusion, when liberated extracellular potassium, myoglobin, and other enzymatic degradation products flood the venous system and create physiologic chaos. This results in myocardial depression and the risk of hyperkalemic cardiac irritability; acute lung injury and the need for ventilatory support; systemic vasodilatation with a septic-shock-like picture; and the major risk of pigment-induced myonephropathic syndrome with the need for renal replacement therapy. Early use of resuscitation fluids that do not contain potassium, cardioprotection with calcium chloride administration, and interventions to control hyperkalemia (e.g., infusion of insulin-dextrose and bicarbonate) are essential. Early dialysis may be required, and inotropic support may be needed if signs of cardiogenic shock are present.[61,62]

Rehabilitation

Early involvement of physical therapists and occupational therapists in the mobilization of the revascularized limb is essential to prevent joint stiffness, muscle atrophy, and contracture development. Prevention of contractures with splinting and the use of dynamic hand splints after upper limb fasciotomy are recommended.[63,64] Psychological and social support for the patient is also essential.[65]

Conclusion

Penetrating vascular trauma of the limbs is a highly morbid and potentially fatal injury pattern. Early identification of the injury and rapid surgical intervention with appropriate imaging, as indicated, will decrease the risk of limb loss. Careful observation and early intervention for the postoperative consequences of injury will reduce the need for amputation. Liberal use of fasciotomy will increase the chances of limb salvage; however, early or late amputation may be required in some circumstances.

Critical actions

- Early surgical access and rapid transfer to definitive care saves limbs.
- Identify catastrophic bleeding. Prehospital tourniquets may be life-saving.
- Comprehensive systematic assessment of the patient with a penetrating limb injury is essential.
- Activate massive hemorrhage protocols early.
- Identify the threatened limb; consider early fasciotomy.
- Consider appropriate use of imaging modalities (most patients need very little imaging): early surgical exploration without imaging is more important.
- Consider the use of damage control techniques and vessel shunting.
- Identify the specific type of injury.
- Military wounds require more extensive attention.
- Identify spasm in children; expect an injury in adults.
- Select the right type of repair or ligation for the right patient.
- Ensure rapid, tension-free repairs with tissue coverage.
- Anticipate local and systemic complications and preserve the kidneys.
- Refer the patient for rehabilitation to the relevant discipline(s).

Clinical approach when resources are limited

Countries with limited resources often have a scourge of penetrating trauma for a variety of reasons. Fortunately, penetrating extremity vascular injuries are usually clinically evident, so simple equipment such as radiology facilities, basic intravenous access, contrast material, and willing trained personnel are sufficient for their management. The majority of vascular injuries can be managed with early open surgical intervention, using autologous tissue for repair, provided that the injury is identified and the patient is transferred early to the best-equipped regional facility. Early fasciotomy, renal prophylaxis, and the use of tourniquets enhance the chance of survival for penetrating trauma victims in these countries. Adoption and implementation of the "Essential Trauma Care" principles of the Violence and Injury Department of the World Health Organization is encouraged.[66] Following basic surgical principles will lead to good outcomes, even with limited resources.

Pearls and pitfalls

- Do not let "obvious" limb injuries distract team from occult life-threatening injuries. Limb injuries seldom cause death!
- Clinical assessment of the limb is essential. Most vascular injuries of immediate significance are fairly obvious.
- Do an unnecessary fasciotomy rather than an unnecessary amputation.
- Dead limbs cannot be resurrected; early amputation may be the treatment of choice.
- Tension-free repairs with a confirmatory on-table angiogram are associated with the best limb survival.
- Do not spend endless time repairing veins that have adequate collaterals.
- Children are best served by a conservative approach; adults do better with aggressive intervention.
- A bruised or "spasmed" vessel is an intimal injury until proven otherwise – explore it!
- CT angiography has a high false-negative rate with penetrating injury. When indicated, imaging is best done with conventional angiography.

- The surgeon must remain with the patient while other orthopedic procedures are undertaken.

References

1. Norman R. *Estimates of Injury Mortality and Disability Based on the Cape Metropole Study*. Cape Town: South African Medical Research Council; 2002.

2. Bondurant FJ, Cotler, HB, Buckle R, *et al.* The medical and economic impact of severely injured lower extremities. *J Trauma* 1988; 28: 1270–3.

3. Boffard KD, ed. *Manual of Definitive Surgical Trauma Care*, 2nd edition. London: Hodder Arnold; 2002.

4. Scalea TM. Optimal timing of fracture fixation: have we learned anything in 20 years? *J Trauma* 2008; 65: 253–60.

5. United Nations Economic and Social Council: Commission on Crime Prevention and Criminal Justice. *Criminal Justice Reform and Strengthening of Legal Institutions Measures to Regulate Firearms* (Report E /CN.15 /1997/4). Vienna: United Nations Commission on Crime Prevention and Criminal Justice; 1997. Available at www.uncjin.org/Documents/6comm/4e.pdf. Accessed on March 30, 2012.

6. Degiannis E, Velmahos GC, Florizone MG, *et al.* Penetrating injuries of the popliteal artery: the Baragwanath experience. *Ann R Coll Surg Engl* 1994; 76: 307–10.

7. Robbs JV, Carrim AA, Kadwa AM, *et al.* Traumatic arteriovenous fistula: experience with 201 patients. *Br J Surg* 1994; 81: 1296–9.

8. Degiannis E, Levy RD, Velmahos GC, *et al.* Penetrating injuries of the femoral artery. *Br J Surg* 1995; 82: 492–5.

9. Degiannis E, Levy RD, Sofianos C, *et al.* Arterial gunshot injuries of the extremities: a South African experience. *J Trauma* 1995; 39: 570–5.

10. Mars M, Hadley GP. Raised intracompartmental pressure and compartment syndrome. *Injury* 1998; 29: 403–11.

11. Nair R, Abdool Carrim AT, Robbs JV. Gunshot injuries of the popliteal artery. *Br J Surg* 2000; 87: 602–7.

12. Bowley DM, Degiannis E, Goosen J, *et al.* Penetrating vascular trauma in Johannesburg, South Africa. *Surg Clin North Am* 2002; 82: 221–35.

13. Zellweger R, Hess F, Nicol A, *et al.* An analysis of 124 surgically managed brachial artery injuries. *Am J Surg* 2004; 188: 240–5.

14. Hardcastle TC, Johnson W. Brachial artery injuries: a seven-year experience with a prospective database. *Eur J Trauma Emerg Surg* 2008; 34: 493–7.

15. Padayachy V, Robbs JV, Mulaudzi TV, *et al.* A retrospective review of brachial artery injuries and repairs – is it still a "training artery"? *Injury* 2010; 41: 843–6.

16. Sobnach S, Nicol A, Nathire H, *et al.* Management of the retained knife blade. *World J Surg* 2010; 34: 1648–52.

17. Borut LT, Acosta CJ, Tadlock LC, *et al.* The use of temporary vascular shunts in military extremity wounds: a preliminary outcome analysis with 2-year follow-up. *J Trauma* 2010; 69: 174–8.

18. Chambers LW, Green DJ, Sample K, *et al.* Tactical surgical intervention with temporary shunting of peripheral vascular trauma during Operation Iraqi Freedom: one unit's experience. *J Trauma* 2006; 61: 824–30.

19. Fox CJ, Gillespie DL, O'Donnell SD, *et al.* Contemporary management of wartime vascular trauma. *J Vasc Surg* 2005; 41: 638–44.

20. Ramsamy A, Hill AM, Clasper JC. Improvised explosive devices: pathophysiology, injury profiles and current medical management. *J R Army Med Corps* 2008; 155: 265–72.

21. Tai NRM, Dickson EJ. Military junctional trauma. *J R Army Med Corps* 2008; 155: 285–92.

22. Hardcastle T, Hoogerboord M, Du Toit DF. The injured femoral vessels [abstract]. *S Afr Med J* 2006; 96: 556.

23. Campbell JE, ed. *International Trauma Life Support for Prehospital Care Providers*, 6th edition. Upper Saddle River, NJ: Prentice-Hall; 2007.

24. Sanders MJ. *Mosby's Paramedic Textbook. Revised Third Edition*. San Diego, CA: Mosby-JEMS; 2007.

25. Ahleart B. *Emergency Medical Technician*, 2nd edition. New York: McGraw-Hill Emergency Care; 2010.

26. Kozen BG, Kirschner SJ, Henao J, *et al.* An alternative hemostatic dressing: comparison of Celox, Hemcon and Quikclot. *Acad Emerg Med* 2008; 15: 74–81.

27. Lawton G, Granville-Chapman J, Parker PJ. Novel haemostatic dressings. *J R Army Med Corps* 2008; 155: 309–14.

28. Mabry J, McManus JG. Prehospital advances in the management of severe penetrating trauma. *Crit Care Med* 2008; 36: S258–66.

29. Lee C, Porter KM, Hodgetts TJ. Tourniquet use in the civilian prehospital setting. *Emerg Med J* 2007; 24: 584–7.

30. Deo SD, Knottenbelt JD, Peden MM. Evaluation of a small trauma team for major resuscitation. *Injury* 1997; 28: 633–7.

31. American College of Surgeons Committee on Trauma. *ATLS Student Course Manual*, 8th edition. Chicago, IL: American College of Surgeons; 2008.

32. Hardcastle TC. Complications of massive transfusion in trauma patients. *ISBT Sci Ser* 2006; 1: 180–4.

33. Hardcastle TC. Massive transfusion in trauma: practicalities and management of complications. *Spec Forum* 2006; 6: 23–9.

34. Juchesne JC, Hunt JP, Wahl G, *et al.* Review of current blood transfusions strategies in a mature level 1 trauma center: were we wrong for the last 60 years? *J Trauma* 2008; 65: 272–8.

35. Frykberg ER, Dennis JW, Bishop K, *et al.* The reliability of physical examination in the evaluation of penetrating extremity trauma for vascular injury: results at one year. *J Trauma* 1991; 34: 502–11.

36. Hardcastle TC, Baatjes KJ, Du Toit DF. Routine arteriogram in Zone-1 penetrating neck trauma: is it required? [abstract 25]. International Surgical Week 2007, Montreal, Canada: International Surgical Society – Societe Internationale de Chirurgie; 2007: 32.

37. Nassoura ZE, Ivatury RR, Simon RJ, *et al.* A reassessment of Doppler pressure indices in the detection of arterial lesions in proximity penetrating injuries of extremities: a prospective study. *Am J Emerg Med* 1996; 14: 151–6.

38. O'Gorman RB, Feliciano DV, Bitondo CG, *et al.* Emergency center arteriography in the evaluation of suspected peripheral vascular injuries. *Arch Surg* 1984; 119: 568–73.

39. Beningfield S, Potgieter H, Nicol A, *et al.* Report on a new type of trauma full-body digital X-ray machine. *Emerg Radiol* 2003; 10: 23–9.

40. Ball CG, Nicol AJ, Beningfield SJ, *et al.* Emergency room arteriography: an updated digital technology. *Scand J Surg* 2007; 96: 67–71.

41. Busquets AR, Acosta JA, Colon E, *et al.* Helical computed tomographic angiography for the diagnosis of traumatic arterial injuries of the extremities. *J Trauma* 2004; 56: 625–8.

42. Shah N, Anderson SW, Vu M, *et al.* Extremity CT-angiography: application to trauma using 64-MDCT. *Emerg Radiol* 2009; 16: 425–32.

43. Anderson SW, Foster BR, Soto JA. Upper extremity CT-angiography in penetrating trauma: use of a 64-section multidetector CT. *Radiology* 2008; 249: 1064–73.

44. Knudson MM, Lewis FR, Atkinson K, *et al.* The role of duplex ultrasound arterial imaging in patients with penetrating extremity trauma. *Arch Surg* 1993; 128: 1033–7.

45. Mill RP, Robbs JV. Pediatric arterial injury: management options at the time of injury. *J R Coll Surg Edinb* 1991; 36: 13–17.

46. De Virgilio C, Mercado PD. Noniatrogenic pediatric vascular trauma: a ten-year experience at a level I trauma center. *Am Surg* 1997; 63: 781–4.

47. Klinker DB, MJ Arca, BD Lewis, *et al.* Pediatric vascular injuries: patterns of injury, morbidity, and mortality. *J Pediatr Surg* 2007; 42: 178–83.

48. Shah SR, Wearden PD, Gaines BA. Pediatric peripheral vascular injuries: a review of our experience. *J Surg Res* 2009; 153: 162–6.

49. St Peter SD, Ostlie DJ. A review of vascular surgery in the pediatric population. *Pediatr Surg Int* 2007; 23: 1–10.

50. Moeng MS, Loveland JA, Boffard KD. Damage control: beyond the limits of the abdominal cavity: a review. *Trauma Care* (ITACCS) 2005; 15: 189–96.

51. Hardcastle TC. Operating on the traumatized patient: the team approach. *Arch Ibadan Med* 2006; 7: 15–8.

52. Hardcastle TC. Ethical and medico-legal aspects of trauma. *S Afr J Bioethics Law* 2010; 3: 25–7.

53. Hoff WS, Bonadies JA, Cachecho R, *et al.* EAST Practice Management Guidelines Workgroup: update to the practice management guidelines for prophylactic antibiotic use in open fractures. *J Trauma* 2011; 70: 751–4.

54. Welling DR, Rich NM, Burris DG, *et al.* Who was William Ray Rumel? *World J Surg* 2008; 32: 2122–5.

55. Feliciano DV, Mattox KL, Graham JM, *et al.* Five-year experience with PTFE grafts in vascular wounds. *J Trauma* 1985; 25: 71–82.

56. Du Toit DF, Leith JG, Strauss DC, *et al.* Endovascular management of traumatic cervicothoracic arteriovenous fistula. *Br J Surg* 2003; 90: 1516–21.

57. Du Toit DF, Strauss DC, Blaszczyk M, *et al.* Endovascular treatment of penetrating thoracic outlet arterial injuries. *Eur J Vasc Endovasc Surg* 2000; 19: 489–95.

58. Du Toit DF, Odendaal W, Lambrechts A, *et al.* Surgical and endovascular management of penetrating innominate artery injuries. *Eur J Vasc Endovasc Surg* 2008; 36: 56–62.

59. Rasmussen TE, Clouse WD, Peck MA, *et al.* Development and implementation of endovascular capabilities in wartime. *J Trauma* 2008; 64: 1169–76.

60. Dennis JW, Frykberg ER, Veldenz HC, *et al.* Validation of nonoperative management of occult vascular injuries and accuracy of physical examination alone in penetrating extremity trauma: 5 to 10-year follow-up. *J Trauma* 1998; 44: 243–52.

61. Brown CVR, Rhee P, Chan L, *et al.* Preventing renal failure in patients with rhabdomyolysis: do bicarbonate and mannitol make a difference? *J Trauma* 2004; 56: 1191–6.

62. Smith WA, Hardcastle TC. A crushing experience: the spectrum and outcome of soft tissue injury and myonephropathic syndrome at an urban South African university hospital. *Afr J Emerg Med (AfJEM)* 2011; 1: 17–24.

63. Ellis E, Lamb S. Physiotherapy following injury. In Langstaff D, Christie J, eds. *Trauma Care – A Team Approach.* Oxford, UK: Butterworth-Heinemann; 2000: 290–7.

64. McDowell H. The role of the occupational therapist in trauma care. In Langstaff D, Christie J, eds. *Trauma Care – A Team Approach.* Oxford, UK: Butterworth-Heinemann; 2000: 298–309.

65. Davidson K. The consequences of altered body image following trauma. In Langstaff D, Christie J, eds. *Trauma Care – A Team Approach.* Oxford, UK: Butterworth-Heinemann; 2000: 262–9.

66. Mock C, Lormand JD, Goosen J, *et al. Guidelines for Essential Trauma Care.* Geneva, Switzerland: World Health Organization; 2004.

Acute mesenteric ischemia

George C. Willis

Acute mesenteric ischemia (AMI) is a life-threatening disease that should be in the differential diagnosis for any patient who presents with complaints of abdominal pain. Over the past several years, physicians' awareness of acute mesenteric ischemia has increased, leading to more successful treatment and better outcomes. Overall, the incidence of AMI is still fairly low, accounting for 1 in every 1,000 hospitalizations.[1,2] However, this number is slowly increasing as the proportion of elderly rises in the United States and throughout the rest of the world. With that rise comes an increase in diseases that predispose the elderly to increased risk of mesenteric ischemia. AMI is associated with a mortality rate as high as 70%.[2–9] The high rate is predominantly due to delays in diagnosis. Misdiagnosis and delays in the management of a patient with AMI can have drastic outcomes. It is incumbent upon the emergency provider to remain vigilant in the diagnosis and management of this lethal condition.

Anatomy

The vasculature of the gastrointestinal tract arises directly off the aorta. The three main arteries supplying arterial flow to the gastrointestinal tract, namely the celiac artery (CA), the superior mesenteric artery (SMA), and the inferior mesenteric artery (IMA), are associated with the organs from their embryologic origins. During the growth of the fetus, a collateral arterial system develops to ensure continued perfusion to the gastrointestinal tract.

The CA provides blood to the organs derived from the embryologic foregut: the esophagus, the stomach, the liver, the spleen, and the top portion of the pancreas and the duodenum. The CA originates at nearly a 90° angle; therefore, occlusion by thrombosis or embolism is very rare.

The SMA originates approximately 1 cm below the CA. It provides blood to the organs derived from the embryologic midgut: the bottom half of the pancreas and duodenum, the entire small intestines, and the first two-thirds of the large intestines. The SMA provides arterial blood to the largest portion of the gastrointestinal tract. It branches off the aorta at an angle of about 30° and is directed inferiorly, which predisposes it to arterial compromise from thrombosis or embolism, making it the most affected artery in mesenteric ischemia.

The IMA originates right above the aortic bifurcation into the common iliac arteries. The IMA provides blood supply to the organs derived from the hindgut, i.e., the last third of the large intestines, the sigmoid colon, and the rectum.

There is also collateral arterial circulation between these three arteries. The CA and SMA have collateral circulation between the superior pancreaticoduodenal artery, which branches off the celiac artery, and the inferior pancreaticoduodenal artery, which branches off the SMA. These provide perfusion to the pancreas and the first part of the duodenum. The SMA and the IMA have collateral circulation by way of the marginal artery of Drummond and the arc of Riolan, which provide arterial perfusion to the large intestines.

Etiology

The most common cause of ischemia is an occlusive event that interrupts the major arterial blood supply to an organ. The three most common causes of acute mesenteric ischemia are SMA embolism, SMA

Vascular Emergencies, ed. Robert L. Rogers, Thomas Scalea, Lee Wallis, and Heike Geduld. Published by Cambridge University Press. © Cambridge University Press 2013.

Table 17.1 Risk factors for SMA embolism

- Cardiac dysrhythmias such as atrial fibrillation.
- Valvular disorders.
- Ventricular aneurysm.
- Ventricular thrombi.
- Cardiomyopathy.
- Right-to-left shunts (e.g., patent foramen ovale).
- History of embolic phenomenon (e.g., stroke, digital ischemia).

Table 17.2 Risk factors for SMA thrombosis

- Hypercholesterolemia.
- Coronary artery disease.
- Diabetes mellitus.
- Hypertension.
- Chronic mesenteric ischemia.
- Aortic atherosclerotic disease.
- Smoking.
- Female gender.

thrombosis, and non-occlusive mesenteric ischemia (NOMI). Superior mesenteric artery embolism and SMA thrombosis account for 50–80% of all cases of AMI in the United States.[1,2] Non-occlusive mesenteric ischemia accounts for about 20% of AMI. The least common cause, mesenteric venous thrombosis (MVT), is discussed separately.

Superior mesenteric artery embolism

Superior mesenteric artery embolus, the most common cause of AMI, is responsible for 35 to 50% of cases worldwide.[1,2,4] Patients with SMA emboli are usually at risk secondary to conditions that predispose them to embolus formation, including cardiac arrhythmias (e.g., atrial fibrillation), valvular heart disease, and ventricular thrombus (Table 17.1). Emboli often form in the left heart circulation, travel to the arterial side, and then enter the systemic circulation, placing end organs, including the gastrointestinal tract, at risk.

Once an embolus forms, it is most likely to enter the SMA because of its width and acute angle of branching. The CA has an obtuse angle and the IMA has a narrow caliber. Also, there is usually sufficient collateral circulation in the organs perfused by these arteries to avoid significant ischemia should an embolus occlude one of them. The SMA, on the other hand, has the largest area of intestines to perfuse but inadequate collateral circulation, predisposing the organs to ischemia. Furthermore, emboli tend to lodge distal to the middle colic artery, which places the small intestines at the highest risk of ischemia.[10] The rest of the organs supplied by the SMA are largely unaffected, owing to collateral circulation.

Patients with SMA emboli have rapid progression of symptoms compared with those with thrombosis. Subsequently, necrosis sets in much faster and is more complete with SMA embolus because of the lack of arterial blood supply. The rapidity of progression leads to a mortality rate of 70%.[2,4]

Superior mesenteric artery thrombosis

Thrombosis of the SMA is the cause of 15 to 30% of cases of mesenteric ischemia.[2,4] Thrombosis occurs in the setting of atherosclerotic disease in the aorta and the mesenteric vasculature. The pathophysiology is similar to that of acute myocardial infarction. Patients who experience an SMA thrombosis usually have an element of chronic mesenteric ischemia, the same way patients who have myocardial infarctions usually have an element of coronary artery disease.[2,11] Risk factors for SMA thrombosis are presented in Table 17.2.

As in acute myocardial infarction, in SMA thrombosis, an atherosclerotic plaque builds up in the artery and then ruptures. Platelets aggregate at the site of the plaque causing a thrombotic occlusion. This occurs most commonly at the origin of the SMA off the aorta. Patients with this condition often experience "intestinal angina," a symptom of decreased perfusion of the gut when eating, which causes abdominal pain and goes away when they are not eating (equivalent to stable angina in cardiac patients). This sensation is caused by atherosclerotic disease of the aorta that transiently diminishes perfusion to the bowel when it is working (i.e., digesting) and returns to adequate flow when at rest. If the pain occurs without eating or if the pain does not stop several hours after eating, it is the equivalent of unstable angina or acute myocardial infarction of the bowel and should be thought of as an emergency.

Patients with SMA thrombosis have a very high mortality rate: up to 90%.[1,4] Although they have built up adequate collateral vessels through the years of chronic ischemia, large areas of bowel are affected by thrombosis because of the widespread atherosclerosis. This condition usually requires a large bowel resection and can lead to multiple postoperative complications such as short gut syndrome, renal insufficiency, and multiple operations.[12]

Non-occlusive mesenteric ischemia

NOMI is an entity of mesenteric ischemia that is not caused by embolism or thrombosis, but by a non-occlusive event that brings about decreased blood flow through the mesenteric vasculature. Most commonly, this is due to a low-flow state such as hypotension, depressed cardiac output, hemodialysis, or cardiac surgery. As a result of this low-flow state, global vaso-constriction occurs, including the mesenteric vessels. Commonly, there is atherosclerotic disease present in these vessels exacerbating the decreased blood flow during low-flow states, leading to ischemia. Other causes include medications such as digoxin, vasopressors, ergot alkaloids, and cocaine, which can bring about splanchnic vasoconstriction leading to NOMI. Twenty-five percent of patients with NOMI may experience no abdominal pain, which can be due to the critical state of the patient, and the diagnosis is suspected due to unexplained abdominal distention or gastrointestinal bleeding.[2,13] Mortality for NOMI is 50 to 90%, often due to delays in diagnosis but also the critical condition of the patient and the difficulty in treating the underlying condition.[2,10]

Disease progression

After arterial blood flow is interrupted to the organs, the artery goes through intense spasm, exacerbating tissue ischemia. Initially this causes bowel wall spasm, leading to gut emptying. Tissue edema sets in and subsequent fluid sequestration out of the vasculature and into the periphery causes shock. Meanwhile, toxins and free radicals combine with gut flora and translocate across the compromised bowel wall and enter the systemic circulation, leading to sepsis. Eventually, the lack of oxygen supply leads to bowel wall necrosis and microperforations, often resulting in frank perforation. The intravascular bacteria and toxins as well as fluid sequestration into the extravascular space eventually lead to shock and circulatory collapse. This cascade of events can transpire very quickly, with irreversible bowel necrosis occurring in as little as eight hours.

Diagnosis

Clinical presentation

A thorough history and physical examination are paramount to making the diagnosis and decreasing adverse outcomes in this patient population. The classic presentation of abdominal pain, signs of gastric emptying, and history of cardiac disease is found in only 30% of patients. Abdominal pain is the most common complaint, present in virtually all patients with mesenteric ischemia.[14,15]

The characteristics of the abdominal pain vary and can be helpful with delineating the possible cause of the ischemia. The pain associated with SMA emboli is usually acute in onset. Patients usually remember exactly when the pain began and exactly what they were doing when it occurred. It tends to be very sharp and unrelenting, and patients become more uncomfortable as its duration increases.

An acute onset of abdominal pain can signal SMA thrombosis as well, but, because of atherosclerotic disease, its onset can be more insidious. Many patients with SMA thrombosis have advanced atherosclerotic disease of the aorta and the mesenteric vessels. As a result, they have chronic mesenteric ischemia and have experienced episodes of "intestinal angina." Therefore, patients often give a history of multiple bouts of abdominal pain that either increased in severity or did not subside.

Other complaints expressed by patients with AMI are non-specific. Nausea is the next most common symptom, seen in around 50 to 60% of patients; while gastrointestinal emptying in the form of vomiting and diarrhea is found in about 30%.[2,5] Bloody diarrhea or emesis is noted less commonly, at around 15%.[5] Altered mental status can occur in patients in shock states or with sepsis, especially the elderly.

Other diagnostic clues lie in the medical history, as they can indicate risk factors for the development of AMI. A history of embolic conditions (e.g., stroke) or cardiac dysrhythmias suggests the possibility of SMA embolism. A history of coronary artery disease or chronic mesenteric ischemia shows risk for SMA thrombosis. The patient's use of medications or non-compliance with medication instructions, such as warfarin for patients with atrial fibrillation, should be ascertained.

Physical examination findings in patients with AMI are equally non-specific. Findings are usually very difficult to link to the diagnosis. Patients usually present with the classic "pain out of proportion," meaning the abdomen will be soft despite the patient's complaints of severe abdominal tenderness. This finding can be helpful if the emergency care provider is considering the diagnosis. However, it can lead the care provider to minimize the patient's complaint because of the absence of a surgical abdomen. Among patients with AMI, a surgical abdomen is often a sign of perforation or significant bowel necrosis. A rectal examination, including a fecal occult blood test, should be performed on all patients in whom mesenteric ischemia is suspected. The presence of occult blood is another late finding, but its presence should alert the emergency physician to pursue the diagnosis. Bowel sounds remain early in the disease, until ischemia progresses, causing the sounds to diminish.

Other physical examination findings are non-specific for mesenteric ischemia but may be helpful in identifying ischemic causes. Auscultation of the heart may reveal an irregular rhythm, murmurs, or other arrhythmias that suggest underlying cardiac conditions. Tachypnea, specifically deep and rapid breathing, may be an underlying sign of metabolic acidosis from lactic acid production. Signs of previous embolic events such as residual neurologic deficits from a previous stroke or amputations necessitated by limb ischemia should clue the provider in to possible SMA embolism. Most patients with AMI have fever and tachycardia, but these signs also can be absent.

The elderly population is most at risk for mesenteric ischemia. Many confounding factors can make this diagnosis much more difficult in this population. The mortality rate associated with mesenteric ischemia increases with age, most likely due to delays in diagnosis. Elderly patients tend to have decreased pain sensation and many patients delay their presentation for treatment. Cognitive impairment may also delay treatment as well as diagnosis, as altered mental status may direct the emergency care provider away from the abdomen altogether. Polypharmacy also plays a significant role in elderly patients' presentation for medical care. Pain medications, such as non-steroidal anti-inflammatory drugs (NSAIDs) and opiates, can blunt the pain response and decrease an already slowed gastrointestinal motility, lessening the likelihood of vomiting and diarrhea. NSAIDs and acetaminophen can mask a fever, and β-adrenergic antagonists can mask tachycardia. Therefore, the provider must maintain a wide differential with the elderly population, especially those with complaints of abdominal pain.

Laboratory studies

Laboratory studies should be obtained in all patients with a suspicion of mesenteric ischemia, with the understanding that reliance on certain values, especially for elderly patients, will likely muddy the picture. Multiple abnormal laboratory values can suggest the diagnosis; however, there are no laboratory tests specific for mesenteric ischemia. Patients with AMI can have a significant leukocytosis, often in excess of $15,000/mm^3$. An elevated hemoglobin and hematocrit showing hemoconcentration might also be present as well as elevated amylase and liver transaminase levels.

An elevated lactic acid concentration is present in most patients with AMI, and this indicator was for a while thought of as an adequate screening test for the diagnosis. Its sensitivity is about 96% for the presence of mesenteric ischemia.[2] However, the presence of lactic acid is a late finding, and the absence of lactic acid in a patient with a high clinical suspicion should not falsely relieve the provider. Some new studies with D-lactate and L-lactate show promise.[2,16] These lactate isomers are released into the circulation by gut flora, which overgrow in the setting of bowel wall ischemia.

Diagnostic imaging

Imaging is the mainstay of the diagnosis of AMI. Multiple imaging modalities can be performed and are chosen depending on what is available.

Plain radiographs are the least helpful modality in the diagnosis of AMI. They miss up to 75% of cases because the findings are non-specific and often very subtle, especially early in the disease course. Early findings include a paucity of bowel gas or an ileus-like pattern. Later findings include portal venous or biliary air, thumbprinting (signs of mural wall necrosis or hemorrhage), pneumatosis intestinalis (air in the bowel wall) and pneumoperitoneum.[2,11,17] Radiographs are helpful in the evaluation of patients with peritoneal signs for pneumoperitoneum.

Ultrasound findings are often non-specific and not helpful. They include decreased peristalsis, dilated loops of bowel, and portal venous or biliary air, all of which are late findings.[18] With the use of Doppler flow, ultrasound can evaluate the mesenteric vessels for signs of occlusion, displaying dilated vessels with clot within the lumen.[1,2,11,17] Its limitation is that it is heavily dependent on the operator's skill and the patient's body habitus. In addition, in AMI, there is often gaseous distention of the bowel, making the visualization of the mesenteric vasculature more problematic. Therefore, this modality is not recommended.

Multidetector computed tomography (MDCT) has become the most frequently used imaging modality in the assessment of patients for mesenteric ischemia. With its higher definition and smaller cuts, as well as the addition of MDCT angiography, this modality is comparable to angiography in the diagnosis of AMI. This imaging is performed with intravenous contrast, and the images are usually obtained in the arterial and venous phases. The advantage of MDCT is that it can evaluate the bowel for signs of ischemia and perforation. Oral contrast is not needed and actually may make the images more difficult to read, but water in the gastrointestinal tract distends the bowel loops, facilitating evaluation of the bowel wall.[17,19,20] MDCT angiography can also allow evaluation of the mesenteric vasculature for signs of occlusion. Findings suggestive of acute mesenteric ischemia include bowel wall edema, diminished contrast enhancement of the bowel wall, pneumatosis intestinalis, and portal venous or biliary air. Findings indicating occlusion include diminished contrast enhancement of affected areas of the bowel wall, cutoff of contrast in the vasculature, and infarcts of organs.[17,20] MDCT can also reveal significant atherosclerotic disease of the vasculature. MDCT does not allow interventions to be performed during the imaging, but it is an important non-invasive screening test for AMI.

MRI is comparable to CT scanning in its ability to diagnose AMI. MRA enhances the diagnostic usefulness. Magnetic resonance imaging should be considered in patients with contraindications to CT or intravenous contrast. The limitations of MRI are that it cannot be used on patients with metallic foreign bodies (iatrogenic or otherwise) and that it is time consuming and costly.

Angiography is the gold standard in diagnosis of AMI. This is the only modality shown to improve survival in patients with AMI if performed before the development of peritoneal signs. However, it requires a large dye load, is invasive, is time consuming, is not always available, and is expensive, making it a poor screening examination, except in the patient for which there is a very high suspicion. Since the advent of CT, especially after new programming allowed CT angiography, 3D reconstructions, and smaller cuts, CT has supplanted this modality as the preferred screening modality.[17,19] Angiography still has a role as the definitive study of choice in patients with positive findings on other imaging modalities, and it is useful for intervening as well. It should also be the imaging method of choice in patients with a high suspicion, as these patients will certainly benefit. Once the lesion is identified, intra-arterial papaverine (a vasodilator) and thrombolytics can be directed right to the problem area. Angiography does not evaluate the bowel for signs of infarction, which forces the provider to rely on other means: usually the clinical examination, other imaging modalities, or laparotomy.[19]

Emergency department management

Initial assessment

The keys to the management of acute mesenteric ischemia are prompt diagnosis, resuscitation and stabilization, and early surgical consultation for prompt revascularization. Unfortunately, in most cases, one of these steps is delayed and it becomes incumbent upon the emergency care provider to ensure that time-effective management occurs. A delay in any of these steps is detrimental to the patient and often results in adverse outcomes.

Begin by placing at least one large-bore line for IV access; two if possible. Administer isotonic fluids intravenously to increase perfusion to the gastrointestinal tract. Because of decreased perfusion in the ischemic portion, the body will attempt to compensate by vasoconstricting the splanchnic vasculature to increase perfusion pressure to the rest of the bowel wall. This can worsen ischemia as well as widen the area of affected bowel, especially if the patient is already hypovolemic. Therefore, address any unstable vital signs early, especially hypotension. Hypotension should be avoided if at all possible. In most circumstances, hypovolemia is secondary to fluid sequestration into the periphery. If medical augmentation is necessary, inotropes such as dobutamine are preferred agents, as vasoconstrictors often worsen bowel ischemia.

Connect the patient to a cardiac monitor and obtain an electrocardiogram to assess for dysrhythmias. Atrial fibrillation is the most common dysrhythmia in a patient with mesenteric ischemia. If the patient is in atrial fibrillation with rapid ventricular response, rate control is still necessary to maximize cardiac output, as the ventricles need time to fill. Calcium channel blockers and β-antagonists are acceptable therapeutic choices for rate control; they will also provide some splanchnic vasodilation. These agents, however, should be avoided in patients with hypotension. Digoxin, used for rate control of atrial fibrillation, should be avoided in AMI patients since it can cause splanchnic vasoconstriction.

Ischemia frequently leads to increased oxygen demand. Therefore, avoid hypoxia at all costs. Administer oxygen to the patient. Maximization of oxygen delivery to the ischemic portion of the gut is certainly beneficial; however, hyperoxia is detrimental. Therefore, maintain the oxygen saturation at an adequate level of greater than 95% and titrate it as deemed necessary. Intubate significantly hypoxic or unstable patients early to decrease oxygen demand.

Initiate adequate pain control. Patients in pain have an increased catecholamine surge, which can worsen ischemia in inadequately perfused portions of bowel. Therefore, controlling their pain should be a priority. Narcotic analgesics are usually necessary. Also, insert a nasogastric tube to decompress the bowel and relieve distention.

First few hours

After the patient is more stabilized, initiate the search for a diagnosis. The differential diagnosis is extensive as the presentation is non-specific, especially in the elderly population. Other disease processes with similar presentations include peptic ulcer disease, pancreatitis, diverticulitis, small bowel obstruction, infectious colitis, appendicitis, and cholecystitis.

Samples for laboratory studies should be drawn and delivered to the lab when the IV line is placed. Request a complete blood count; lactic acid level; electrolyte panel, including liver function tests; amylase; lipase; and urinalysis, including a pregnancy test if the patient is a woman of child-bearing age. In addition to diagnostic laboratory tests, preoperative laboratory studies should be obtained as well as a type and screen for blood products to be made available to the operating room.

Patients with stable vital signs and no signs of peritoneal irritation should undergo CT scanning with IV contrast to allow evaluation of the mesenteric vasculature. If CT is contraindicated, consider alternative modalities such as MRI or ultrasound with Doppler. If the patient has unstable vital signs or peritoneal signs, obtain an upright chest radiograph or abdominal radiograph to evaluate for free air, indicating potential perforation. Once perforation has been ruled out, more definitive studies can be performed. However, involve surgical consultants early if peritoneal signs are present. Angiography is warranted if peritoneal signs are present and/or the clinical suspicion is high.

Early surgical consultation is necessary once the diagnosis is confirmed. The early involvement of a surgeon is associated with improved outcomes.[21–23] Consultation with a vascular surgeon is helpful for a disposition. Once the diagnosis is considered, he/she can facilitate angiography and intervention as needed.

Anticoagulation is also paramount in the early management phase. As with any other acute thrombotic event, the initiation of heparin therapy will prevent clot propagation and additional thrombosis. Unfractionated heparin is preferred over low-molecular-weight heparin, as it can be titrated and is reversible.[1,2,9,24] The risks of not initiating heparin far outweigh the risks of initiating it.

Ischemic bowel tissue has the ability to translocate normally benign gut bacteria across ischemic bowel wall into the periphery.[1,2] Although this translocation has not been shown to worsen outcomes, it certainly can increase the risk of post-surgical wound infections and intra-abdominal abscesses. Therefore, administer broad-spectrum antibiotics to AMI patients. Antimicrobial agents should be directed against Gram-negative organisms and anaerobes.

Once treatment has begun and the options for revascularization are weighed, disposition should be considered. Most surgeons ask that patients with acute mesenteric ischemia be managed in an intensive care setting for frequent monitoring. The small percentage of stable patients who have uneventful revascularization and remain stable after intervention can be managed on the surgical floor.

Clinical approach when resources are limited

Making the diagnosis of acute mesenteric ischemia is difficult in hospitals with advanced technology. The difficulty is, of course, exacerbated in clinical facilities without access to a CT scanner, an angiography suite, or the expertise of a vascular surgeon. In terms of management, the strategies are similar in resource-rich and resource-limited settings.

Patients who are at risk for mesenteric ischemia require initial resuscitation of vital signs, especially restoration of blood pressure and oxygenation. Laboratory studies should be requested. Imaging studies can reveal subtle signs of mesenteric ischemia such as pneumatosis intestinalis or air in the portal vein. Anticoagulation is recommended, especially in patients with cardiac dysrhythmias or in whom AMI is highly suspected. Antimicrobial therapy should be initiated as well.

A general surgeon, if available, should be consulted early, especially for any patient with peritoneal signs or signs of perforation. The surgeon can undertake damage control procedures, including resecting infarcted bowel and making sure the retained bowel is functional. Most operative interventions for AMI warrant a second-look operation. The nearest vascular surgeon should be contacted and might recommend transferring the patient for definitive treatment, including revascularization.

Definitive treatment

Superior mesenteric artery embolus

Patients with SMA emboli almost inevitably require an open operative intervention. The transition from embolus to infarction happens quickly. The resultant infarcted bowel usually must be resected because the damage is irreversible. An open technique allows evaluation of the bowel for infarction, surgical embolectomy, and evaluation of post-revascularization blood flow. After vascularization has been restored and necrotic bowel has been resected, a second-look operation is scheduled to assess for further ischemia.[24]

Endovascular techniques for revascularization through local thrombolysis or embolectomy have been successful. A number of studies have shown endovascular techniques to be associated with fewer complications and a lower mortality rate than open techniques.[12,25,26] If a revascularization cannot be completed with this approach, the approach can be converted to an open operation; bypass grafting is usually necessary.

Regardless of which technique is implemented, intra-arterial papaverine should be administered. Infusion of this phosphodiesterase inhibitor into the arterial system maximizes perfusion to the bowel, even the ischemic portions. The infusion is usually maintained for 24 hours.

Superior mesenteric artery thrombosis

Because of the atherosclerotic disease present throughout the mesenteric vessels, endovascular techniques allow the surgeon to evaluate the vasculature to see if any other vessels are at risk and to undertake any interventions that are warranted. Thrombectomy is most often performed, and stents are placed in areas of significant stenosis or occlusion to prevent recurrence of disease.[12,25–27] Open techniques are used if signs of bowel infarction are present on imaging and resection of infarcted bowel is necessary. If disease is extensive and revascularization is not possible with stenting, bypass grafting is performed. Second-look operations are performed to assess the viability of bowel after intervention. Papaverine is utilized to maintain bowel perfusion following the intervention.

Complications

Unfortunately, the incidence of post-management complications is high: around 50%.[12] The majority of complications involve renal insufficiency and cardiopulmonary complications such as myocardial infarction. Another frequent complication is the need for further bowel resection on second-look operation. The mechanism behind these complications is debatable. A common thought is that the reperfusion injury sends toxic free radicals and bacteria to other organs and heightens the likelihood of complications.[2] Advanced age and prolonged duration of symptoms are the highest risk factors for complications.[23] Endovascular techniques decrease the complication rate significantly, as well as the mortality rate.[25,26]

Summary

Acute mesenteric ischemia continues to be a dismal diagnosis fraught with complications and poor survivability. However, improvements in clinical technology and an increased awareness of this medical emergency may enable care providers to turn the outcomes around. Through early diagnosis and aggressive management, we can improve survival rates and overall patient outcomes.

Pearls

- Consider the diagnosis of AMI early, especially in high-risk patients, in order to direct diagnosis and treatment regimens.

- Manage hypotension and hypoxia early.
- Computed tomography has largely supplanted angiography as a screening test for acute mesenteric ischemia except in high-risk patients.
- Unless contraindicated, initiate heparin therapy and antimicrobial therapy once the diagnosis is confirmed.
- Consult surgeons early in the care of the patient to improve outcomes.

Pitfalls

- Do not rely on the lack of physical examination findings to rule out acute mesenteric ischemia.
- Do not rely on substandard imaging studies such as radiographs.
- Do not rely on the absence of abdominal pain, especially in the elderly, who may have cognitive impairments or altered mental status as their presenting complaint.

Critical actions

- Consider the diagnosis in patients with risk factors.
- Avoid hypoxia and hypotension at all costs.
- Confirm the diagnosis with imaging.
- Consult a surgeon early (specifically, a vascular surgeon if one is available).
- Initiate anticoagulation and antimicrobial therapy.

References

1. Herbert GS, Steele SR. Acute and chronic mesenteric ischemia. *Surg Clin North Am* 2007; 87: 1115–34.

2. Martinez JP, Hogan GJ. Mesenteric ischemia. *Emerg Med Clin North Am* 2004; 22: 909–28.

3. Brandt LJ, Boley SJ. AGA technical review on intestinal ischemia. *Gastroenterology* 2000; 118: 954–68.

4. Schoots IG, Koffeman GI, Legemate DA, *et al.* Systematic review of survival after acute mesenteric ischaemia according to disease aetiology. *Br J Surg* 2004; 91:17–27.

5. Park WM, Gloviczki P, Cheery KJ Jr, *et al.* Contemporary management of acute mesenteric ischemia: factors associated with survival. *J Vasc Surg* 2002; 35: 445–52.

6. Oldenburg WA, Lau LL, Rodenberg TJ, *et al.* Acute mesenteric ischemia: a clinical review. *Arch Intern Med* 2004; 164: 1054–62.

7. Lock G. Acute intestinal ischemia. *Best Pract Res Clin Gastroenterol* 2001; 15: 83–98.

8. Cho JS, Carr JA, Jacobsen G, *et al.* Long-term outcome after mesenteric artery reconstruction: a 37-year experience. *J Vasc Surg* 2002; 35: 453–60.

9. Falkensammer J, Oldenburg WA. Surgical and medical management of mesenteric ischemia. *Curr Treat Options Cardiovasc Med* 2006; 8: 137–43.

10. Cangemi JR, Picco MF. Intestinal ischemia in the elderly. *Gastroenterol Clin North Am* 2009; 38: 527–40.

11. Ozden N, Gurses B. Mesenteric ischemia in the elderly. *Clin Geriatr Med* 2007; 23: 871–87.

12. Schermerhorn ML, Giles KA, Hamdan AD, *et al.* Mesenteric revascularization: management and outcomes in the United States, 1988–2006. *J Vasc Surg* 2009; 50: 341–8.

13. Burns BJ, Brandt LJ. Intestinal ischemia. *Gastroenterol Clin North Am* 2003; 32: 1127–43.

14. Lewiss RE, Egan DJ, Shreves A. Vascular abdominal emergencies. *Emerg Med Clin North Am* 2011; 29: 253–72.

15. Hirsch AT, Haskal ZJ, Hertzer NR, *et al.* ACC/AHA 2005 guidelines for the management of patients with peripheral arterial disease (lower extremity, renal, mesenteric, and abdominal aortic): executive summary: a collaborative report from the American Association for Vascular Surgery/Society for Vascular Surgery, Society for Cardiovascular Angiography and Interventions, Society for Vascular Medicine and Biology, Society of Interventional Radiology, and the ACC/AHA Task Force on Practice Guidelines (Writing Committee to Develop Guidelines for the Management of Patients With Peripheral Arterial Disease) endorsed by the American Association of Cardiovascular and Pulmonary Rehabilitation; National Heart, Lung, and Blood Institute; Society for Vascular Nursing; TransAtlantic Inter-Society Consensus; and Vascular Disease Foundation. *J Am Coll Cardiol* 2006; 47: 1239–312.

16. Nielsen C, Lindholt JS, Erlandsen EJ, *et al.* d-lactate as a marker of venous-induced intestinal ischemia: an experimental study in pigs. *Int J Surg* 2011; 9: 428–32.

17. Gore RM, Yaghmai V, Thakrar KH, *et al.* Imaging in intestinal ischemic disorders. *Radiol Clin North Am* 2008; 46: 845–75.

18. Kim AY, Ha HK. Evaluation of suspected mesenteric ischemia: efficacy of radiologic studies. *Radiol Clin North Am* 2003; 41: 327–42.

19. Horton KM, Fishman EK. Multidetector CT angiography in the diagnosis of mesenteric ischemia. *Radiol Clin North Am* 2007; 45: 275–88.

20. Levy AD. Mesenteric ischemia. *Radiol Clin North Am* 2007; 45: 593–9.

21. Eltarawy IG, Etman YM, Zenati M, *et al.* Acute mesenteric ischemia: the importance of early surgical consultation. *Am Surg* 2009; 75: 212–19.

22. Wadman M, Syk I, Elmstahl S. Survival after operations for ischaemic bowel disease. *Eur J Surg* 2000; 166: 872–7.

23. Kougias P, Lau D, El Sayed HF, *et al.* Determinants of mortality and treatment outcome following surgical interventions for acute mesenteric ischemia. *J Vasc Surg* 2007; 46: 467–74.

24. Bingol H, Zeybek N, *et al.* Surgical therapy for acute superior mesenteric artery embolism. *Am J Surg* 2004; 188: 68–70.

25. Arthurs ZM, Titus J, Bannazadeh M, *et al.* A comparison of endovascular revascularization with traditional therapy for the treatment of acute mesenteric ischemia. *J Vasc Surg* 2011; 53: 698–705.

26. Block TA, Acosta S, Bjorck M. Endovascular and open surgery for acute occlusion of the superior mesenteric artery. *J Vasc Surg* 2010; 52: 959–66.

27. Wyers MC, Powell RJ, Nolan BW, *et al.* Retrograde mesenteric stenting during laparotomy for acute occlusive mesenteric ischemia. *J Vasc Surg* 2007; 45: 269–75.

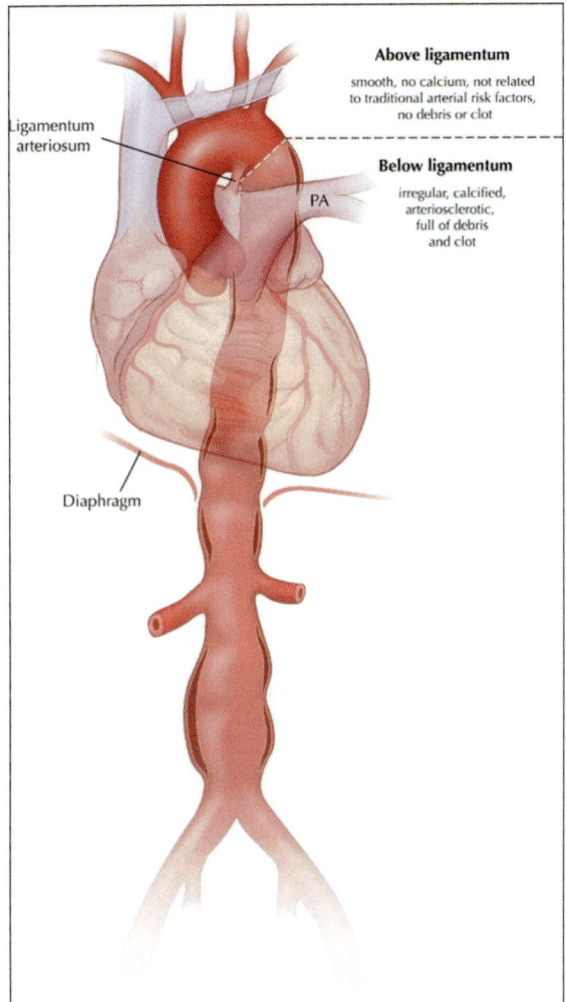

Above ligamentum

smooth, no calcium, not related to traditional arterial risk factors, no debris or clot

Below ligamentum

irregular, calcified, arteriosclerotic, full of debris and clot

Ligamentum arteriosum

PA

Diaphragm

Figure 11.2 Aortic aneurysm is really two diseases: ascending disease differs markedly from descending/abdominal disease. Note that thoracic aneurysm disease divides naturally into two patterns, separated at the ligamentum. Above the ligamentum, the aorta is thin, but not atherosclerotic; below the ligamentum, as with abdominal aortic aneurysms, heavy arteriosclerosis and calcification predominate. PA, pulmonary artery. (Figure illustration by Rob Flewell.).

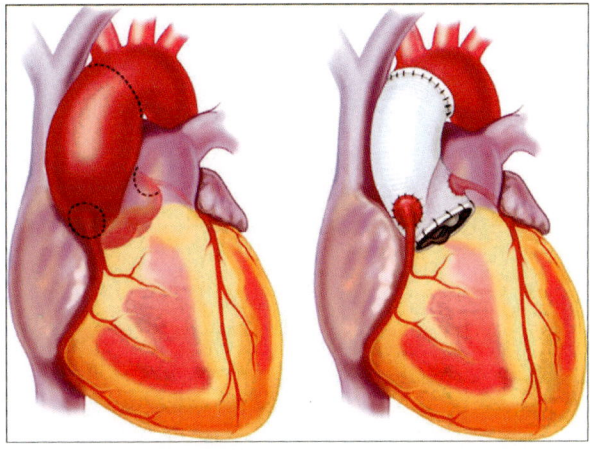

Figure 11.10 Composite graft replacement of ascending aorta and aortic valve, with reimplantation of coronary artery "buttons." (Reprinted from Isselbacher.[25] Used with permission ©Massachusetts General Hospital Thoracic Aortic Center.)

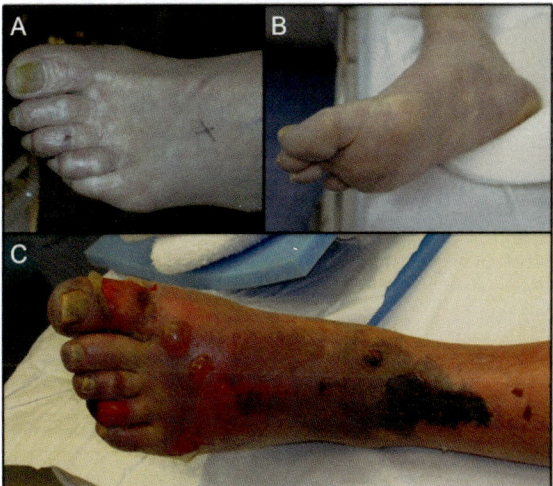

Figure 13.2 Appearance of acutely ischemic lower extremities. The limb in panel A, Rutherford IIa, is marginally threatened. Note the significant pallor. The limb in panel B, Rutherford IIb, is immediately threatened. The first signs of mottling are present. Note the areas of blanching over the forefoot. These areas represent significantly delayed capillary refill. The limb in panel C, Rutherford III, suffers from irreversible ischemia. This limb demonstrates fixed mottling. Also present is blistering and rigor (not apparent in the photograph). It is important to understand that the difference between marginally and immediately threatened limbs is not obvious based on appearance alone.

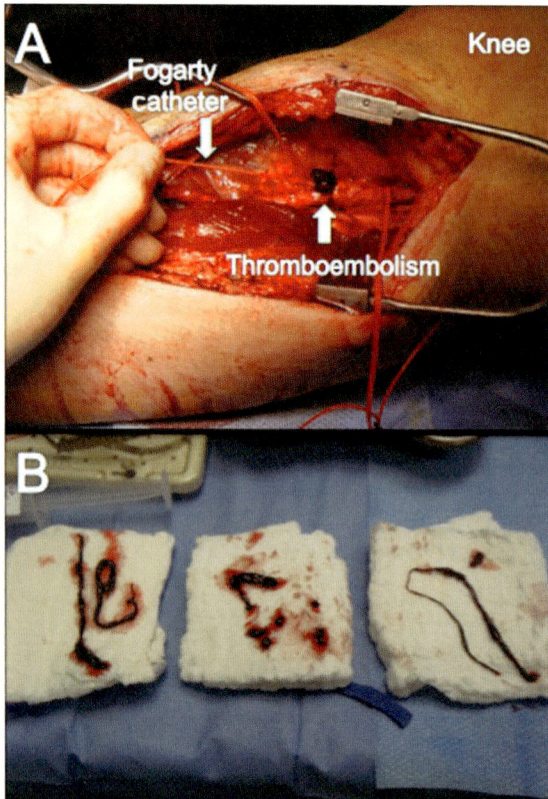

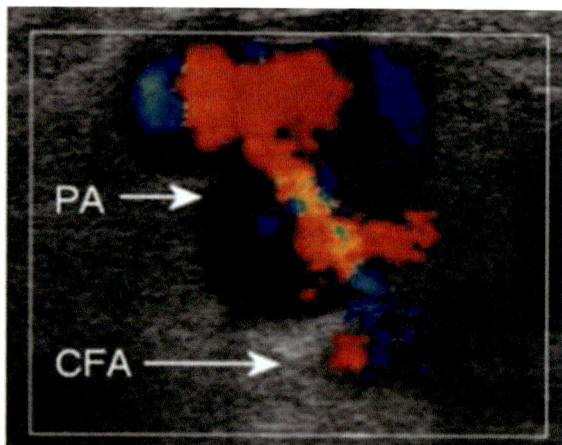

Figure 14.1 Peripheral pseudoaneurysm with characteristic to and fro Doppler flow pattern. PA, pseudoaneurysm; CFA, common femoral artery.

Figure 13.5 Surgical embolectomy. To perform an open embolectomy, exposure of the affected vessel is obtained. The vessel is controlled and a transverse arteriotomy is made. A Fogarty catheter is directed toward the embolism, inflated and swept toward the arteriotomy (A). The Fogarty catheter is repeatedly inserted until no more thromboembolism is retrieved. Thrombus will form in a vessel after an embolism occurs. Panel B depicts acute thrombus associated with an embolic event.

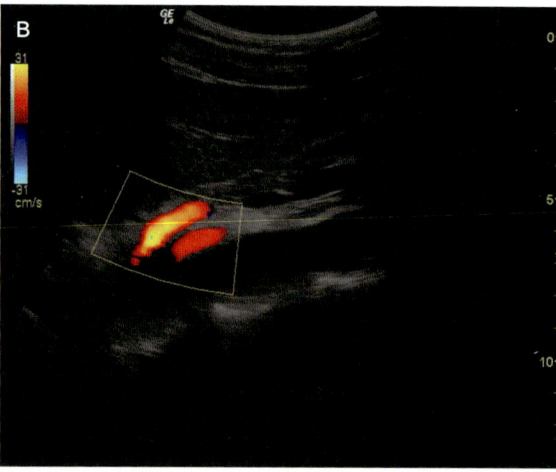

Figure 25.12B Duplex Doppler of celiac and superior mesenteric arteries. Normal flow is present. Complete occlusion of either vessel would appear as an absence of color in the vessel.

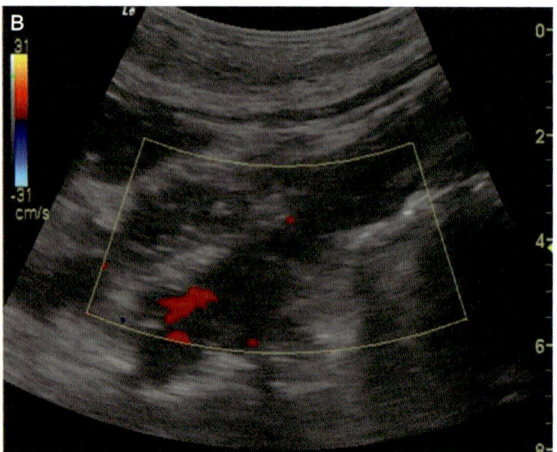

Figure 25.11 Aortic occlusion. (B) In longitudinal, there is an absence of color flow. (Reprinted from Roxas et al.,[5] with permission from Elsevier.)

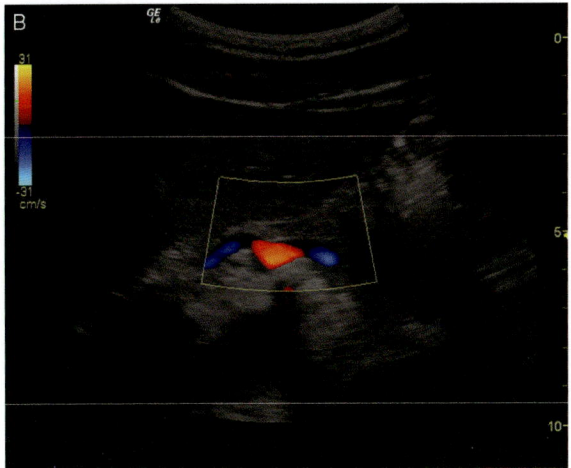 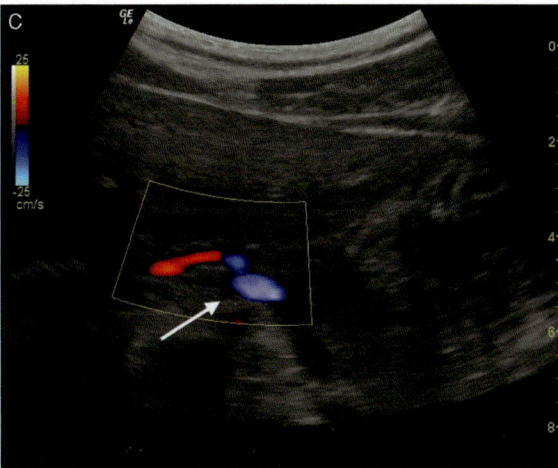

Figure 25.13 Branches of the celiac artery. (B) Normal color Doppler flow through the celiac branches. Flow toward the ultrasound probe (upward on screen) is colored red, and flow away (downward on screen) is colored blue. Blood flows anteriorly through the celiac artery, then posteriorly through the HA and SA. Note that the wingtips of the "seagull" are the same color. (C) Retrograde flow through the hepatic artery. The HA is red due to flow from posterior to anterior, toward the celiac artery (arrow). Note that the wingtips of the "seagull" are different colors.

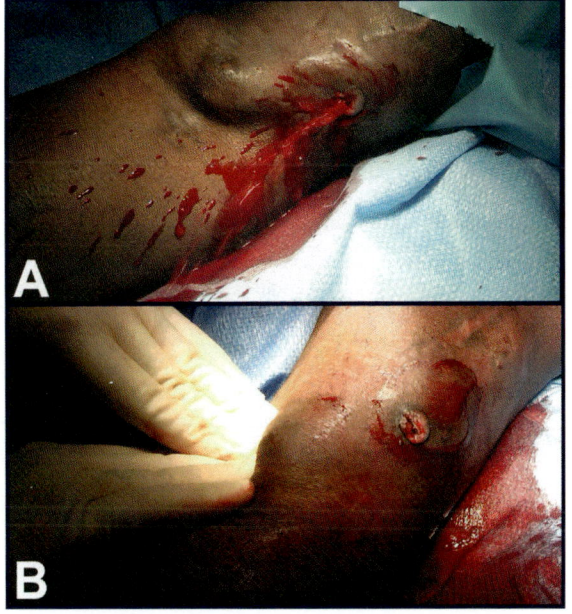

Figure 26.3 (A) Vigorous bleeding from a brachial-cephalic AV fistula buttonhole that spontaneously broke open. (B) Technique of hemorrhage control by digital compression of arterial end of fistula.

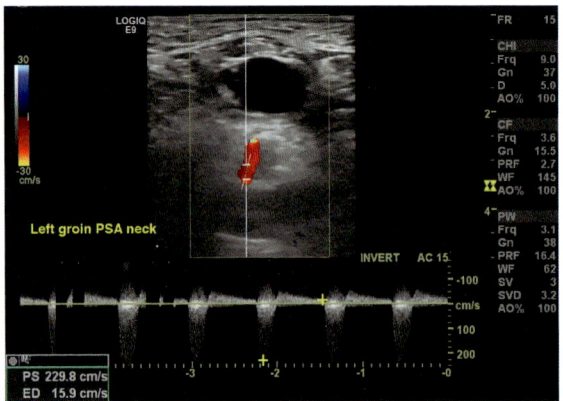

Figure 28.1 Duplex showing pseudoaneurysm (PSA) neck with "to and fro" Doppler flow pattern. (Image courtesy of Sarah Rust, RVT.)

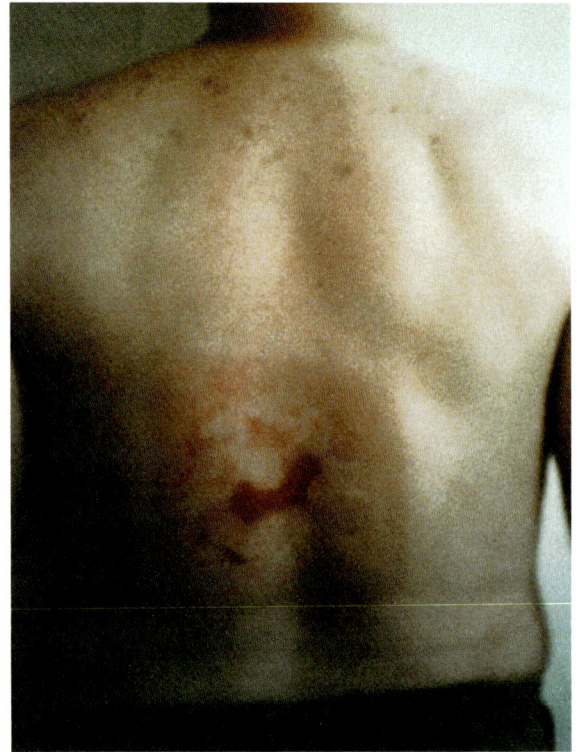

Figure 28.8 Radiation-induced skin burn. (Downloaded from: http://www.fda.gov/Radiation-EmittingProducts/ RadiationEmittingProductsandProcedures/MedicalImaging/ MedicalX-Rays/ucm116682.htm.)

Chapter

18

Acute visceral venous disease

Matthew K. Folstein, Karan Chopra, and Kapil Gopal

Acute visceral venous disease occurs within the superior mesenteric, inferior mesenteric, splenic, portal, and renal veins. These conditions have distinct pathophysiologic and treatment goals from corresponding arterial occlusions. Mesenteric vein thrombosis was first recognized as a separate disease process in 1935 by Warren and Eberhard.[1] Of the visceral venous vessels, thrombosis of the superior mesenteric vein is the most lethal, with mortality rates reported as high as 23%.[2] The natural history of the disease remains difficult to delineate due to its insidious onset and vague symptoms, and diagnosis being made at exploratory laparotomy or autopsy. Incidence of mesenteric vein thrombosis remains extremely rare in the adult at 0.1%, while incidence of renal vein thrombosis is even lower at 0.05%.[2,3] However, approximately 15% of acute mesenteric ischemia patients were diagnosed with acute visceral venous thrombosis in the population-based study by Acosta *et al.* from Malmo, Sweden.[2]

Patients at increased risk for mesenteric venous thrombosis exhibit Virchow's triad with conditions that lead to stasis (i.e., congestive heart failure, portal hypertension, etc.), injury (i.e., post-surgical, blunt, and penetrating abdominal trauma), or hypercoagulability (i.e., thrombophilias, oral contraceptive use, etc.) (Table 18.1[4]). Inherited thrombophilias have been reported in up to 55% of patients with mesenteric venous thrombosis.[5] The underlying commonality is that acute visceral venous thrombosis is usually secondary to another pathological entity that can lead to end-organ ischemia. The body's tolerance of this ischemia is dependent upon the circulation affected and extent of collateral flow. Most often, renal vein thrombosis may not be diagnosed from vague flank or abdominal pain, as the functional contralateral kidney

Table 18.1 Risk factors for visceral venous thrombosis[4]

Direct injury

Abdominal trauma (post-surgical, penetrating, or blunt)

Intra-abdominal inflammation (pancreatitis or inflammatory bowel disease)

Intra-abdominal abscess or peritonitis

Stasis

Portal venous hypertension or cirrhosis

Congestive heart failure

Hypersplenism

Obesity

Abdominal compartment syndrome

Thrombophilia

Protein C and S deficiency

Antithrombin III deficiency

Factor V Leiden

Presence of 20210A prothrombin gene

Neoplasms

Oral contraceptive use

Polycythemia vera

Lupus anticoagulant

Extramesenteric venous thromboembolism

will compensate for any damage to the kidney with the thrombosed vein. Portal vein thrombosis can be compensated through collaterals from the stomach, esophagus, and spleen. Inferior mesenteric vein thrombosis can be compensated via hemorrhoidal venous collaterals. The most devastating vessel to be thrombosed is the superior mesenteric vein, as it serves as the major vessel for intestinal venous drainage.

The sequelae of venous thrombosis vary according to the degree of end-organ ischemia: loss of

Vascular Emergencies, ed. Robert L. Rogers, Thomas Scalea, Lee Wallis, and Heike Geduld. Published by Cambridge University Press. © Cambridge University Press 2013.

kidney function; splenic abscess in an infarcted spleen, or need for splenectomy; portal venous hypertension; intestinal ischemia requiring intestinal resection; and death due to widespread intestinal ischemia. Death is rarely the result from infarcted spleen or kidney. The primary goal of treatment is to halt thrombosis, resect any necrotic tissue causing physiologic abnormalities, and treat the underlying cause of the venous thrombosis.

Diagnosis

Symptomatology

This disease is typically seen in middle-aged patients who present to the emergency department with a history of vague abdominal discomfort evolving over days to weeks. This is because mesenteric venous thrombosis can lead to a prolonged ileus in the initial stages. In arterial occlusion, the progression of abdominal pain and symptoms is much quicker: over hours to a few days. Other gastrointestinal symptoms of nausea, vomiting, constipation, and gastrointestinal bleeding may also be present. These symptoms can evolve as the degree of intestinal ischemia increases, and the patient can develop an acute abdomen from intestinal infarction. In cases of prolonged portal vein thrombosis, patients may present with bloody vomiting, and patients with renal vein thrombosis may have microscopic hematuria. Patients with an intra-abdominal abscess may have fevers. A thorough history may reveal a predisposing risk factor from Table 18.1 that might raise suspicion of acute visceral venous thrombosis, as 75% of cases are considered to be secondary mesenteric venous thrombosis.

Special attention should be paid to previous history in the patient or family of venous thrombosis, such as lower extremity deep vein thrombosis, pulmonary embolism, or history of blood relatives that were told of having hypercoagulable states, which can be present in 50% of patients with visceral venous thrombosis. The diagnosis of primary mesenteric venous thrombosis remains a diagnosis of exclusion.

Physical examination

The *sine qua non* of intestinal mesenteric ischemia is pain out of proportion to examination in the early presentation. This is described as a patient having diffuse abdominal pain in all quadrants, despite not having other findings of increased abdominal tenderness to palpation, distension, rebound, or guarding. As the ischemia progresses to transmural infarction, these patients may present with a distended abdomen, guaiac-positive stool, and peritoneal signs. If the patient has an underlying intra-abdominal infection, peritoneal signs may be elicited and a palpable abdominal mass may be felt.

Patients with renal vein thrombosis, splenic vein thrombosis, or portal vein thrombosis may present with vague back or flank dull ache, or right and left upper quadrant abdominal pain without gastrointestinal symptoms or physical findings. If there is an abscess, there may be an ileus that develops and associated nausea, vomiting, and abdominal distension.

Laboratory studies

Laboratory analysis is unfortunately not very useful in the emergency department diagnosis of mesenteric venous thrombosis. In the setting of high clinical suspicion, therapy should not be delayed to perform laboratory tests. A D-dimer blood test can be ordered if available, which will be elevated in the presence of acute venous thrombosis anywhere in the body. Thus, D-dimer is sensitive for venous thrombosis presence but not a specific test for visceral venous thrombosis.[6] Patterns of laboratory abnormalities are related to end-organ ischemia. In the acute setting, the emergency physician should order prothrombin time (PT), an activated partial thromboplastin time (aPTT), complete blood count (CBC), hepatic function panel, and chemistries. These may reveal a leukocytosis, hemoconcentration, and metabolic acidosis. These are highly non-specific findings in patients with longstanding ischemia. Other important tests should include hypercoagulable panel (protein C and S, antithrombin III, anticardiolipin antibodies, factor V Leiden) in patients with a high index of suspicion for having hypercoagulable state or in patients without a clearly defined cause.

Imaging

Abdominal X-rays in upright and decubitus positions should be ordered, paying particular attention for any findings of acute abdomen such as free air or gas in the portomesenteric system that may necessitate urgent surgical evaluation. However, the majority of the time, there will be non-specific findings with possible presence of ileus or small bowel obstruction. CTA with intravenous contrast injection with venous phase is the most important and sensitive diagnostic test.[7,8] The findings can reveal the status of multiple vessels, showing thrombosis in portal vein, superior mesenteric vein, splenic vein, or the renal veins. Furthermore, a CT scan may show generalized small bowel edema, mesenteric edema, small bowel dilatation, and presence of gas in the portomesenteric venous system. In centers with angiographic capabilities, it is important that the mesenteric vessels be studied in the venous phase as well as the arterial phase. Angiogram can reveal possible arterial vasospasm; lack of venous vasculature visualization and absent flow will represent necrotic bowel areas.

In a center with ultrasound capability, a duplex can be obtained of the superior mesenteric, splenic, portal, hepatic, and renal veins. This test requires highly skilled technologists with experience in vascular lab imaging, and the results can be highly variable as presence of abdominal bowel gas can prevent visualization of the vessels. However, the advantages of duplex scans are that they can be performed at the bedside (useful in an unstable patient), or without use of intravenous contrast – important in a renal failure patient. In a situation with prolonged abdominal pain suspicious for intestinal ischemia from mesenteric venous thrombosis and no availability of these imaging modalities, exploratory laparoscopy and laparotomy remain viable options for treatment and diagnosis.

Emergency department management

Initial assessment

The list of differential diagnoses for patients with abdominal pain and associated gastrointestinal symptoms is long. It is imperative to initially assess the patient's overall physiologic status, as the patient may be in critical condition if there is peritonitis with hemodynamic instability. Resuscitation with intravenous fluids and urgent surgical evaluation should be obtained in this setting. However, the majority of patients with mesenteric or renal vein thrombosis present with a history of vague abdominal discomfort progressively worsening over days to weeks. These patients are frequently dehydrated, and establishment of intravenous access with appropriate resuscitation is imperative. The patients are able to be interviewed to elicit history of any recent traumas, previous medical history, and family history that may raise suspicions of

acute visceral venous thrombosis. Of note in endemic areas, particular attention should be paid to the possibility of parasites that may cause liver abscesses and can lead to portal vein thrombosis with distal extension into the superior mesenteric or splenic veins.

Physical examination with pain out of proportion to examination should be suspicious for mesenteric ischemia. Any presence of non-pulsatile abdominal masses or peri-rectal masses can be suspicious for intra-abdominal abscesses. Blood work focusing on infection, bleeding, hepatic dysfunction, metabolic derangement, renal function, and coagulation status should be requested. In settings where D-dimer can be checked, it can help to determine if there is the presence of venous thrombosis in the body. Put together with the constellation of symptoms, D-dimer can be extremely helpful in increasing suspicion of this disease state. Urinanalysis can show microscopic hematuria in cases of renal vein thrombosis.

Imaging should be obtained as described above, with an initial abdominal X-ray to rule out signs of free air until an appropriate CT scan with intravenous contrast in venous phase can be obtained to assess the intra-abdominal vessels and structures. Further imaging can be obtained with mesenteric venous duplex in centers that have this technology available, which can prove to be invaluable in patients with renal failure. However, in patients suspected of having an acute abdomen which is life threatening, and where CT is available, it should be performed with intravenous contrast regardless of renal function status.

With no evidence of peritonitis and no other explanation for abdominal pain or flank pain, or with past patient history suspicious for superior mesenteric or renal vein thrombosis, the patient should be anticoagulated with intravenous unfractionated heparin bolus and infusion to achieve therapeutic levels (aPTT time of 50–70 seconds). If recent gastrointestinal bleeding has occurred, the benefit of anticoagulation and the possibility of averting bowel infarction may still warrant anticoagulation despite the risk of bleeding. If needed, heparin anticoagulation can be reversed with use of protamine. Intravenous antibiotics are not required unless there is confirmed bowel perforation or peritonitis. A surgical evaluation should be obtained should the patient become unstable and require a laparotomy. A nasogastric tube for decompression may be necessary if the patient is actively having nausea and vomiting, which will also allow for the performance of a lavage to assess for upper gastrointestinal bleeding. It is important to make a distinction here: that superior mesenteric vein thrombosis presents with lower gastrointestinal bleeding or guaiac-positive stool. Upper gastrointestinal bleeding is likely related to portal vein hypertension or portal vein thrombosis. Anticoagulation is not as urgent for portal vein or splenic vein thrombosis.

Admission and level of care

The patient should be admitted for observation in a monitored setting, paying particular attention to hemodynamic stability or signs of worsening intestinal ischemia. The patient should remain on continued hydration with fasting and serial abdominal examinations and strict urine output monitoring. Any change in status should prompt another CT scan, or if unavailable then consider surgical intervention for diagnosis and treatment. CT scans can show extension of venous thrombosis or worsening ischemia of the bowel.

Definitive care and outcome

Medical treatment

The mainstay of therapy remains anticoagulation, in both the initial period and afterwards for life, with conversion of unfractionated heparin therapy to oral warfarin, as there is a recurrence rate of as high as 36%.[9] Low-molecular-weight heparin is expensive, but can be used to bridge the patient until appropriate levels of INR are achieved, or can be used indeterminately if the patient has liver dysfunction and contraindication to warfarin and conservative medical therapy.[10] Anticoagulation remains the mainstay of therapy even if there is surgical intervention, with or without bowel resection. The overall 30-day survival with recent series was 80% in 51 patients, with 5-year survival of 70%.[5] The natural progression of the mesenteric venous system is not well delineated after long-term anticoagulation because it is not routinely evaluated with serial CT scans. It has been noted that there seems to be no change or regression after a short period of treatment. Long-term sequelae are related to gastrointestinal (stricture, bleeding), or renal complications (nephropathy, renal failure), or portal venous hypertension (esophageal or gastric varices, ascites).

Surgical treatment

Indications for surgical intervention are peritonitis, severe gastrointestinal bleeding, or bowel perforation in the acute setting. On laparotomy or laparoscopy, the bowel appears hyperemic and edematous. The bowel should be inspected for frank necrosis with appropriate areas resected. Primary bowel anastomosis can be performed after bowel resection. However, if there are areas of the bowel with questionable viability, the patient can be brought back for a second-look laparotomy in 24 to 48 hours to reassess the bowel.[4] It is essential that the patient be maintained on anticoagulation throughout the perioperative periods to prevent further venous thrombosis. The patient should be maintained on bowel rest with parenteral nutrition support, with transition to lifelong oral anticoagulation as bowel function returns.

There is little role for open thrombectomy of the visceral venous vessels, due to the high recurrence rate. A splenectomy may be required for splenic abscess, a nephrectomy for infarcted kidney with uncontrolled hypertension, and a transjugular intrahepatic portosystemic shunt for complications of portal venous hypertension. There are few if any data regarding the incidence of these complications after mesenteric venous thrombosis. There are isolated reports of the use of endovascular therapies that include percutaneous thrombectomy, and thrombolysis; however if the patient requires a laparotomy, the patient cannot undergo catheter-directed thrombolysis. There can also be development of short-term complications related to the surgery such as wound infection, sepsis, and bleeding.[4] The survival rate over two years showed no difference between groups undergoing surgery or medical treatment.[10]

Clinical approach when resources are limited

1. Identify acutely ill patients by examination and begin intravenous resuscitation with urgent surgical consultation.
2. In hemodynamically stable patients, obtain a good history of present illness, previous medical, and family history.
3. Obtain abdominal X-rays to assess for any signs of bowel perforation.
4. Initiate systemic anticoagulation with unfractionated heparin.

5. Admit for observation with bowel rest, serial abdominal examination, and laboratory data.

Pearls and pitfalls

Pearls

1. Diagnosis of exclusion and high suspicion based on history and physical examination.
2. Obtain a CT scan with intravenous contrast in venous phase as gold standard.
3. Obtain D-dimer if available, as it is highly sensitive for a venous thrombotic event.
4. Obtain surgical consultation early.
5. Initiate systemic anticoagulation early; the anticoagulation can be stopped if there is a new concrete diagnosis or if CT scan does not show mesenteric venous thrombosis.

Pitfalls

1. Not recognizing abdominal pain out of proportion to examination as a sign of mesenteric ischemia.
2. Not beginning anticoagulation early when there is no other explanation for symptoms.
3. Not utilizing the resources available.

Critical actions

- Intravenous fluid resuscitation
- Determination of acuteness of symptoms
- Obtain surgical evaluation
- Obtain medical and family history
- Initiate heparin anticoagulation

References

1. Warren S, Eberhard TP. Mesenteric venous thrombosis. *Surg Gynecol Obstet* 1935; 61: 102–21.

2. Acosta S, Ögren M, Sternby N-H, *et al*. Mesenteric venous thrombosis with transmural intestinal infarction: a population-based study. *J Vasc Surg* 2005; 41: 59–63.

3. van Bockel JH, Hamming, JF. Renovascular disease: acute occlusive events. In Cronenwett JL, Johnston KW, eds. *Rutherford's Vascular Surgery*, 7th edition. Philadelphia: Saunders Elsevier; 2010: 2253.

4. Acosta S, Björck M. Mesenteric vascular disease: venous thrombosis. In Cronenwett JL, Johnston KW, eds. *Rutherford's Vascular Surgery*, 7th edition. Philadelphia: Saunders Elsevier; 2010: 2304–10.

5. Acosta S, Alhadad A, Svensson P, Ekberg O. Epidemiology, risk and prognostic factors in mesenteric venous thrombosis. *Br J Surg* 2008; 95: 1245–51.

6. Acosta S, Nilsson TK, Björck M. D-Dimer testing in patients with suspected acute thromboembolic occlusion of the superior mesenteric artery. *Br J Surg* 2004; 91: 991–4.

7. Horton K, Fishman E. Multidetector CT angiography in the diagnosis of mesenteric ischemia. *Radiol Clin North Am* 2007; 45: 275–88.

8. Levy A. Mesenteric ischemia. *Radiol Clin North Am* 2007; 45: 593–9.

9. Rhee Ry, Gloviczki P, Mendonca CT, *et al*. Mesenteric venous thrombosis: still a lethal disease in the 1990s. *J Vasc Surg* 1994; 20: 688–97.

10. Brunaud L, Antunes L, Collinet-Adler S, *et al*. Acute mesenteric venous thrombosis: case for nonoperative management. *J Vasc Surg* 2001; 34: 673–9.

Upper extremity deep venous thrombosis

Majid Afshar and Nirav G. Shah

Upper extremity deep venous thrombosis (UEDVT) is a clinical entity with increasing incidence and considerable morbidity and mortality. This chapter will focus on upper extremity DVT and what emergency care providers should know about it in order to take care of patients in the emergency department.

The upper extremity veins are divided into the deep venous system and the superficial venous system. The deep veins of the upper extremity are the radial, ulnar, brachial, axillary, subclavian, internal jugular, and brachiocephalic veins. The superficial veins include the cephalic, basilic, median antebrachial, median antecubital, and accessory cephalic veins. The cephalic and basilic veins, the more common superficial veins, drain directly into the axillary vein and have fewer complications from thrombosis than their complementary deep veins.

Upper extremity deep venous thrombosis is characterized as primary or secondary. Primary UEDVT includes patients with idiopathic UEDVT (in whom no underlying disease may be found) and venous thoracic outlet syndrome, also called "effort-induced thrombosis" or Paget–Schroetter syndrome.[1,2] Paget–Schroetter syndrome was named after James Paget, who first proposed the idea of venous thrombosis causing upper extremity pain and swelling, and Leopold von Schroetter, who later linked the clinical syndrome to thrombosis of the axillary and subclavian veins.[3] Secondary UEDVT develops in patients with predisposing risk factors such as central venous catheters (CVCs), malignancy, or insertion of wires or other devices.

Clinical significance

Although the incidence of UEDVT is less than that of lower extremity deep venous thrombosis (LEDVT),

its significance should not be underappreciated. Since the 1970s, following the introduction of transvenous pacers and CVCs, more thromboses in upper extremities have been documented.[4–6] The increased use of CVCs is associated with the increased use of hemodialysis, parenteral nutrition, and chemotherapy worldwide.

Pathophysiology

Primary UEDVT caused by venous thoracic outlet syndrome has a combination of predisposing and precipitating factors. The predisposition is an anatomic abnormality involving one or more structures at the costoclavicular junction (first rib, clavicle, subclavius muscle, costoclavicular ligament, or anterior scalene muscle), which causes a narrowing of the subclavian and jugular veins near the region where they form the innominate vein.[7] The precipitating factor that leads to thrombosis is excessive activity of the arm; repetitive microtrauma causes inflammation, venous intima hyperplasia, and fibrosis. Venous stretching and microtrauma activate the coagulation cascade and cause local hypercoagulability with subsequent thrombosis.[8]

Secondary UEDVT from CVCs occurs as two types: thrombin sheath and mural thrombi (also called, respectively, fibrin sleeve thrombosis and vascular occlusive thrombosis). Predisposing factors for thrombin sheath formation are catheter-induced vessel wall damage and venous blood flow impedance. The thrombin sheath can develop as early as 24 hours after insertion of a CVC. It is asymptomatic but becomes clinically apparent when blood cannot be withdrawn from or fluids infused into the catheter. The thrombin sheath may become colonized with bacteria, especially *Staphylococcus* species, potentially causing an infection. The more common cause of secondary UEDVT is a mural thrombus, which is larger and completely occludes the vein.

In comparison with the lower extremity venous system, the upper extremity veins are less affected by gravitational stress or stasis. Patients confined to bed continue to move their upper extremities, resulting in less stasis. Additionally, upper extremity veins are shorter and have less surface area for thrombosis than those in the lower extremities.

Epidemiology

About 5 to 10% of venous thromboembolism involves the upper extremities.[9] The three-month mortality rates for patients with UEDVT is about 7%.[8] Compared with patients with LEDVT, patients with UEDVT are statistically more likely to be younger, to be male, to have a lower body mass index, and to have a diagnosis of cancer, and are less likely to have hereditary thrombophilia.[10] Among patients with UEDVT, those with cancer are at greatest risk for recurrent deep venous thrombosis (DVT), symptomatic pulmonary embolism (PE), and major bleeding from therapy.[11] Approximately 20% of cases of UEDVT are primary (60% of which are caused by venous thoracic outlet syndrome). The remaining 80% have secondary causes, and an ongoing or previous episode of lower extremity deep venous thrombosis can be found in 10 to 20%.[12]

Risk factors

In primary UEDVT, risk factors include anatomic abnormalities at the costoclavicular junction and microtrauma from repetitive arm movements or overhead activities. Individuals engaged in work activities (such as painting and car repair) or sports activities (such as tennis, baseball, swimming, lifting weights, wrestling, and volleyball) that involve strenuous arm exercise can develop primary UEDVT.[13] Common risk factors for secondary UEDVT are listed below:

- central venous catheters;
- chemotherapy, parenteral nutrition, blood products administration, hemodialysis;
- malignancy;
- pacemakers or defibrillator leads;
- radiation therapy of the chest;
- hereditary or acquired thrombophilia;

Table 19.1 A clinical prediction score for upper extremity deep vein thrombosis

Clinical feature	Score
"Venous material," including catheter or access device in the deep vein of upper extremity or a pacemaker wire	1
Localized pain in the affected extremity	1
Unilateral pitting edema of the extremity	1
Other diagnosis at least as likely	−1

Total score: 0, low probability; 1, intermediate probability; 2 or 3, high probability.
Based on information supplied in Constans *et al.*[21]

- upper extremity surgery within the past two months;
- trauma with injury or compression of upper extremity veins;
- immobilization (e.g., plaster cast);
- pregnancy;
- hormonal contraception use.

CVCs and malignancy are the most common risk factors in secondary UEDVT.[14–17] Hereditary thrombophilia, including factor V Leiden mutation; prothrombin G20210A; or antithrombin III, protein C, or protein S deficiency, have a five- to sixfold increase in the risk for UEDVT.[18]

Peripherally inserted central venous catheters (PICCs) offer a relatively safe and cost-effective method of providing long-term intravenous access for extended antibiotic therapy, chemotherapy, and total parenteral nutrition. The placement of a PICC in a superficial vein can cause a superficial thrombophlebitis, but the course of disease is self-limited once the catheter is removed.[19,20]

Initial emergency department management

Patients arriving with signs or symptoms of UEDVT should be evaluated for risk factors. A simple pretest clinical prediction score has been developed to assist the physician with this evaluation. Derived and validated with ultrasound confirmation from a cohort of patients with suspected UEDVT, four factors were identified for scoring (Table 19.1). Total scores of 0 as "unlikely UEDVT" and ≥ 1 as "likely DVT" have a sensitivity and specificity of 78% and 64%, respectively.[21]

Table 19.2 Treatment for upper extremity deep venous thrombosis

Indication	Recommendation
Initial treatment	Therapeutic doses of LMWH
Long-term treatment	Vitamin-K agonist for three months
In association with a CVC	CVC should not be removed if it is functional and if there is a continued need for it
In association with a removed CVC	Duration of anticoagulation treatment for three months
Initial treatment in patients with a low risk of bleeding and severe symptoms of recent onset	Catheter-directed thrombolysis if appropriate resources and expertise are available
Failure of anticoagulant or thrombolytic treatment and severe persistent symptoms	Catheter extraction, surgical thrombectomy, angioplasty by interventional or surgical procedure

CVC, central venous catheter; LMWH, low-molecular-weight heparin.
Based on information supplied in Kearon et al.[9]

Compression ultrasonography currently constitutes the standard approach for diagnosis of UEDVT and has 97% sensitivity and 96% specificity.[22] Anticoagulation should be initiated prior to confirmation of the diagnosis if no contraindications exist. Acute management is summarized in Table 19.2. If the diagnosis remains unclear after ultrasound but suspicion remains high, other modalities of imaging can be utilized, including CT and contrast venography. Other than the special circumstances described in Table 19.2, it is not recommended to routinely use systemic or catheter-directed thrombolysis (CDT), catheter extraction, surgical thrombectomy, transluminal angioplasty, stent placement, systemic thrombolysis, or superior vena cava (SVC) filter placement in the acute management of UEDVT. Management strategies are discussed in the Treatment section of this chapter.

Diagnosis

History

Discomfort, pain, paresthesias, and weakness in the arm are common symptoms in patients with UEDVT. Caval tumor infiltration may lead to superior vena cava syndrome, manifesting as facial swelling, headache, nausea, and dyspnea. However, nearly two-thirds of patients reveal no symptoms suggestive of UEDVT, making diagnosis difficult.[21]

Physical examination

The most common presenting sign is edema of the affected extremity, caused by obstruction of the major thoracic veins. This can be distinguished from fluid retention by noting asymmetry and the absence of lower extremity edema. Other signs can include discoloration, swelling, and visible venous collaterals. Tenderness and erythema from phlebitis are encountered less frequently. The most common site for UEDVT is the internal jugular vein.[23] Nearly two-thirds of patients have devices that are an identifiable source of thrombosis.[18]

A variety of catheter characteristics and circumstances heighten the risk of thrombosis.[14,15,23–26] The thrombosis rates for 5-French and 6-French catheters are 6 to 10%, compared with a rate of approximately 1% for catheters that are less than or equal to 4 French.[23] Central venous catheters come in a variety of materials. Silicone, silastic, and polyurethane are less likely to cause thrombosis than materials such as latex, polyethylene, and polyvinyl.[27] The risk is also higher for multiple-lumen and open-ended catheters. Placement of the catheter tip at the junction of the superior vena cava and innominate vein or more peripherally poses a higher risk for thrombosis than appropriate placement at the junction of the right atrium and superior vena cava (where blood flow is more rapid). If the catheter is misplaced, it should be replaced using sterile technique.[15,28] A history of requiring multiple attempts to insert the catheter is associated with higher risk, as is a history of CVC placement, and the presence of infection at the insertion site.

Laboratory data

When LEDVT is suspected, a rapid quantitative enzyme-linked immunosorbent assay test (D-dimer) is sometimes performed after the pretest clinical probability has been determined. Only one small study evaluated D-dimer in the exclusion of UEDVT. The negative predictive value was 100%, but the specificity was only 14% using a diagnostic cutoff value of 500 μg/L.[29] Although it may seem that these results for UEDVT are similar to the high sensitivity and negative predictive value demonstrated in patients with suspected LEDVT or PE, they are not clinically applicable, given the limited evidence and poor specificity.[22] Patients with UEDVT have a high prevalence of cancer and/or permanent catheter placement, which can contribute to an elevated D-dimer and misguide the physician. Basic laboratory data, such as a complete blood count or comprehensive metabolic panel, can aid in the evaluation of malignancy and help assess thrombosis risk factors in UEDVT.

Imaging

Ultrasonography. Compression ultrasonography and duplex ultrasonography have replaced conventional venography in diagnosing UEDVT. The technique is non-invasive, safe, simple, and reliable, with high sensitivity and specificity (97% and 96%, respectively). The addition of color Doppler has not been shown to improve accuracy.[22] Deep venous thrombosis is confirmed by compression ultrasonography when a segment of the vein cannot be compressed, when an abnormal flow pattern is present (absent flow or absence of a phasic flow pattern, indicating outflow obstruction), or when an intraluminal thrombus is visualized.[30] The overlying bony structures (acoustic shadowing from the clavicle in the visualization of a short segment of the subclavian vein) and the inability to visualize the central intrathoracic venous system are challenges in imaging studies for UEDVT.

Venography. Despite the increased use of ultrasonography, contrast venography remains the gold standard for diagnosis of UEDVT. After introduction of contrast material into the basilic vein, visualization of an intraluminal defect can confirm the presence of thrombus. This test can identify extrinsic compression and delineate any collateral circulation. Venography is indicated in patients who have flow abnormalities and a strong clinical suggestion of UEDVT but negative results from ultrasound.[31] It is also used prior to CDT and surgical procedures. Technical challenges arise in patients with edematous arms and in patients unable to abduct the affected arm. Relative contraindications are renal dysfunction and allergies to contrast agents.

CT venography. Although CT and MRI are potential diagnostic tests for UEDVT, limited evidence exists to guide their use.[22] Computed tomography has the advantage of directly imaging central veins. It can diagnose other sources of venous obstruction caused by external compression from adjacent structures and allows the simultaneous diagnosis of PE. Spiral multidetector CT venography, with 3D reconstructions, allows upper extremity venous anatomy to be mapped in reference to adjacent anatomy.[32]

Magnetic resonance angiography (MRA). Although MRA is an alternative, non-invasive option, its cost makes it fairly unreasonable. MRA findings have been shown to correlate well with those of venography, and this imaging study allows complete evaluation of collaterals and visualization of the surrounding soft tissues.[33]

Treatment

The approach to effective treatment of UEDVT is not well established and resembles the recommendations for LEDVT treatment. The aims of treatment are listed below:

- to alleviate the signs and symptoms of UEDVT;
- to prevent thrombus progression and PE;
- to prevent early recurrence;
- to prevent post-thrombotic syndrome (PTS).

Treatment strategies are divided into initial and long-term phases.

Initial therapy. Patients with acute UEDVT require prompt treatment with unfractionated or low-molecular-weight heparin (enoxaparin and fondaparinux).[9] Instructions for their administration are presented in Chapter 20, Lower extremity deep venous thrombosis. Unfractionated heparin is preferred in patients with renal dysfunction and in those for whom thrombolytics are being considered, otherwise low-molecular-weight heparin (LMWH) is preferred. Removal of an extant catheter does not need to be routine in patients with little risk of recurrence and progression of thrombosis. However, catheter removal is necessary in patients with contraindications to anticoagulation therapy, persistent signs or symptoms of thrombosis after three days of anticoagulation therapy, catheter malfunction, or infection from the catheter and when the catheter is no longer indicated.[9] Removal of the catheter does not eliminate the risk of extension or embolization of the thrombus, and it does not change the duration of anticoagulation therapy.[9]

Long-term therapy. Patients with symptomatic UEDVT require long-term treatment with anticoagulants following initial treatment. A process similar to the one for LEDVT should be used to determine the optimal duration. However, there are no data to support indefinite anticoagulant therapy for a first episode of unprovoked UEDVT.[9] Long-term treatment requires a vitamin-K antagonist for three months in patients with and without malignancies, with a target INR of 2.0 to 3.0.[18] In patients with malignancy, LMWH is considered superior and is recommended over vitamin-K antagonists, given the decreased risk of rethrombosis and bleeding.[9] Mechanical therapies such as compression bandages or sleeves have not been shown to be effective and are not recommended except in patients who develop PTS. Patients with persistent arm swelling and pain may derive symptomatic relief from elastic bandages or compression sleeves, with little risk of harm.[9]

CDT. In patients with extensive swelling and less than 14 days of functional impairment, low risk of bleeding, good functional status, and life expectancy $\geq$ 1 year, CDT may be considered for initial treatment if appropriate expertise and resources are available.[9,34] Catheter-directed thrombolysis with streptokinase, urokinase, or recombinant tissue plasminogen activator can restore venous patency early, with symptom resolution. It remains unclear whether thrombolysis, compared with anticoagulation alone, reduces the risk of recurrent thrombosis, PE, or PTS in patients with UEDVT. Systemic thrombolysis can be utilized alone, although this has not been well studied and should be considered only in selected patients with acute DVT, a low risk of bleeding, and severe onset of symptoms.[9] Complications from bleeding have been reported in as many as 15% of patients.[35]

Surgery. In patients with extensive swelling, functional impairment, and a low risk of bleeding who have failed anticoagulation or thrombolytic therapy, surgical procedures can be considered when appropriate expertise and resources are available.[36] In patients with venous thoracic outlet syndrome, surgery requires resection of the first rib, with occasional resection of the costoclavicular ligament, anterior scalenectomy, and venolysis, depending on patient characteristics and surgeon preference.[37] Venous patency rates after decompression of the thoracic outlet are good; up to 85% of patients have no evidence of PTS at follow-up.[38] Surgical decompression of the thoracic outlet with optional percutaneous balloon angioplasty is usually performed if PTS is present. Postoperative complications can include hemopneumothorax, injury of the long thoracic or the phrenic nerve, wound hematoma, and recurrent subclavian thrombosis.[39]

SVC filter and stent. SVC filter placement should be limited to patients with contraindications to anticoagulation therapy, thrombus progression, or symptomatic PE despite adequate treatment with anticoagulants. Very little is known regarding appropriate follow-up in patients with SVC filters. In one small study, long-term follow-up revealed less than a 3% incidence of PE and no incidence of PTS.[40] The risks of SVC filters include filter migration, filter dislodgment, filter fracture, and precipitation of the SVC syndrome.[27] Stents should not be used to treat subclavian vein stenosis within the costoclavicular junction because of the unacceptably high rates of stent deformation, stent fractures, and recurrent thrombosis.[41]

Complications

Upper extremity deep venous thrombosis may lead to complications such as recurrence of thrombosis, PE, bleeding, and PTS of the arm. Less than 2% of patients have recurrence after treatment with LMWH, and there are even fewer cases of PE.[42–44] At the time of diagnosis of UEDVT, concurrent PE is found in nearly 5% of patients; whereas in LEDVT, the percentage is considerably higher.[45,46] Recurrence of DVT at 12 months is twice as likely in the lower extremity as the upper extremity.[18,47,48] The risk of major bleeding while on anticoagulation for UEDVT is 2 to 4%.[42,43]

Post-thrombotic syndrome develops in nearly 20% of patients with UEDVT at one year and nearly 30% by two years.[44] Patients with thrombosis of the axillary and subclavian veins have a threefold higher incidence of PTS.[3] Post-thrombotic syndrome can decrease quality of life and present as any of the following symptoms: chronic swelling with or without pain, extremity heaviness, venous collaterals, erythema, skin induration, or hyperpigmentation of the affected extremity.

In severe cases, venous stasis increases arm girth, with skin ulceration and superimposed infection.

Disposition

Patients receiving effective treatment should be monitored for complications associated with UEDVT for three months following the diagnosis. Evidence of disease resolution with no further sequelae of thrombosis after completion of three months of anticoagulation therapy is adequate for discontinuation of therapy unless the thrombosis is secondary to CVC, in which case anticoagulation should continue for as long as the CVC is in place. Some practitioners advocate follow-up ultrasonography to confirm resolution of disease; however, this assessment is not necessary.[9]

Prevention

Routine pharmacologic prophylaxis in patients with CVCs is not indicated, and no formal recommendations currently exist. Several randomized trials have shown no significant reduction in symptomatic thrombosis in patients with cancer or CVCs when LMWH or unfractionated heparin was compared with placebo.[49] Confirming proper catheter placement with a chest radiograph should be routine practice and may help avoid UEDVT and its associated morbidity. Catheter infection leading to thrombosis can be prevented with appropriate sterile technique during insertion and timely removal of indwelling catheters. Ultimately, prompt removal of a CVC once it is no longer indicated is the best prevention for thrombosis.

Clinical approach when resources are limited

The gold standard for diagnosing UEDVT is contrast venography, but the associated expense and need for specialized expertise are significant limitations in settings with a paucity of resources. Under these circumstances, ultrasound becomes the preferred imaging modality. Although the operating characteristics of compression ultrasonography are excellent, the test might not detect thrombosis that is restricted to veins obscured by the ribs. When ultrasonography is not available or is inconclusive in patients with persistent pain and swelling near the CVC site, UEDVT can be diagnosed with the clinical prediction score.[22] In circumstances of likely UEDVT using the clinical prediction score and an inconclusive ultrasound image, anticoagulation should be started, with the intent to treat for three months.

Conclusion

Over the past several decades, UEDVT has accounted for an increasing proportion of venous thromboembolic disease. The clinical presentation varies from asymptomatic to severe symptoms; therefore, evaluating risk factors and predisposing conditions is essential. In asymptomatic patients, a high index of suspicion, coupled with a thorough personal history and ultrasound, can reveal an accurate diagnosis. Management with invasive methods for UEDVT remains controversial and requires a multidisciplinary approach with vascular and thoracic surgery, interventional radiology, and hematology/oncology. Because of the limited number of studies on UEDVT management, current anticoagulation recommendations stem from data surrounding LEDVT.

Clinical pearls

- Nearly two-thirds of patients with UEDVT have no presenting symptoms.
- The greatest risk factors for development of UEDVT are CVC placement and malignancy.
- When UEDVT is suspected, duplex ultrasonography is the screening test of choice.
- Superficial thrombosis from PICCs does not need to be treated with anticoagulation.
- Anticoagulation for UEDVT is recommended for three months.
- Compared with anticoagulation treatment, there is insufficient evidence to suggest that thrombolysis improves outcomes.
- There is no role for prophylactic anticoagulation in patients with CVCs.
- UEDVT morbidity and mortality rates are lower than those associated with LEDVT.

References

1. Lindblad B, Tengborn L, Berqvist D, *et al.* Deep vein thrombosis of the axillary-subclavian veins: epidemiologic data, effects of different types of treatment and late sequelae. *Eur J Vasc Surg* 1988; 2: 161–5.

2. Sanders RJ, Hammond SL, Rao NM. Thoracic outlet syndrome. *Neurologist* 2008; 14(6): 365–73.

3. Elman E, Kahn S. The post-thrombotic syndrome after upper extremity deep venous thrombosis in adults: a systematic review. *Thromb Res* 2006; 117(6): 609–14.

4. Joffe HV. Upper-extremity deep vein thrombosis: a prospective registry of 592 patients. *Circulation* 2004; 110(12): 1605–11.

5. Spencer FA, Emery C, Lessard D, *et al.* Upper extremity deep vein thrombosis: a community-based perspective. *Am J Med* 2007; 120(8): 678–84.

6. Isma N, Svensson PJ, Gottsäter A, *et al.* Upper extremity deep venous thrombosis in the population-based Malmö thrombophilia study (MATS): epidemiology, risk factors, recurrence risk, and mortality. *Thromb Res* 2010; 125(6): e335–8.

7. Kucher N. Deep-vein thrombosis of the upper extremities. *N Engl J Med* 2011; 364(9): 861–9.

8. Sajid MS, Ahmed N, Desai M, *et al.* Upper limb deep vein thrombosis: a literature review to streamline the protocol for management. *Acta Haematologica* 2007; 118(1): 10–18.

9. Kearon C, Aki EA, Comerota AJ, *et al.* Antithrombotic therapy for VTE disease: antithrombotic therapy and prevention of thrombosis, 9th ed. American College of Chest Physicians Evidence-Based Clinical Practice Guidelines. *Chest* 2012; 141(2 suppl): e419S–94S.

10. Linnemann B, Meister F, Schwonberg J, *et al.* Hereditary and acquired thrombophilia in patients with upper extremity deep-vein thrombosis: results from the MAISTHRO registry. *Thromb Haemost* 2008; 100(3): 440–6.

11. Munoz FJ, Mismetti P, Poggio R, *et al.* Clinical outcome of patients with upper-extremity deep vein thrombosis: results from the RIETE Registry. *Chest* 2008; 133(1): 143–8.

12. Prandoni P, Polistena P, Bernardi E, *et al.* Upper extremity deep vein thrombosis. *Arch Intern Med* 1997; 157(1): 57–62.

13. van Stralen KJ, Blom JW, Doggen CJM, *et al.* Strenuous sport activities involving the upper extremities increase the risk of venous thrombosis of the arm. *J Thromb Haemost* 2005; 3: 2110–1.

14. Lee AYY. Incidence, risk factors, and outcomes of catheter-related thrombosis in adult patients with cancer. *J Clin Oncol* 2006; 24(9): 1404–8.

15. Verso M, Agnelli G, Kamphuisen PW, *et al.* Risk factors for upper limb deep vein thrombosis associated with the use of central vein catheter in cancer patients. *Intern Emerg Med* 2008; 3(2): 117–22.

16. Lobo BL, Vaidean G, Broyles J, *et al.* Risk of venous thromboembolism in hospitalized patients with peripherally inserted central catheters. *J Hosp Med* 2009; 4(7): 417–22.

17. Anderson AJ, Krasnow SH, Boyer MW, *et al.* Thrombosis: the major Hickman catheter complication in patients with solid tumor. *Chest* 1989; 95(1): 71–5.

18. Martinelli I, Battaglioli T, Bucciarelli P, *et al.* Risk factors and recurrence rate of primary deep vein thrombosis of the upper extremities. *Circulation* 2004; 110(5): 566–70.

19. Bonizzoli M, Batacchi S, Cianchi G, *et al.* Peripherally inserted central venous catheters and central venous catheters related thrombosis in post-critical patients. *Intensive Care Med* 2010; 37(2): 284–9.

20. Evans RS, Sharp JH, Linford LH, *et al.* Risk of symptomatic DVT associated with peripherally inserted central catheters. *Chest* 2010; 138(4): 803–10.

21. Constans J, Salmi L-R, Sevestre-Pietri M-A, *et al.* A clinical prediction score for upper extremity deep venous thrombosis. *Thromb Haemost* 2007; 99(1): 202–7.

22. Di Nisio M, Van Sluis GL, Bossuyt PMM, *et al.* Accuracy of diagnostic tests for clinically suspected upper extremity deep vein thrombosis: a systematic review. *J Thromb Haemost* 2010; 8(4): 684–92.

23. Grove J, Pevec W. Venous thrombosis related to peripherally inserted central catheters. *J Vasc Interv Radiol* 2000; 11(7): 837–40.

24. Fabri P, Mirtallo J, Ebbert M, *et al.* Clinical effect of nonthrombotic total parenteral nutrition catheters. *JPEN J Parenter Enteral Nutr* 1984; 8(6): 705–7.

25. Eastridge BJ, Lefor AT. Complications of indwelling venous access devices in cancer patients. *J Clin Oncol* 1995; 13: 233–8.

26. van Rooden CJ. Infectious complications of central venous catheters increase the risk of catheter-related thrombosis in hematology patients: a prospective study. *J Clin Oncol* 2004; 23(12): 2655–60.

27. Spiezia L, Simioni P. Upper extremity deep vein thrombosis. *Intern Emerg Med* 2009; 5(2): 103–9.

28. Luciani A, Clement O, Hallmi P, *et al.* Catheter-related upper extremity deep venous thrombosis in cancer patients: a prospective study based on Doppler US. *Radiology* 2001; 220: 655–60.

29. Merimond T, Pellicciotta S, Bounameaux H. Limited usefulness of D-dimer in suspected deep vein thrombosis of the upper extremities. *Blood Coagul Fibrinolysis* 2006; 17(3): 225–6.

30. Fraser JD, Anderson DR. Deep venous thrombosis: recent advances and optimal investigation with US. *Radiology* 1999; 211(1): 9–24.

31. Baarslag HJ, van Beek EJ, Koopman MM, *et al.* Prospective study of color duplex ultrasonography

compared with contrast venography in patients suspected of having deep venous thrombosis of the upper extremities. *Ann Intern Med* 2002; 136(12): 865–72.

32. Goodman LR, Stein PD, Matta F, *et al.* CT venography and compression sonography are diagnostically equivalent: data from PIOPED II. *Am J Roentgenol* 2007; 189(5): 1071–6.

33. Joffe HV. Upper-extremity deep vein thrombosis. *Circulation* 2002; 106(14): 1874–80.

34. Mewissen MW, Seabrook GF, Meissner MH, *et al.* Catheter-directed thrombolysis for lower extremity deep venous thrombosis: report of a national multi-center registry. *Radiology* 1999; 211: 39–49.

35. Sabeti S, Schillinger M, Mlekusch W, *et al.* Treatment of subclavian–axillary vein thrombosis: long-term outcome of anticoagulation versus systemic thrombolysis. *Thromb Res* 2002; 108(5-6): 279–85.

36. Oderich GSC, Treiman GS, Schneider P, *et al.* Stent placement for treatment of central and peripheral venous obstruction: a long-term multi-institutional experience. *J Vasc Surg* 2000; 32(4): 760–9.

37. Illig KA, Doyle AJ. A comprehensive review of Paget–Schroetter syndrome. *J Vasc Surg* 2010; 51(6): 1538–47.

38. Lee JT, Karwowski JK, Harris EJ, *et al.* Long-term thrombotic recurrence after nonoperative management of Paget–Schroetter syndrome. *J Vasc Surg* 2006; 43(6): 1236–43.

39. Schneider DB, Dimuzio PJ, Martin ND, *et al.* Combination treatment of venous thoracic outlet syndrome: open surgical decompression and intraoperative angioplasty. *J Vasc Surg* 2004; 40(4): 599–603.

40. Spence LD, Gironta MG, Malde HM, *et al.* Acute upper extremity deep venous thrombosis: safety and effectiveness of superior vena caval filters. *Radiology* 1999; 210: 53–8.

41. Meier GH, Pollak JS, Rosenblatt M, *et al.* Initial experience with venous stents in exertional axillary-subclavian vein thrombosis. *J Vasc Surg* 1996; 24: 81–3.

42. Kovacs MJ, Kahn SR, Rodger M, *et al.* A pilot study of central venous catheter survival in cancer patients using low-molecular-weight heparin (dalteparin) and warfarin without catheter removal for the treatment of upper extremity deep vein thrombosis (The Catheter Study). *J Thromb Haemost* 2007; 5: 1650–3.

43. Savage KJ, Wells PS, Schulz V, *et al.* Outpatient use of low molecular weight heparin (Dalteparin) for the treatment of deep vein thrombosis of the upper extremity. *Thromb Haemost* 1999; 82: 1008–10.

44. Prandoni P, Bernardi E, Marchiori A, *et al.* The long term clinical course of acute deep vein thrombosis of the arm: prospective cohort study. *Br Med J* 2004; 329(7464): 484–5.

45. Kucher N, Tapson VF, Goldhaber SZ. Risk factors associated with symptomatic pulmonary embolism in a large cohort of deep vein thrombosis patients. *Thromb Haemost* 2005; 93(3): 494–8.

46. Stein PD, Matta F, Musani MH, Diaczok B. Silent pulmonary embolism in patients with deep venous thrombosis: a systematic review. *Am J Med* 2010; 123(5): 426–31.

47. Flinterman LE, van Hylckama Vlieg A, Rosendaal FR, *et al.* Recurrent thrombosis and survival after a first venous thrombosis of the upper extremity. *Circulation* 2008; 118(13): 1366–72.

48. Heit JA, Mohr DN, Silverstein MD, *et al.* Predictors of recurrence after deep vein thrombosis and pulmonary embolism: a population-based cohort study. *Arch Intern Med* 2000; 160: 761–8.

49. Akl EA, Kamath G, Yosuico V, *et al.* Thromboprophylaxis for patients with cancer and central venous catheters. *Cancer* 2008; 112(11): 2483–92.

Lower extremity deep venous thrombosis

Leann L. Silhan and Robert M. Reed

Lower extremity deep venous thrombosis (LEDVT) refers to a blood clot located in the external or internal iliac, deep femoral, superficial femoral, popliteal, or posterior tibial vein. The superficial femoral vein (a.k.a. great saphenous vein) is considered a deep vein for therapeutic purposes. Therapeutic implications differ according to whether a vein is deep (i.e., accompanied by an artery) or superficial (i.e., subcutaneous, which includes the dorsal venous foot vein, posterior arch vein, perforator veins, and the Giaccomini vein), and whether it is proximal (i.e., above the knee) or distal (i.e., below the knee).[1]

Clinical significance

The two major complications of DVT include pulmonary embolism (PE) and post-thrombotic syndrome (PTS). Causing more than 650,000 deaths in the United States each year, PE is the third most common cause of death in hospitalized patients.[2] Half of patients presenting with LEDVT have concomitant PE, and many of these emboli are asymptomatic.[2] Conversely, about 79% of patients who present with PE have evidence of LEDVT.[2]

Post-thrombotic syndrome occurs in 20 to 50% of patients within one or two years after a diagnosed DVT, and is associated with substantial long-term disability. PTS is a clinical diagnosis consisting of chronic, persistent pain; edema; and, in 5 to 10% of patients, non-healing venous ulcers.[3] The greatest risk factor for DVT is a previous episode of DVT, especially when the cause is idiopathic.[1]

Pathophysiology

In 1856, German physician Rudolf Virchow described what is now known as Virchow's triad. This triad describes the three main pathophysiologic risk factors for the development of DVT: venous stasis, hypercoagulability, and endothelial injury.[4]

Epidemiology

The annual incidence of *diagnosed* DVT is approximately 80 cases per 100,000 patients (i.e., 1 person per 1,250).[5] It is estimated that only half of incident cases are diagnosed, so true burden of disease may exceed 600,000 cases annually in the United States.[6] Approximately half of the documented cases of DVT are complicated by PE,[6] which results in up to 300,000 deaths per year.[7]

Risk factors

A thorough assessment of risk factors is important in the initial evaluation of DVT. These include the following:
- recent orthopedic surgery of the knee or hip;
- prolonged bed rest or immobility;
- estrogen replacement therapy or oral contraception;
- prolonged sitting (e.g., during a long car or plane ride);
- cancer;
- peripartum period;
- inherited hypercoagulability (e.g., factor V Leiden, prothrombin gene mutation);
- acquired hypercoagulability (e.g., antiphospholipid syndrome);
- trauma;
- nephrotic syndrome;
- obesity;
- recent myocardial infarction or heart failure;

- some respiratory diseases (e.g., chronic obstructive pulmonary disease);
- family history of clotting;
- presence of a central venous catheter.

Determining whether DVT is idiopathic or results from an identifiable transient or "provoked" risk factor (e.g., following surgery) helps determine the optimal duration of therapy. For DVT resulting from a cause with an anticipated resolution, the likelihood of recurrence is low, and a three-month course of anticoagulation is generally adequate. An idiopathic DVT has a much higher risk of recurrence, more than twofold that of a provoked DVT. A prospective cohort study, published out of the University of Padua in Italy, enrolled 1,626 patients with any-cause first occurrence DVT or PE and followed them up to 10 years after discontinuance of anticoagulation. They found a total recurrence of DVT or PE of 11% after 1 year, 29.1% after 5 years, and 39.9% after 10 years. However, when broken down between idiopathic and "provoked," the hazard ratio of idiopathic venous thromboembolism (VTE) was 2.3 (95% CI 1.82–2.90). At one year, the recurrence rate was 15.0% in the idiopathic VTE group vs. 6.6% in the secondary VTE group. By 10 years, the recurrence rate was 52.6% in the idiopathic group vs. 22.5% in the secondary group.[8] The rate of recurrence in this study is consistent with a previous registry of over 1,700 patients in Olmsted County, Minnesota.[9] Due to the high risk of recurrence in idiopathic DVT, experts now argue that anticoagulation be continued indefinitely in this subset of patients.[10] A careful history should therefore include any findings that would help characterize the event as provoked DVT, in which case duration of anticoagulation can be limited to three to six months.

Initial emergency department management

Diagnosis

History. Although often asymptomatic, patients with LEDVT may present with leg edema and pain in the affected extremity.

Physical examination. The physical examination is unreliable to definitively make the diagnosis of LEDVT, but some signs may be present:

- edema, usually pitting;
- warmth;

- tenderness of the affected extremity;
- increased tissue turgor;
- palpable cord;
- Homan's sign (pain on passive dorsiflexion of the ankle) has virtually no clinical value, as evidenced by its sensitivity of 60 to 88% and specificity of 30 to 72%.[11]

  - *phlegmasia alba dolens* or *phlegmasia cerulea dolens:* when a large thrombus or a complete occlusion of the ileo-femoral venous system is present, two signs warranting concern may be present: phlegmasia alba dolens ("painful white edema") or phlegmasia cerulea dolens ("painful blue edema"). Classically associated with malignancy or pregnancy,[12] these rare manifestations of an acute massive thrombus may mimic an arterial thrombus (i.e., acute severe edema, initial skin blanching, and eventual limb ischemia and cyanosis). Despite anticoagulation, limb necrosis may occur and the risk of PE is high.

Laboratory data

D-dimer. D-dimer levels are elevated in plasma in the presence of an acute thrombus because of simultaneous activation of coagulation and fibrinolysis. Therefore, a normal D-dimer level makes acute DVT unlikely, i.e., the negative predictive value (NPV) of D-dimer is high. Although D-dimer is very specific for fibrin, the specificity of fibrin for VTE is poor because fibrin is produced in a variety of conditions, such as cancer, inflammation, infection, and dissection of the aorta, and the positive predictive value (PPV) of D-dimer is low. Therefore, D-dimer is not useful for confirming a diagnosis of DVT.[13] The Wells scoring system for clinical pretest probability of DVT is presented in Table 20.1.[14,15] If the clinical suspicion for LEDVT is high based on the Wells model or other clinical scoring system, the D-dimer level has no diagnostic significance and further testing should be pursued. There are D-dimer assays of high sensitivity (> 95%, e.g., ELISA) and moderate sensitivity (85–90%, e.g., latex-derived assay SimpliRED or whole blood agglutination assays). When using a high-sensitivity D-dimer assay, a negative result can

Table 20.1 Wells clinical model for predicting pretest probability for deep venous thrombosis[14] (left); modified Wells clinical model[15] (right)

Wells clinical model		Modified Wells clinical model	
Clinical feature	Score	Clinical feature	Score
Active cancer (treatment ongoing or within the past six months)	1	Clinical signs and symptoms of deep vein thrombosis (minimum of leg swelling and pain with palpation of the deep veins)	3.0
Paralysis, paresis, or recent plaster immobilization of the leg	1	Alternative diagnosis less likely than pulmonary embolism	3.0
Recently bedridden for more than three days or major surgery within four weeks	1	Heart rate > 100 bpm	1.5
Localized tenderness along the distribution of the deep venous system	1	Immobilization (more than three days) or surgery in the previous four weeks	1.5
Entire leg swollen	1	Previous pulmonary embolism or deep vein thrombosis	1.5
Calf swelling by > 3 cm compared with the asymptomatic leg (measured 10 cm below the tibial tuberosity)	1	Hemoptysis	1.0
Pitting edema (greater in the symptomatic leg)	1	Malignancy (receiving treatment, treated in the last six months or palliative)	1.0
Collateral superficial veins (non-varicose) (suggests chronic rather than acute)	1		
Alternative diagnosis at least as likely as that of deep venous thrombosis	−2		
0 = low probability, 1–2 = moderate probability, ≥ 3 = high probability		4 or less points = clinical probability of PE unlikely; 5 or more points = clinical probability of PE likely	

rule out both low and moderate probability VTE. However, if you are using a moderately sensitive D-dimer assay, only low-probability VTE can be ruled out.[13] Although each institution has its own diagnostic threshold, the usual value for a "positive D-dimer" is > 500 or 750 ng/mL.[16]

D-dimer testing can also help determine the duration of anticoagulation. Palareti *et al.* demonstrated that patients treated with warfarin for three months who had an abnormal D-dimer level one month after completion of warfarin therapy had an increased rate of recurrent thromboembolism (hazard ratio, 2.27) whereas those without elevated D-dimer could be continued safely off anticoagulation.[17] Among patients with an abnormal post-treatment D-dimer level who resumed anticoagulation, the risk of recurrent thromboembolism was decreased (hazard ratio, 4.26).[17]

Hypercoagulable evaluation. We do not favor the routine performance of a hypercoagulable workup for several reasons.[18] First, acute thrombosis and heparin therapy can independently alter key

anticoagulant and procoagulant protein levels, limiting the diagnostic accuracy of the test during initial diagnosis.[3,19] Second, a growing consensus in the literature suggests that, even if properly performed, this evaluation has little clinical utility.[3,4] Several large cohorts have demonstrated that the diagnosis of thrombophilia does not significantly alter DVT recurrence rates.[2,20] Committing a patient to prolonged courses of anticoagulation based upon hypercoagulable studies rather than clinical context is unwarranted. Despite these data, factor V Leiden remains the most commonly ordered genetic test worldwide. Finally, the cost of the comprehensive hypercoagulable evaluation exceeds $4,500 in our institution. Based on these considerations, we believe that the routine evaluation for thrombophilia in patients with idiopathic DVT should be discouraged.[21]

Imaging

Ultrasonography. Doppler compression ultrasonography is considered the best non-invasive diagnostic method for proximal LEDVT. Compared with the gold standard, venography, ultrasonography has a sensitivity and specificity of 97%. However, its sensitivity is only ~75% for identification of distal (i.e., below the knee) LEDVT. When a distal DVT is found, anticoagulation is not necessary, but a repeat ultrasound in five to seven days is recommended because about a quarter of such thromboses eventually extend into the proximal deep veins.[22] If suspicion for LEDVT exists despite a negative ultrasound or a negative D-dimer, it is reasonable to repeat the ultrasound in five to seven days or pursue further definitive testing.[22]

Several methods exist to examine the deep venous system sonographically. With compression ultrasound, the lumen of normal veins should compress completely, whereas veins with a thrombus are either partially or entirely non-compressible. Duplex and color Doppler sonography enhance blood flow patterns to permit differentiation between normal (phasic with respiratory phase) and abnormal (continuous) flow in the venous system.[1]

Ultrasound is an extremely valuable bedside tool for diagnosing venous system disease, and it can be used effectively by physicians with minimal training. After a three-day course, participating intensivists showed considerable expertise in diagnosing proximal LEDVT by compression ultrasonography. In this study, the prevalence of DVT was 20%, and the examination had a sensitivity of 86%, a specificity of 96%, and an accuracy of 95% compared with formal vascular studies performed by ultrasonography technicians and interpreted by radiologists.[23]

Plethysmography. This is the measurement of changes in volume within a given body part, such as a vein. In the venous system this enables amount of blood flow to be determined. Patients can be assessed for LEDVT by various methods of plethysmography, including digital photoplethysmography, computerized strain-gage plethysmography, and impedence plethysmography. All methods record changes in size of the limb caused by tissue fluid or pooled blood in the veins. Although this may be used as a relatively easy, non-invasive, rapid diagnostic study, its sensitivity and specificity are 80% and 95%, respectively. Now that ultrasonography is so readily available and has a much higher sensitivity and specificity, plethysmography is no longer used frequently.[1]

Lower extremity venogram. The venogram is considered the gold standard in definitively diagnosing an LEDVT. However, it is invasive and carries a risk of dye allergy and thrombus formation.

Computed tomography venogram with contrast dye. Computed tomography (CT) venogram, compared against invasive venography, has a sensitivity of 100% and specificity of 96%,[1] and it requires 80% less contrast dye. Studies looking at contrast-induced nephropathy (defined as a 25% rise in creatinine), from either CT scanning with intravenous contrast or angiography, show approximately an 8% incidence in patients with a normal creatinine level ($<$ 1.5 mg/dL) and up to 16% incidence in patients with an elevated creatinine level.[24] When CT venogram was compared with ultrasound for clinically significant ileo-femoral thrombi, there was no difference in sensitivity. CT venography does increase the sensitivity over ultrasonography alone for detecting distal thrombi. The role of a CT venogram can be limited by inadequate timing of contrast dye, risk of anaphylaxis to dye, exposure to radiation in the gonadopelvic area, and inability to differentiate acute from chronic thrombi. Some centers incorporate a limited examination of the proximal deep veins while minimizing radiation to the gonadopelvic area through the addition of two or three CT cuts to a PE protocol CT scan.

Magnetic resonance imaging/MR venogram. Studies have shown that magnetic resonance venography for thrombi is equivalent to invasive venography without the risks of IV contrast or venous access.[25] Although limited by cost and availability, magnetic resonance venography is an alternative that can be used in the now rare case when an invasive venogram would otherwise be considered.

Acute management

The main short-term goal of therapy for LEDVT is limiting progression of DVT to PE, whereas longer-term goals include reducing the risk for DVT recurrence and PTS development. The suspicion of a DVT should trigger two urgent considerations: the presence of contraindications to anticoagulation and the likelihood of concomitant PE. If PE is suspected, anticoagulation should ideally begin prior to diagnostic confirmation and thrombolysis should be considered in hemodynamically unstable patients. However, if absolute contraindications to anticoagulation exist, timely insertion of an inferior vena cava filter may be considered.

Deep venous thrombi detected above the knee need to be treated. DVT below the knee should be monitored periodically for two weeks and treated if any progression is observed, even if progression remains below the knee. It is also reasonable to treat below the knee thrombosis if severe symptoms are present. Superficial thrombus of the greater saphenous vein should be treated with anticoagulation because the risk of progression to DVT is high.

Treatment

Either low-molecular-weight heparin (LMWH) or unfractionated heparin (UFH) should be administered. The two currently approved LMWHs for treatment of DVT are enoxaparin (Lovenox) and fondaparinux (Arixtra). LMWH is preferred in the general population. UFH is preferred only for patients with renal impairment or severe obesity or when thrombolytics are being considered. The dosages are described below:

- Heparin intravenous infusion: 70 to 100 IU/kg bolus, then 10 to 15 IU/kg·h. Adjust to aPTT of 1.5 to 2 times baseline.
- Enoxaparin (Lovenox) subcutaneous injection: 1 mg/kg twice daily or 2 mg/kg daily (latter preferred). Cost-effective analysis found LMWH to be superior to UFH.[26]
- Fondaparinux (Arixtra) subcutaneous injection: 7.5 mg daily if the patient weighs 50 to 100 kg (5 mg if < 50 kg; 10 mg if > 100 kg). Its advantage over enoxaparin is that it does not appear to be associated with an increased risk of heparin-induced thrombocytopenia (HIT).

After adequate anticoagulation with either LMWH or UFH has been initiated, an oral vitamin-K inhibitor should be initiated.[25] Dosing needs to be adjusted to a goal INR of 2.0 to 3.0. However, if the thrombus is associated with malignancy, evidence supports chronic treatment with LMWH rather than oral warfarin.[27]

Duration of therapy

The optimal duration of anticoagulation is an area of ongoing research and subject to change. A study comparing three versus six months of anticoagulation in patients with no ongoing risk factors found no difference in cumulative incidence of subsequent DVT or PE.[28] Similar rates of recurrence were seen in patients with idiopathic DVT who were treated with either 3 or 12 months of anticoagulation. However, in studying 3 versus 24 months of anticoagulation for first-time DVT, the group treated for 24 months had a significantly lower rate of recurrence.

Recommendations for length of therapy are presented below:[29]

- DVT with transient risk factor (e.g., complicating surgery or pregnancy): three months.
- Unprovoked or idiopathic DVT: 3–12 months followed by evaluation of risks versus benefits of indefinite therapy and low risk for bleeding "when consistent with patient's preference."[30] We favor 12 months to lifetime therapy given the high risk of recurrence in idiopathic DVT.
- Recurrent DVT: indefinite therapy.
- Active or recent cancer and DVT: treatment with LMWH as long as cancer is active.[22]
- Elastic compression stocking use for two years is recommended for all patients diagnosed with LEDVT.[13,31] A Cochrane Review of randomized controlled trials regarding the use of compression stockings in patients with LEDVT found that the number-needed-to-treat was four or five to prevent one episode of PTS. Most of the studies involved knee-high stockings.[32]

Surgical options/thrombolysis

Studies involving large ileo-femoral thrombi have focused on catheter-directed thrombolysis (CDT), systemic thrombolysis, percutaneous venous thrombectomy, and operative venous thombectomy for acute DVT. A recent randomized controlled trial in Norway of 209 patients randomized to CDT plus standard care vs. standard treatment alone for acute ilio-femoral deep vein thrombosis (the CaVenT study) found an absolute risk reduction in post-thrombotic syndrome of 14.4% in the CDT group. The number-needed-to-treat was seven. There were five major bleeding complications in the CDT group, none of which were fatal.[33] The use of catheter-directed thrombolysis for large ilio-femoral DVTs is increasing as more studies have shown its effectiveness in preventing PTS. Current ACCP (American College of Chest Physicians) guidelines recommend CDT over percutaneous venous thrombectomy or systemic thrombolysis in patients who have had symptoms for less than 14 days, have a low risk of bleeding, and are being treated in a medical center with expertise in these procedures.[29] If risk of bleeding is unacceptably high, operative venous thrombectomy is preferable. Any patient who undergoes one of these procedures still requires anticoagulation for the recommended duration.[29]

Inferior vena cava (IVC) filters

The role of IVC filters is controversial, and currently they should be considered only in patients with absolute contraindications to anticoagulation. The PREPIC study randomized 400 patients with proximal DVT to IVC filter placement in addition to standard anticoagulation and showed increased rates of secondary DVT without any improvement in the mortality rate when an IVC filter was inserted.[34] We recommend against routine placement of IVC filters in patients with PE who have concomitant DVT, as procedural complications can make anticoagulation problematic and lead to contraindication to thrombolysis if the patient deteriorates. While modern IVC filters are retrievable to minimize the risk of recurrent DVT, it should be understood that in clinical practice most removable filters are never removed. Filters should be retrieved when duration of treatment for a thrombotic event has been met, the risk of an embolism is no longer high, and/or there is no longer an absolute contraindication to anticoagulation.

Ambulation

There is a lack of data regarding the optimal time to start physical therapy or ambulation after a diagnosis of DVT, but the ACCP consensus is that it may begin 24 hours after anticoagulation is achieved.[29] There is no evidence concerning the benefit of immobilization for the clinical outcome of patients with pulmonary embolism. In these patients with DVT, studies have demonstrated similar incidence of new PE on repeat pulmonary vascular imaging, for early ambulation and leg compression compared to immobilization.[13]

Prevention

Guidelines issued by the ACCP[31] recommend prophylaxis with UFH (5000 IU subcutaneously three times per day), LMWH daily, or fondaparinux daily for acutely ill, hospitalized medical and surgical patients who have congestive heart failure or severe pulmonary disease and for those confined to bed. Such therapy prevents over 50% of in-hospital cases of DVT.[13,31] Most hospitals have a system in place for risk assessment and recommendations for prophylaxis. Compression stockings should be given for all moderate-to-high-risk patients, and medical prophylaxis for those patients who do not have contraindications (active bleeding or high risk for bleeding).

Admission criteria/disposition

In the emergency department, several factors should be considered when deciding whether to admit a patient with a diagnosis of LEDVT. LEDVT not complicated by PE does not always require inpatient treatment. There are, however, practical aspects to keep in mind. First, the patient needs to receive either UFH or LMWH soon after confirming the diagnosis of DVT. Then a vitamin-K inhibitor (warfarin) should be administered, with the goal of achieving an INR of 2 or 3 over the following few days. Before the advent of LMWH, patients were admitted to the hospital for three or four days of intravenous infusion of UFH. But LMWH has been shown to be superior to UFH in most patients. If administration of LMWH can be initiated in the emergency department, with subsequent discharge and close primary care physician follow-up within four to five days, then the patient can be treated as an outpatient. However, the likelihood of bleeding as a complication of anticoagulation is greatest shortly after initiation, so admission for observation is reasonable. Indications for inpatient therapy are listed in Table 20.2.

Clinical approach when resources are limited

Ultrasonography has made the diagnosis of many diseases more feasible. Because of its portability, sonography can be used to diagnose LEDVT even in facilities in remote areas with limited resources. Compression ultrasonography is a skill that clinicians can master with relatively minimal time and effort. Monitoring coagulation levels (INR) in a patient on warfarin

Table 20.2 Indications for inpatient therapy[14,15]

- Co-diagnosis of PE;
- Inability to obtain LMWH as an outpatient (not always covered by insurance);
- Inability to administer the injections;
- Ileo-femoral DVT;
- Pregnancy;
- Renal failure, creatinine > 2;
- Morbid obesity (UFH preferred).

is often challenging, especially when resources are limited. Direct thrombin inhibitors have the advantage of not needing any blood monitoring to correctly dose the anticoagulant. As new medication developments emerge, treatment may become easier as medications which do not need frequent monitoring become available. However, even in wealthy countries, direct thrombin inhibitors will be expensive for many years.

Clinical pearls

- Patients with LEDVT may be asymptomatic, so maintain a high level of suspicion.
- A negative high-sensitivity D-dimer rules out DVT in all but the highest pretest probability subjects.
- Wells criteria can be used to formally determine pretest probability.
- Lower extremity Doppler ultrasound is the most efficient way to diagnose a thrombus in the emergency department.
- A hypercoagulability workup should not be routine.
- Patients with above the knee DVT need anticoagulation.
- Patients with below the knee DVT should be followed with ultrasound for two weeks.
- Thrombus of the superficial femoral vein should be treated with anticoagulation because risk of progression to DVT is high.
- IVC filters should not be placed routinely.
- Compression stockings should be prescribed for at least 24 months following diagnosis and possibly should be recommended for the rest of the patient's life.
- The standard course for anticoagulation is three months for a first episode of DVT.
- Patients with idiopathic, recurrent, or cancer-associated LEDVT should receive 12 months to lifelong therapy unless at high bleeding risk.

- Patients with LEDVT associated with cancer should receive treatment with low-molecular-weight heparin rather than warfarin.
- Idiopathic DVT is more likely to recur than post-surgical or post-traumatic DVT.

References

1. Tovey C, Wyatt S. Diagnosis, investigation, and management of deep vein thrombosis. *BMJ* 2003; 326: 1180–4.

2. Tapson V. Acute pulmonary embolism. *N Engl J Med* 2008; 358: 1037–52.

3. Kahn SR, Ginsberg JS. The post-thrombotic syndrome: current knowledge, controversies, and directions for future research. *Blood Rev* 2002; 16: 155–65.

4. Dickson BC. Venous thrombosis: on the history of Virchow's triad. *Univ Toronto Med J* 2004; 81: 166–71.

5. Silversein MD, Heit JA, Mohr DN, *et al.* Trends in the incidence of deep vein thrombosis and pulmonary embolism: a 25-year population-based study. *Arch Intern Med* 1998; 158: 585–93.

6. Anderson FA Jr, Wheeler HB, Goldberg RJ, *et al.* A population-based perspective of the hospital incidence and case-fatality rates of deep vein thrombosis and pulmonary embolism. The Worcester DVT Study. *Arch Intern Med* 1991; 151: 933–8.

7. Heit JA, Cohen AT Jr, Frederick A. On Behalf of the VTE Impact Assessment Group. Estimated annual number of incident and recurrent, non-fatal and fatal venous thromboembolism (VTE) events in the the US [abstract]. *Blood* 2005; 106: 267a.

8. Prandoni P, Noventa F, Ghirarduzzi A, *et al.* The risk of recurrent venous thromboembolism after discontinuing anticoagulation in patients with acute proximal deep vein thrombosis or pulmonary embolism. A prospective cohort study in 1,626 patients. *Haematologica* 2007; 92: 199–205.

9. Heit JA, Mohr DN, Silverstein MD, *et al.* Predictors of recurrence after deep vein thrombosis and pulmonary embolism: a population-based cohort study. *Arch Intern Med* 2000; 160: 761–8.

10. Goldhaber SZ. Prevention of recurrent idiopathic venous thromboembolism. *Circulation* 2004; 110(suppl IV): IV-20–4.

11. Joshua AM, Celermajer DS, Stockler MR. Beauty is in the eye of the examiner: reaching agreement about physical signs and their value. *Intern Med J* 2005; 35: 178–87.

12. Reams G, Rosner M. Phlegmasia cerulea dolens: a case report with a review of the literature. *Arch Intern Med* 1960; 106: 647–52.

13. Torbicki A, Perrier A, Konstantinides S, *et al.* Guidelines on the diagnosis and management of acute pulmonary embolism. The task force for the diagnosis and management of acute pulmonary embolism of the European Society of Cardiology. *Eur Heart J* 2008; 29: 2276–315.

14. Wells PS, Anderson DR, Bormanis J, *et al.* Value of assessment of pretest probability of deep-vein thrombosis in clinical management. *Lancet* 1997; 350: 1795–8.

15. van Belle A, Büller HR, Huisman MV, *et al.* Effectiveness of managing suspected pulmonary embolism using an algorithm combining clinical probability, D-dimer testing, and computed tomography. *JAMA* 2006; 295(2): 172–9.

16. Wells PS, Anderson DR, Rodger M, *et al.* Evaluation of D-dimer in the diagnosis of suspected deep-vein thrombosis. *N Engl J Med* 2003; 349: 1227–35.

17. Palareti G, Cosmi B, Leganani C, *et al.* D-Dimer testing to determine the duration of anticoagulation therapy. *N Engl J Med* 2006; 355: 1780–90.

18. Haemostasis and Thombosis Task Force, British Committee for Standards in Haematology. Investigation and management of heritable thrombophilia. *Br J Haematol* 2001; 114: 512–28.

19. Baglin T, Luddington R, Brown K, Baglin C. Incidence of recurrent venous thromboembolism in relation to clinical and thrombophilic risk factors: prospective cohort study. *Lancet* 2003; 362: 523–6.

20. Christiansen S, Cannegieter S, Koster T, *et al.* Thrombophilia, clinical factors, and recurrent venous thrombotic events. *JAMA* 2005; 293: 2352–61.

21. Middeldorp S, van Hylckama Vlieg A. Does thrombophilia testing help in the clinical management of patients? *Br J Haematol* 2008; 143: 321–35.

22. Bernardi E, Prandoni P, Lensing AW, *et al.* D-dimer testing as an adjunct to ultrasonography in patients with clinically suspected deep vein thrombosis: prospective cohort study. The Multicentre Italian D-dimer Ultrasound Study Investigators Group. *BMJ* 1998; 317: 1037–40.

23. Kory PD, Pellecchia CM, Shiloh AL, *et al.* Accuracy of ultrasonography performed by critical care physicians for the diagnosis of DVT. *Chest* 2011; 139: 538–42.

24. Barrett BJ, Parfrey PS. Preventing nephropathy induced by contrast media. *N Engl J Med* 2006; 354: 379–86.

25. Carpenter JP, Holland GA, Baum RA, *et al.* Magnetic resonance venography for the detection of deep venous thrombosis: comparison with contrast venography and duplex Doppler ultrasonography. *J Vasc Surg* 1993; 18(5): 734–41.

26. Gould MK, Dembitzer AD, Sanders GD, Garber AM. Low-molecular-weight heparins compared with unfractionated heparin for treatment of acute deep venous thrombosis. A cost-effectiveness analysis. *Ann Intern Med* 1999; 130: 789–99.

27. Lee AY, Levine MN, Baker C, *et al.* Low-molecular-weight heparin versus a coumarin for the prevention of recurrent venous thromboembolism in patients with cancer. *N Engl J Med* 2003; 349: 146–53.

28. Kearon C, Gent M, Hirsh J, *et al.* A comparison of three months of anticoagulation with extended anticoagulation for a first episode of idiopathic venous thromboembolism. *N Engl J Med* 1999; 340: 901–7.

29. Kearon C, Kahn SR, Agnelli G, *et al.* Antithrombotic therapy for venous thromboembolic disease: American College of Chest Physicians Evidence-Based Clinical Practice Guidelines (8th Edition). *Chest* 2008; 133: 454S–545S.

30. Guyatt GH, Akl EA, Crowther M, *et al.* Executive summary: antithrombotic therapy and prevention of thrombosis, 9th ed: American College of Chest Physicians Evidence-Based Clinical Practice Guidelines. *Chest* 2012; 141(2 suppl): 7S–47S.

31. Geerts WH, Bergqvist D, Pineo GF, *et al.* Prevention of venous thromboembolism: American College of Chest Physicians Evidence-Based Clinical Practice Guidelines (8th Edition). *Chest* 2008; 133(6 suppl): 381S–453S.

32. Kolbach D, Sandbrink MW, Hamulyak K, *et al.* Non-pharmaceutical measures for prevention of post-thrombotic syndrome. *Cochrane Database Syst Rev* 2004; (1): CD004174.

33. Enden T, Haig Y, Kløw NE, *et al.* Long-term outcome after additional catheter-directed thrombolysis versus standard treatment for acute iliofemoral deep vein thrombosis (the CaVenT study): a randomised controlled trial. *Lancet* 2012; 379: 31–8.

34. Decousus H, Leizorovicz A, Parent F, *et al.* A clinical trial of vena caval filters in the prevention of pulmonary embolism in patients with proximal deep-vein thrombosis. Prévention du Risque d'Embolie Pulmonaire par Interruption Cave Study Group. *N Engl J Med* 1998; 338: 409–15.

Chapter

Pulmonary embolism

Samantha L. Wood and Robert M. Reed

Pulmonary embolism (PE) and deep venous thrombosis (DVT) constitute the venous thromboembolic disorders and refer, respectively, to a blood clot in the pulmonary vasculature and a clot in the deep veins. The two are closely related; PE is usually a consequence of DVT.

Clinical significance

Pulmonary embolism has both respiratory and cardiovascular effects. Obstruction of blood flow to the affected lung region results in ventilation–perfusion mismatch and subsequent hypoxia. In patients with limited ventilatory reserve, the increased dead space causes hypercarbia. Clot burden may result in acute pulmonary hypertension and right heart failure.

Pathophysiology and etiology

Virchow's triad comprises the classic risk factors for venous thromboembolic disease: venous stasis, hypercoagulability, and vascular injury. Within these categories, risk factors may be hereditary or acquired. Common hereditary factors include factor V Leiden, protein C or S deficiency, and antithrombin III deficiency. Acquired risk factors include reduced mobility, malignancy, recent surgery, and estrogen use.

Epidemiology

Pulmonary embolism most commonly originates from venous thrombosis of the deep leg veins. Symptomatic PE is found in 40% of people diagnosed with DVT,[1] and 79% of patients with PE are found to have evidence of DVT.[2]

Decompensation in the patient with PE can be precipitous, and it is estimated that, for as many as a quarter of patients, the initial presentation is sudden death.[3] Rates of missed PE are frequently quoted as being quite high, with the implication of significant morbidity and mortality as a result. Such statistics are generally based on decades-old data from inpatient populations, so their validity for extrapolation to an ambulatory emergency department (ED) population has been questioned.[4] Nonetheless, physicians should have a very low threshold to evaluate for PE, a dangerous yet treatable condition.

Initial emergency department management

Diagnosis

The classic history for PE is pleuritic chest pain with shortness of breath in the context of one or more risk factors for venous thromboembolism (VTE). However, the presentation is variable: in one registry, 82% of patients presented with dyspnea, 49% with chest pain, 20% with cough, 14% with syncope, and 7% with hemoptysis.[5] The chest pain associated with PE is classically described as pleuritic, a consequence of distal embolism causing pulmonary infarction and pleural irritation. However, a large central pulmonary embolus with hemodynamic consequences causing right heart ischemia may provoke substernal chest pain that mimics angina. Isolated syncope is another important presentation of PE.

Physical examination

Physical examination should focus on evidence of VTE as well as exclusion of alternative diagnoses. Abnormal vital signs in a patient with PE may include tachycardia, tachypnea, or hypoxia. Fever may be present. Physical examination may reveal lower

Table 21.1 Pulmonary embolism probability scoring systems

Wells criteria for pulmonary embolism		Revised Geneva Score for pulmonary embolism		Pulmonary Embolism Rule-Out Criteria (apply to patients determined to be low risk by scoring system or gestalt)
Clinical signs/symptoms of DVT	3	Pain on lower limb palpation and unilateral edema	4	Age < 50
Alternative diagnosis less likely than PE	3	Unilateral lower limb pain	3	Heart rate < 100 bpm
Heart rate > 100 bpm	1.5	Heart rate 75–94 bpm	3	Oxygen saturation > 94% on room air
Immobilization/surgery in past four weeks	1.5	Heart rate ≥ 95 bpm	5	No hemoptysis
Previous DVT/PE	1.5	Surgery or fracture in past one month	2	No estrogen use
Hemoptysis	1	Previous DVT/PE	3	No prior venous thromboembolism
Malignancy	1	Hemoptysis	2	No unilateral leg swelling
		Active malignancy	2	No surgery or trauma requiring hospitalization in past four weeks
		Age > 65	1	
< 2 = low, 2–6 = moderate, > 6 = high probability		0–3 = low, 4–10 = intermediate, ≥ 11 = high probability		If all criteria apply in a low-risk patient, probability of PE is < 2%
Adapted from references [12–17].				

extremity swelling or redness consistent with deep venous thrombosis. A normal lung examination in the patient with hypoxia raises concern for PE. The physical examination should also focus on evaluation of alternative causes of chest pain and dyspnea, such as pneumothorax or pneumonia.

Laboratory data

Laboratory studies play a minimal role in ruling in PE. D-dimer, a product of degraded cross-linked fibrin, has very good sensitivity for acute thrombus[6] and may be used in a patient with low pretest probability to exclude PE.[7,8] Additional laboratory studies that are commonly obtained include B-type natriuretic peptide (BNP) and troponin to evaluate for right heart strain, as discussed below, and baseline assessment of renal function and coagulation status.

Clinical prediction rules

The diagnostic approach to PE begins with estimation of pretest probability for the diagnosis. Clinical opinion, not guided by a particular scoring system, is fairly accurate in identifying patients at low or high risk of having PE. Such estimates are still suboptimal, with reported rates of PE in patients considered by physician gestalt to be low or high risk of 8 to 9% and 64 to 68%, respectively.[9–11] Several clinical decision rules aimed at improving accuracy have been developed and evaluated. They seem to perform little better than gestalt opinion in assessing patients with possible PE, and there is insufficient evidence to recommend one over the other.[7] Clinical decision rules are most useful in combination with diagnostic testing; the accuracy of laboratory and imaging studies to diagnose PE depends greatly on pretest probability.

The Wells criteria, shown in Table 21.1, categorize patients into low, moderate, or high probability for PE. In the original studies, overall rates of PE by group were 3.4 to 3.6%, 20.5 to 27.8%, and 66.7 to 78.4%, respectively.[12,13]

The Revised Geneva Score, shown in Table 21.1, also classifies patients into low, moderate, and high probability for PE. Rates of PE by group were 7.9 to 9%, 27.5 to 28.5%, and 71.7 to 73.7%, respectively.[14,15]

The Pulmonary Embolism Rule-Out Criteria (PERC) (Table 21.1) constitute a clinical prediction rule that can be applied to patients with a low clinical suspicion for PE. In contradistinction to the other clinical prediction rules, the PERC is not used to generate a pretest probability, but rather to risk stratify after pretest probability has been determined by other methods. In studies by Kline and colleagues, the prevalence of PE was less than 2% in patients who were considered low risk and were PERC negative.[16,17]

Table 21.2 Imaging modalities for pulmonary embolism

Imaging modality	Findings	Advantages	Disadvantages	Comments
Plain radiography	Focal oligemia (Westermark's sign) or peripheral wedge-shaped density (Hampton's hump); classic but rarely seen	Available rapidly and at bedside Can rule in/rule out alternative diagnoses	Poor sensitivity and specificity for PE[5]	Normal chest radiograph in the presence of hypoxia strongly suggests PE
CT angiography	Filling defect of pulmonary vasculature Can compare right (RV)/left ventricular size to evaluate RV strain	Study of choice in most EDs Rapidly obtainable	Quality of scan influences sensitivity/specificity Contrast dye poses risk for renal failure	Can include lower extremity CT venogram to evaluate for DVT and increase sensitivity, but this increases radiation exposure to gonadal-pelvic region[18]
Ventilation–perfusion (VQ) scan	Result may be normal, low, intermediate, or high probability	Normal VQ scan excludes clinically significant PE[19] A high-probability result in a high-probability patient is very specific for PE No dye load	Less useful in patients with underlying lung disease Not always immediately available	A completely normal study can virtually always stop the workup for PE irrespective of pretest likelihood assessment
Lower extremity duplex ultrasound	Deep venous thrombosis	If positive, patient can be treated for VTE without further studies Safe in pregnancy and renal failure	If negative, patient still needs evaluation for PE	Patients with negative CT angiogram plus negative lower extremity ultrasound are at extremely low risk of VTE
Angiography	Visualization of clot in vasculature	Long considered the gold standard for diagnosis	Requires arterial puncture and contrast dye administration	Infrequently has a role when alternative imaging modalities are inconclusive
Magnetic resonance imaging	Filling defect of pulmonary vasculature	Good specificity, sensitivity ranges from 75 to 93%[20]	Time consuming, requires sending potentially unstable patient out of the ED for a lengthy period Cannot be performed in patients with indwelling metallic devices	
Echocardiography	Right heart strain Visualization of intracardiac clot	Useful in unstable patients to evaluate for right heart strain Can evaluate alternative diagnoses such as tamponade and myocardial infarction with focal wall motion abnormality Can be performed at bedside Useful for risk stratification of patients with PE Safe in pregnancy and renal failure	Poor sensitivity[20]	If right atrial clot and patent foramen ovale are identified, strong indication for thrombolysis or thrombectomy

Chapter 21: Pulmonary embolism

Imaging

Accurate diagnosis or exclusion of PE in the stable patient starts with an assessment of its likelihood. Based on this assessment, the appropriate diagnostic tests can then be ordered. In stable patients, discordance between the pretest likelihood of PE and the results of diagnostic testing usually should be evaluated with further tests. Table 21.2 provides a review of diagnostic modalities for pulmonary embolism. The unstable patient with suspected PE represents a special case, as there is both diagnostic urgency and limited diagnostic options due to lack of immediate availability of test results and logistic limitations in managing such patients in testing areas outside the ED.

The unstable patient with high probability of PE. Diagnostic strategies in the unstable patient with suspected PE are limited. It may be inappropriate or impossible to send such a patient out of the ED for time-consuming studies. Echocardiography is a particularly useful diagnostic study in this patient group. It has the advantages of being available at the bedside, providing real-time information, and evaluating alternative causes of hypotension (such as cardiac tamponade, hypovolemia, and myocardial infarction [MI] resulting in segmental wall motion abnormality). Electrocardiography and portable chest radiography are immediately available studies that may provide information to support PE or an alternative diagnosis in the unstable patient. However, the emergency physician confronted with the unstable patient with suspected PE will be in the position of having to intervene and treat based on limited information. In that event, the only possible strategy may be to assess risk of bleeding and, if no contraindications are identified, to give an empiric trial of thrombolysis. When this strategy is employed, it is critical to involve the patient and family in the decision as much as possible.

The stable high-probability patient. In a patient with a high pretest probability of PE, a positive CT scan, lower extremity ultrasound, MRI, or high-probability ventilation–perfusion (VQ) scan are all sufficient for confident diagnosis.[21] If the initial test is negative in a high-probability patient, suspicion for PE must remain high and additional testing must be pursued.

The low-probability patient. If a patient is determined to have low probability for PE,

application of the PERC rule or D-dimer testing is an appropriate next step. The critical action in this group is to interpret the PERC or D-dimer result *after* the pretest probability has been assessed, as physicians who are aware of a negative D-dimer result are more likely to misclassify a patient as low probability. A negative D-dimer test in a high-probability patient should not exclude the diagnosis of PE.[22]

Risk stratification and prognostic evaluation

Diagnosed PE can be categorized based on severity, and these definitions may be used to guide management.[23] Categorization of PE is not related to clot size; rather, it reflects the patient's hemodynamic stability or instability.

Massive PE is defined as acute pulmonary embolism with sustained hypotension (systolic blood pressure < 90 mmHg for at least 15 minutes or requiring inotropic support, not due to a cause other than PE), pulselessness, or sustained bradycardia with heart rate < 40 bpm, and signs or symptoms of shock.

Submassive PE is acute PE without systemic hypotension but with either right ventricular dysfunction or signs of myocardial necrosis. Right ventricular dysfunction can be assessed by echocardiogram, BNP level, electrocardiographic changes, or right ventricular size relative to left ventricular size on CT scan. Myocardial necrosis is indicated by an elevated troponin level.

Low-risk PE is acute PE in the absence of the clinical markers of adverse prognosis that define massive or submassive PE.

Evaluation of right heart strain

Once PE is diagnosed, patients can be risk stratified by evaluating for signs of right heart strain. Echocardiography is a direct and intuitive way of evaluating right heart function and may reveal akinesia of the mid-free wall of the right ventricle (McConnell's sign). Right ventricular overload can also be evaluated by comparing the ratio of the diameter of the right ventricle (RV) with that of the left ventricle (LV) on CT scan, with an RV : LV ratio > 0.9 considered consistent with RV dilation. Elevated troponin and BNP levels are reflective of right heart strain. Electrocardiographic findings that indicate right heart strain include complete or partial right bundle branch block, an S1Q3T3 pattern, and septal T-wave inversions.

Outcomes

Large registries show that patients with PE complicated by hemodynamic instability have far worse outcomes than those who are hemodynamically stable. In one study, the three-month mortality rate was 58.3% in patients who presented with PE and hemodynamic instability versus 15.1% in those who were stable.[5] Another registry found an in-hospital mortality rate of 65% in patients with PE who needed cardiopulmonary resuscitation (CPR) vs. 8.1% in those who were hemodynamically stable.[24]

Submassive PE is associated with worse outcome than low-risk PE. Any signs of right ventricular dysfunction by echocardiography,[5] biomarkers,[25,26] CT,[27] or electrocardiography[28] are associated with higher risk of death.[29]

The long-term sequelae of PE include chronic thromboembolic pulmonary hypertension (CTEPH), which occurs in 2 to 4% of patients.[30] This condition presents months to years after PE, with dyspnea and fatigue, and may progress to right heart failure and death.

Acute management

As with all patients presenting to the ED, treatment of the patient with suspected PE who appears critically ill begins with a rapid assessment of clinical stability. Alternative critical diagnoses that could cause similar presentation, such as MI, aortic dissection, and pneumothorax, should be considered and evaluated simultaneously. A focused history and physical examination will help narrow the differential diagnosis and provide information regarding the risk of anticoagulation or thrombolysis (see Chapter 22, Thrombolytic therapy for venous thromboembolism).

An electrocardiogram can be obtained quickly and provides information pertinent to alternative diagnoses such as myocardial infarction. Its sensitivity and specificity for PE are poor, but electrocardiographic signs of right heart strain such as the S1Q3T3 pattern and partial or complete right bundle branch block suggest greater clot burden when present in a patient with PE. Similarly, troponins and BNP levels can either suggest alternate diagnoses or provide information

important in risk stratification once PE is confirmed. Chest radiography should also be performed in the initial evaluation of suspected PE. Abnormalities on radiographs are rarely diagnostic of PE, but alternate diagnoses including heart failure, aortic dissection, pneumonia, and pneumothorax may be apparent. Additionally, in the setting of severe hypoxia with an acute onset, a clear chest radiograph is highly suggestive of PE.

Routine laboratory studies can inform management decisions. Assessment of renal function is necessary, because low-molecular-weight heparin may be preferable to unfractionated heparin when renal function is normal, and abnormal coagulation studies can factor into the assessment of risk of both anticoagulation and clot lysis. Measurement of D-dimer is primarily useful in low-risk patients but not in those who are hypoxic, tachycardic, or in respiratory distress.

Resuscitation

Hypoxemia associated with PE often responds to supplemental oxygen. Refractory hypoxemia suggests a large embolus and reflects either intrapulmonary shunt or pulmonary hypertension leading to intracardiac shunting through a patent foramen ovale. If mechanical ventilation is required, the emergency physician should anticipate a drop in blood pressure, as positive intrathoracic pressure typically worsens pulmonary hypertension and right ventricular failure. Low tidal volume ventilation is unnecessary in PE, and the "open lung" strategy that is of critical value in acute lung injury should be avoided. Positive end-expiratory pressure (PEEP) should be minimized because it worsens pulmonary hypertension and is unlikely to improve oxygenation in patients with PE. During intubation, the emergency physician should be prepared to give intravenous fluids, administer vasopressors, and consider thrombolytics if the patient's hemodynamic instability is sustained.

Attention to crystalloid resuscitation is important. Patients with acute right heart failure are typically preload dependent and usually respond initially to intravenous fluids. The amount of fluids required is much less than in resuscitation of septic shock. An excessive volume may decrease systemic cardiac output through mechanisms of ventricular interdependence. We recommend limiting the volume to 2 L of crystalloid, after which pressors and lytics should be considered. Few high-quality data exist to guide the selection of vasopressor in PE.

Empiric anticoagulation

The emergency physician should be aggressive in empirically treating suspected PE, because early anticoagulation decreases the mortality rate. This is one of the most critical and effective interventions the emergency physician can make. In one study, patients who received heparin in the ED for diagnosed or suspected PE had an in-hospital mortality rate of 1.4% versus 6.7% for those who received heparin after admission, with 30-day mortality rates of 5.6% versus 14.8%.[31] Therapeutic anticoagulation should be administered during diagnostic workup to patients with no contraindication and an intermediate or a high clinical probability of PE.[23]

Thrombolysis in cardiac arrest

Empiric thrombolytics have not been shown to have any benefit in undifferentiated cardiac arrest.[32] However, administration of thrombolytics to patients with cardiac arrest secondary to known or strongly suspected PE has been reported to improve outcome,[33,34] and the most recent American Heart Association guidelines state that it is reasonable to administer thrombolytics in this situation.[35] Dosing recommendations vary, but an appropriate choice would be 100 mg of recombinant tissue plasminogen activator (rtPA) infused over 15 minutes.[33] If thrombolytics are given during cardiac arrest, CPR should be continued long enough to allow the medication time to work. Fifteen minutes of continued CPR has been suggested.[33]

Thrombolysis in massive PE

Data on the effect of thrombolysis on the mortality rate among patients with massive PE are limited but suggest a benefit. A single randomized controlled trial of heparin plus streptokinase versus heparin alone in patients with massive PE has been performed; the four patients who received thrombolytics all survived, and the four who did not died.[36] Meta-analysis suggests a benefit to thrombolytics in trials that included patients with massive PE, with a decrease in death or recurrent PE from 19 to 9.4%.[37] Guidelines generally support administration of thrombolytics to hemodynamically unstable patients without contraindications.[23,38]

For further discussion of thrombolysis, including contraindications and side effects, please refer to Chapter 22, Thrombolytic therapy for venous thromboembolism.

Definitive treatment

Anticoagulation

Anticoagulation is the cornerstone of treatment of PE and confers a clear survival benefit. As discussed above, empiric anticoagulation is indicated during the evaluation of patients in whom suspicion of PE is high.

Subcutaneous administration of low-molecular-weight heparin is as safe and effective as intravenous (IV) administration of unfractionated heparin (UHF) in the treatment of PE[39] and is recommended over IV UFH unless the patient has severe renal failure, the physician has concerns about subcutaneous absorption, or thrombolysis is planned.[40]

The synthetic thrombolytic fondaparinux is at least as effective and safe as UFH in treatment of pulmonary embolism.[41] Additionally, it is an appropriate choice for patients with heparin-induced thrombocytopenia.

Thrombolysis in non-massive PE

Thrombolysis in submassive PE is controversial. Although thrombolytics reduce clot burden in the short term compared with anticoagulation alone, it is unclear whether they improve mortality rate or prevention of long-term complications. Data are limited, and the one randomized controlled trial revealed no difference in: mortality rate, need for CPR, need for intubation, pressor administration, or surgical or catheter-based interventions, between patients with submassive PE who received alteplase and those who did not.[42] Although rates of chronic thromboembolic pulmonary hypertension following PE are low, it is possible that patients with submassive PE may be at higher risk for it and that thrombolysis in patients with submassive PE may decrease its long-term rate of occurrence.[43] However, administration of thrombolytics for this indication can be delayed for up to several days. Current recommendations regarding the administration of thrombolytics to patients with submassive PE rely heavily on physician judgment on a case-by-case basis. However, unlike the management of massive PE, a decision regarding thrombolytics in submassive PE can generally be postponed for a matter of hours to days and is usually not necessary to make in the ED. For further discussion, please see Chapter 22.

Inferior vena cava filters

The placement of an inferior vena cava (IVC) filter can be considered in patients with PE who have a contraindication to anticoagulation, for patients who develop new PE while on therapeutic anticoagulation, and as a temporary measure in patients with known DVT who might decompensate if any additional clot burden is transmitted to the lungs. However, no proven mortality benefit exists with IVC filter placement, and, although IVC filters reduce rates of PE, they increase the risk of DVT.[44] We recommend against routine placement of IVC filters in the ED.

Thrombectomy

The risks of surgical thrombectomy have declined dramatically over the past several decades, with mortality rates now in the 6% range at centers with significant experience with this procedure.[45] This approach is an option in patients with massive PE and a contraindication to thrombolysis. It has been proposed as a treatment option in patients with submassive PE as well; however, we recommend against this as a routine intervention, given its unproven effect on outcomes, the risks associated with surgical intervention, and the lack of experience with this treatment at most institutions.

Catheter-based interventions

Catheter-directed therapy can be used in patients with massive PE and contraindication to thrombolysis or as rescue therapy when thrombolysis has failed. It has a success rate of 87%.[46] However, as with surgical thrombectomy, favorable outcome depends heavily on available expertise and experience.

Admission criteria/disposition

Patients with low-risk PE may generally be admitted to a regular floor bed or even sent home if arrangements can be made for self-administration of low-molecular-weight heparin and close follow-up.[47] Patients with submassive PE are at high risk for decompensation and should be admitted to a monitored setting. Any patient who has been hemodynamically unstable in the ED or has received thrombolytics should be admitted to a monitored unit.

Special cases

Pregnancy

The relative risk of VTE is fourfold greater in pregnant women than in non-pregnant women of child-bearing age, and fivefold higher in the postpartum period than during pregnancy.[3] The increased risk is thought to stem from a combination of a hypercoagulable state and compression of the IVC and pelvic veins, causing increased stasis.

The initial test of choice for suspected PE in a pregnant woman is lower extremity ultrasound. If positive, therapeutic anticoagulation should be initiated or continued without a need for further imaging. If negative, further diagnostic imaging is indicated, including a chest film and either VQ scan or CTA. Both studies expose mother and fetus to radiation. A ventilation–perfusion scan is associated with higher fetal radiation exposure than CT and an increased risk of childhood cancer (1 in 280,000 vs. less than 1 in 1 million). CTA is associated with a 13% greater relative risk of maternal breast cancer.[48] MRI is another option for diagnosis of PE in the pregnant patient. However, gadolinium has an unknown effect on the fetus and is rated pregnancy class C; the inability to use it in the pregnant patient may mean a reduction in sensitivity of MRI from the reported 75 to 93%.[20]

Pediatrics

Venous thromboembolic disease in children is uncommon and in most cases associated with an underlying condition, such as the presence of a central venous catheter, malignancy, or nephrotic syndrome.[49] Clinical decision rules have not been validated in children. Recommendations for evaluation and treatment generally parallel those for adults.[50] However, D-dimer testing is likely to be less useful than in adults, as most children with PE have an underlying disorder.

Clinical approach when resources are limited

- If echocardiography is not available, look for clues of right ventricular dysfunction on CT scan or an electrocardiogram.
- Use bedside echo to evaluate for right ventricular dysfunction.
- Initiate anticoagulation before transferring the patient to a higher level of care.
- In the patient with suspected PE and clinically or ultrasonographically apparent DVT, no further testing is needed and treatment for VTE should be initiated.

Pearls and pitfalls

- A negative test result does not rule out PE in a high-probability patient. The diagnosis of PE hinges on pretest probability. Discordance between that probability and test results must be pursued further.
- The PERC rule and D-dimer testing should be applied only after an assessment of pretest probability for PE.
- PE often presents atypically; consider this diagnosis in patients with isolated syncope.

Critical actions in the emergency department

- Recognize and aggressively treat massive PE with thrombolysis if there is no contraindication.
- Start anticoagulation early – give it empirically during workup if the patient is at intermediate or high probability for PE.
- Choose low-molecular-weight heparin unless the patient has renal failure, the physician has concern about subcutaneous absorption, or thrombolysis is planned.

References

1. Moser KM, Fedullo PF, LitteJohn JK, Crawford R. Frequent asymptomatic pulmonary embolism in patients with deep venous thrombosis. *JAMA* 1994; 271(3): 223–5.

2. Tapson VF. Acute pulmonary embolism. *N Engl J Med* 2008; 358(10): 1037–52.

3. Roger VL, Go AS, Lloyd-Jones DM, *et al.* Heart disease and stroke statistics – 2011 update: a report from the American Heart Association. *Circulation* 2011; 123(4): e18–209.

4. Calder KK, Herbert M, Henderson SO. The mortality of untreated pulmonary embolism in emergency department patients. *Ann Emerg Med* 2005; 45(3): 302–10.

5. Goldhaber SZ, Visani L, De Rosa M. Acute pulmonary embolism: clinical outcomes in the International Cooperative Pulmonary Embolism Registry (ICOPER). *Lancet* 1999; 353(9162): 1386–9.

6. Di Nisio M, Squizzato A, Rutjes AW, *et al.* Diagnostic accuracy of D-dimer test for exclusion of venous thromboembolism: a systematic review. *J Thromb Haemost* 2007; 5(2): 296–304.

7. Fesmire FM, Brown MD, Espinosa JA, *et al.* Critical issues in the evaluation and management of adult patients presenting to the emergency department with suspected pulmonary embolism. *Ann Emerg Med* 2011; 57(6): 628–52.

8. Qaseem A, Snow V, Barry P, *et al.* Current diagnosis of venous thromboembolism in primary care: a clinical practice guideline from the American Academy of Family Physicians and the American College of Physicians. *Ann Intern Med* 2007; 146(6): 454–8.

9. Value of the ventilation/perfusion scan in acute pulmonary embolism. Results of the prospective investigation of pulmonary embolism diagnosis (PIOPED). The PIOPED Investigators. *JAMA* 1990; 263(20): 2753–9.

10. Perrier A, Miron MJ, Desmarais S, *et al.* Using clinical evaluation and lung scan to rule out suspected pulmonary embolism: is it a valid option in patients with normal results of lower-limb venous compression ultrasonography? *Arch Intern Med* 2000; 160(4): 512–6.

11. Perrier A, Desmarais S, Miron MJ, *et al.* Non-invasive diagnosis of venous thromboembolism in outpatients. *Lancet* 1999; 353(9148): 190–5.

12. Wells PS, Anderson DR, Rodger M, *et al.* Derivation of a simple clinical model to categorize patients' probability of pulmonary embolism: increasing the model's utility with the SimpliRED D-dimer. *Thromb Haemost* 2000; 83(3): 416–20.

13. Wells PS, Ginsberg JS, Anderson DR, *et al.* Use of a clinical model for safe management of patients with suspected pulmonary embolism. *Ann Intern Med* 1998; 129(12): 997–1005.

14. Le Gal G, Righini M, Roy PM, *et al.* Prediction of pulmonary embolism in the emergency department: the revised Geneva score. *Ann Intern Med* 2006; 144(3): 165–71.

15. Klok FA, Mos IC, Nijkeuter M, *et al.* Simplification of the revised Geneva score for assessing clinical probability of pulmonary embolism. *Arch Intern Med* 2008; 168(19): 2131–6.

16. Kline JA, Mitchell AM, Kabrhel C, *et al.* Clinical criteria to prevent unnecessary diagnostic testing in emergency department patients with suspected pulmonary embolism. *J Thromb Haemost* 2004; 2(8): 1247–55.

17. Kline JA, Courtney DM, Kabrhel C, *et al.* Prospective multicenter evaluation of the pulmonary embolism rule-out criteria. *J Thromb Haemost* 2008; 6(5): 772–80.

18. Stein PD, Fowler SE, Goodman LR, *et al.* Multidetector computed tomography for acute pulmonary embolism. *N Engl J Med* 2006; 354(22): 2317–27.

19. Worsley DF, Alavi A. Comprehensive analysis of the results of the PIOPED study. *J Nucl Med* 1995: 36(12): 2380–7.

20. Clemens S, Leeper KV. Newer modalities for detection of pulmonary emboli. *Am J Med* 2007; 120(10b): S2–12.

21. Roy PM, Colombet I, Durieux P, *et al*. Systematic review and meta-analysis of strategies for the diagnosis of suspected pulmonary embolism. *BMJ* 2005; 331(7511): 259.

22. Gibson NS, Sohne M, Gerdes VE, *et al*. The importance of clinical probability assessment in interpreting a normal D-dimer in patients with suspected pulmonary embolism. *Chest* 2008; 134(4): 789–93.

23. Jaff MR, McMurtry MS, Archer SL, *et al*. Management of massive and submassive pulmonary embolism, ileofemoral deep vein thrombosis, and chronic thromboembolic pulmonary hypertension: a Scientific Statement from the American Heart Association. *Circulation* 2011; 123(16): 1788–830.

24. Kasper W, Konstantinides S, Geibel A, *et al*. Management strategies and determinants of outcome in acute major pulmonary embolism: results of a multicenter registry. *J Am Coll Cardiol* 1997; 30(5): 1165–71.

25. Cavallazzi R, Nair A, Vasu T, Marik PE. Natriuretic peptides in acute pulmonary embolism: a systematic review. *Intensive Care Med* 2008; 34(12): 2147–56.

26. Becattini C, Vedovati MC, Agnelli G. Prognostic value of troponins in acute pulmonary embolism: a meta-analysis. *Circulation* 2007; 116(4): 427–33.

27. Schoepf UJ, Kucher N, Kipfmueller F, *et al*. Right ventricular enlargement on chest computed tomography: a predictor of early death in acute pulmonary embolism. *Circulation* 2004; 110(20): 3276–80.

28. Vanni S, Polidori G, Vergara R, *et al*. Prognostic value of ECG among patients with acute pulmonary embolism and normal blood pressure. *Am J Med* 2009; 122(3): 257–64.

29. Sanchez O, Trinquart L, Colombet I, *et al*. Prognostic value of right ventricular dysfunction in patients with haemodynamically stable pulmonary embolism: a systematic review. *Eur Heart J* 2008; 29(12): 1569–77.

30. Pengo V, Lensing AW, Prins MH, *et al*. Incidence of chronic thromboembolic pulmonary hypertension after pulmonary embolism. *N Engl J Med* 2004; 350(22): 2257–64.

31. Smith SB, Geske JB, Maguire JM, *et al*. Early anticoagulation is associated with reduced mortality for acute pulmonary embolism. *Chest* 2010; 137(6): 1382–90.

32. Bottiger BW, Arntz HR, Chamberlain DA, *et al*. Thrombolysis during resuscitation for out-of-hospital cardiac arrest. *N Engl J Med* 2008; 359(25): 2651–62.

33. Perrott J, Henneberry RJ, Zed PJ. Thrombolytics for cardiac arrest: case report and systematic review of controlled trials. *Ann Pharmacother* 2010; 44(12): 2007–13.

34. Bailen MR, Cuadra JA, Aguayo De Hoyos E. Thrombolysis during cardiopulmonary resuscitation in fulminant pulmonary embolism: a review. *Crit Care Med* 2001; 29(11): 2211–19.

35. Vanden Hoek TL, Morrison LJ, Shuster M, *et al*. Part 12: cardiac arrest in special situations: 2010 American Heart Association Guidelines for Cardiopulmonary Resuscitation and Emergency Cardiovascular Care. *Circulation* 2010; 122(18 suppl 3): S829–61.

36. Jerjes-Sanchez C, Ramirez-Rivera A, de Lourdes Garcia M, *et al*. Streptokinase and heparin versus heparin alone in massive pulmonary embolism: a randomized controlled trial. *J Thromb Thrombolysis* 1995; 2(3): 227–9.

37. Wan S, Quinlan DJ, Agnelli G, Eikelboom JW. Thrombolysis compared with heparin for the initial treatment of pulmonary embolism: a meta-analysis of the randomized controlled trials. *Circulation* 2004; 110(6): 744–9.

38. Torbicki A, Perrier A, Konstantinides S, *et al*. Guidelines on the diagnosis and management of acute pulmonary embolism: the Task Force for the Diagnosis and Management of Acute Pulmonary Embolism of the European Society of Cardiology (ESC). *Eur Heart J* 2008; 29(18): 2276–315.

39. Quinlan DJ, McQuillan A, Eikelboom JW. Low-molecular-weight heparin compared with intravenous unfractionated heparin for treatment of pulmonary embolism: a meta-analysis of randomized, controlled trials. *Ann Intern Med* 2004; 140(3): 175–83.

40. Kearon C, Kahn SR, Agnelli G, *et al*. Antithrombotic therapy for venous thromboembolic disease: American College of Chest Physicians Evidence-Based Clinical Practice Guidelines (8th Edition). *Chest* 2008; 133(6 suppl): 454S–545S.

41. Buller HR, Davidson BL, Decousus H, *et al*. Subcutaneous fondaparinux versus intravenous unfractionated heparin in the initial treatment of pulmonary embolism. *N Engl J Med* 2003; 349(18): 1695–702.

42. Konstantinides S, Geibel A, Heusel G, *et al*. Heparin plus alteplase compared with heparin alone in patients with submassive pulmonary embolism. *N Engl J Med* 2002; 347(15): 1143–50.

43. Kline JA, Steuerwald MT, Marchick MR, *et al*. Prospective evaluation of right ventricular function and functional status 6 months after acute submassive pulmonary embolism: frequency of persistent or

subsequent elevation in estimated pulmonary artery pressure. *Chest* 2009; 136(5): 1202–10.

44. Decousus H, Leizorovicz A, Parent F, *et al.* A clinical trial of vena caval filters in the prevention of pulmonary embolism in patients with proximal deep-vein thrombosis. Prevention du Risque d'Embolie Pulmonaire par Interruption Cave Study Group. *N Engl J Med* 1998; 338(7): 409–15.

45. Samoukovic G, Malas T, deVarennes B. The role of pulmonary embolectomy in the treatment of acute pulmonary embolism: a literature review from 1968 to 2008. *Interact Cardiovasc Thorac Surg* 2010; 11(3): 265–70.

46. Kuo WT, Gould MK, Louie JD, *et al.* Catheter-directed therapy for the treatment of massive pulmonary embolism: systematic review and meta-analysis of modern techniques. *J Vasc Interv Radiol* 2009; 20(11): 1431–40.

47. Aujesky D, Roy PM, Verschuren F, *et al.* Outpatient versus inpatient treatment for patients with acute pulmonary embolism: an international, open-label, randomised, non-inferiority trial. *Lancet* 2011; 378(9785): 41–8.

48. Marik PE, Plante LA. Venous thromboembolic disease and pregnancy. *N Engl J Med* 2008; 359(19): 2025–33.

49. Andrew M, David M, Adams M, *et al.* Venous thromboembolic complications (VTE) in children: first analyses of the Canadian Registry of VTE. *Blood* 1994; 83(5): 1251–7.

50. Babyn PS, Gahunia HK, Massicotte P. Pulmonary thromboembolism in children. *Pediatr Radiol* 2005; 35(3): 258–74.

Chapter

22

Thrombolytic therapy for venous thromboembolism

Sa'ad Lahri

Thrombolysis is approved for the treatment of massive pulmonary embolism (PE) and submassive PE in patients with evidence of right ventricular (RV) strain or myocardial injury.[1–3] The use of thrombolytic agents in patients with submassive PE remains controversial. Anticoagulation with heparin prevents clot extension, whereas thrombolysis dissolves existing clot, ultimately improving hemodynamics.[2] When successful, treatment of massive PE with thrombolytic therapy results in rapid resolution of the pulmonary arterial clot burden, decreased pulmonary artery pressure, and improvements in cardiac output and pulmonary circulation.[1–3] One small study demonstrated a mortality benefit with thrombolysis for massive PE,[4] but most of the data supporting its use are derived from subgroup analysis from large registries of patients with PE in Europe and the United States.[1–4] The benefits of thrombolytic therapy in the treatment of massive PE and submassive PE in RV strain subgroups are countered by an increased risk of major bleeding events and, of greatest concern, intracerebral hemorrhage (ICH). Armed with a solid decision-making approach to thrombolytic therapy, the emergency physician can limit the morbidity and mortality associated with this condition. This chapter will tackle this very important topic in vascular emergencies.

Clinical approach in select subgroups

Patients with PE can present with a wide variety of clinical features, ranging from cardiac arrest to an incidental diagnosis in an asymptomatic patient. The probability of thrombolysis resulting in either harm or benefit in any specific patient depends on a multitude of variables that need to be considered carefully in

Table 22.1 Thrombolysis recommendations

Indicated	Massive acute PE and cardiac arrest due to suspected PE Acceptable risk of bleeding complications
Consider it	Submassive acute PE with clinical evidence of adverse prognosis (new hemodynamic instability, worsening respiratory insufficiency, severe RV dysfunction, or major myocardial necrosis) and low risk of bleeding complications
Not recommended	Low-risk PE Submassive acute PE with minor RV dysfunction Undifferentiated cardiac arrest

every case. It is important to employ a patient-centered approach to thrombolytic therapy, as each patient's risk factors, clinical presentation, and bleeding risk are unique. The use of thrombolytics in hemodynamically stable patients with PE and RV dysfunction is controversial, but their use is well supported in the hemodynamically unstable patient (Table 22.1).[1–3]

Obtaining diagnostic confirmation of PE is clearly preferred before initiating thrombolysis.[2] However, in a patient with a high clinical pretest probability for massive PE and when imaging is not feasible because a CT scanner is not available, or if the patient is too unstable for transport, thrombolysis is a reasonable initial treatment approach.[1,5] Treating patients in undifferentiated cardiac arrest with thrombolysis is generally not recommended because it does not offer clinical benefit.[1,4,5]

Cardiac arrest

The cardiac arrest subgroup deserves special consideration. The immediate use of intravenous alteplase may be lifesaving for patients in cardiac arrest caused

Vascular Emergencies, ed. Robert L. Rogers, Thomas Scalea, Lee Wallis, and Heike Geduld. Published by Cambridge University Press. © Cambridge University Press 2013.

by *suspected PE*,[6] but it is not recommended for *undifferentiated* cardiac arrest[1,3] because a survival benefit has not been demonstrated. The longstanding fear of increased bleeding complications with thrombolytic use after prolonged and vigorous cardiopulmonary resuscitation efforts has been dispelled.[7,8] Therefore, return of spontaneous circulation following cardiac arrest itself is not a contraindication to thrombolytic therapy.[5]

Massive pulmonary embolism

Massive PE is defined as acute PE with sustained hypotension (systolic blood pressure < 90 mmHg for at least 15 minutes or requiring inotropic support, not caused by a condition other than PE, such as dysrhythmia, hypovolemia, sepsis, or left ventricular [LV] dysfunction) or persistent profound bradycardia (heart rate < 40 bpm with signs or symptoms of shock).[3] In the absence of contraindications, this subgroup clearly benefits from thrombolytic therapy.[3,5,6] Because of ethical concerns, few clinical trials have assessed the true efficacy of thrombolytic therapy in patients with massive PE. Jerjes-Sanchez *et al.* sought to randomize 40 patients with massive PE to streptokinase plus heparin or heparin alone.[4] The study was terminated after the enrollment of eight patients – the four patients who received streptokinase survived and the four who received heparin alone died. Wan *et al.*[9] performed a meta-analysis of five randomized controlled trials that included patients with massive PE (including the study by Jerjes-Sanchez and associates[4]). Wan *et al.* showed that the number-needed-to-treat (NNT) was 10 to reduce recurrent PE or death.[9] For patients who have a high likelihood of PE but are too unstable for a radiographic confirmation study (i.e., massive PE is suspected), consideration of thrombolytic therapy is warranted.[1–3] The finding of RV dysfunction on bedside echocardiography may be used as indirect evidence for the presence of PE.[10] Mortality benefit from thrombolytic therapy in this high-risk subgroup is unclear.[1,5]

Submassive PE

Submassive PE is acute PE without systemic hypotension (SBP ≥ 90 mmHg) but with either RV dysfunction or myocardial necrosis.

RV dysfunction is indicated by the presence of at least one of the following:

- Echocardiography: RV dilation (apical four-chamber RV diameter divided by LV diameter > 0.9) or RV systolic dysfunction.
- McConnell's sign: right ventricular (RV) free wall hypokinesis with normal apical contraction on echocardiography. The presence of McConnell's sign has been associated with submassive and massive PE when moderate to high clinical suspicion exists. The sensitivity, specificity, positive predictive value, and negative predictive value of McConnell's sign for diagnosing PE have been estimated at 70, 33, 67, and 36%, respectively.[11]
- Computed tomography: RV dilation (four-chamber RV diameter divided by LV diameter > 0.9).
- B-type natriuretic peptide (BNP) > 90 pg/mL.
- N-terminal pro-BNP > 500 pg/mL.
- Electrocardiographic changes: sinus tachycardia, new complete or incomplete right bundle branch block, anteroseptal ST elevation or depression, or anteroseptal T-wave inversion and S1Q3T3.

Myocardial necrosis is defined as either of the following:[3]

- troponin I > 0.4 ng/mL;
- troponin T > 0.1 ng/mL.

RV dysfunction is a poor prognostic indicator, even in the hemodynamically stable patient. Patients with RV dysfunction may initially appear to be clinically stable but rapidly progress to frank RV failure.[10,12]

Watchful waiting for patients with PE and RV dysfunction is a potential pitfall and can lead to irreversible deterioration and increased morbidity and mortality.[13,14] These patients can be reclassified as having "impending hemodynamic instability" and be managed aggressively with early intubation and thrombolysis.

The goal of caring for patients with PE is to select those who are at high risk for death and disability and who might benefit from thrombolysis. Although studies may not demonstrate significant differences in mortality rates with the administration of lytics for submassive PE, such treatment may improve quality of life.[4,5,15] With fibrinolytic therapy, there is more rapid clot lysis, which leads to quicker improvement in pulmonary perfusion and cardiovascular function,[3–5] eliminates venous thrombi, and thus eliminates the risk of recurrent PE.[5] Lysis may thus prevent

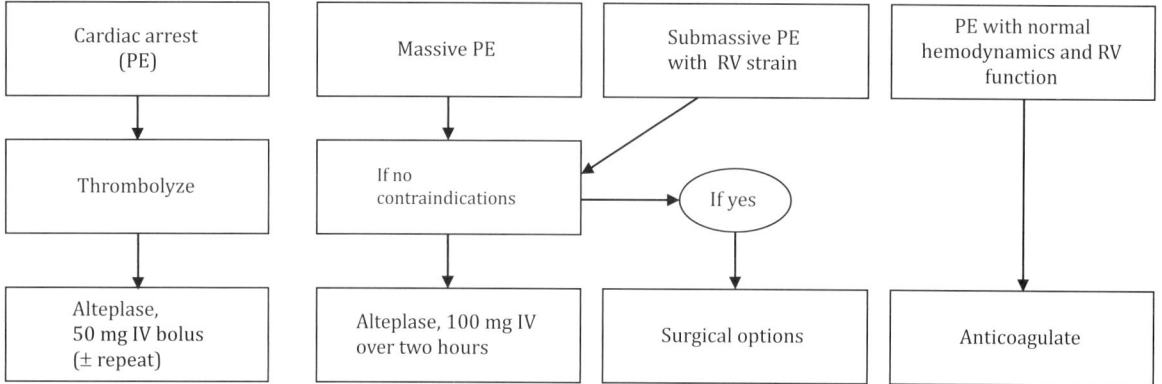

Figure 22.1 Thrombolysis in the acute management of pulmonary embolism. Systemic delivery of the thrombolytic agent is often used for treatment of PE; whereas peripheral arterial thrombi and thrombi in the proximal deep veins of the leg are most often treated using a catheter-directed approach. The choice of surgical thrombectomy or catheter-directed procedures is strongly influenced by available expertise and resources.

the development of persistent pulmonary hypertension.[4–6] Therefore, thrombolytic therapy should be considered in this group in the absence of increased bleeding risk.[1,2]

Respiratory failure

Hypoxemia from PE is caused by ventilation and perfusion (VQ) mismatch and shunting. The mortality rate also is worse in hypoxic patients.[2–4] The presence of severe hypoxemia necessitating mechanical ventilation may be an indication for thrombolysis, despite the absence of circulatory compromise. Thrombolysis might also allow avoidance of mechanical ventilation and its inherent risks.[13]

Low-risk PE: hemodynamically stable PE with normal RV function

Patients with PE who are normotensive with normal biomarker levels and no RV dysfunction on imaging have the lowest short-term mortality rate.[3] This subgroup does well with anticoagulation alone, and thrombolysis is not indicated (Figure 22.1).[1,2]

Clinical approach when resources are limited

In an unstable patient in whom PE is strongly suspected, consider thrombolytic therapy if the diagnosis of PE cannot be confirmed because of the patient's instability or because laboratory testing is not available.[5] The finding of RV dysfunction on bedside

ultrasound can be used as indirect evidence for the presence of PE.[1,10] Not all units have access to ultrasound or the expertise to perform and interpret the scan. Cardiac biomarkers offer a sensitive and specific way to identify hemodynamically stable patients who present with PE and need further testing of RV function with ultrasound. Elevation of troponins T and I is significantly associated with RV dysfunction on echocardiography and correlates significantly with a complicated hospital course and death.[1,2] If measurement of cardiac biomarkers and ultrasound are available, both should be performed.

Selection of thrombolytics and heparin

Thrombolytics, sometimes referred to as plasminogen activators, are divided into two categories. Fibrin-specific agents (e.g., alteplase, reteplase, and tenecteplase) produce limited plasminogen conversion in the absence of fibrin. Non-fibrin-specific agents (such as streptokinase) catalyze systemic fibrinolysis.[16] The common goal of thrombolytic agents is the generation of plasmin that lyses the clot. The plasminogen activator system forms plasminogen that binds to the clot and achieves lysis.[16]

Three thrombolytic agents have been approved by the US Food and Drug Administration (FDA): streptokinase, urokinase, and alteplase.[16] They have comparable rates of efficacy.[17] Streptokinase is not widely used in the United States but continues to be used in low-resource environments because of its lower cost. Streptokinase therapy has two major drawbacks: first, prior administration is a contraindication because of the risk of anaphylaxis, and, second, its thrombolytic actions are non-specific and can cause systemic fibrinolysis, potentially leading to severe hemorrhagic complications.

Since endothelial cells produce recombinant tissue plasminogen activator (rtPA), it is not antigenic and causes more selective thrombolysis than streptokinase.[3,16] Recombinant tissue plasminogen activator binds to fibrin and converts plasminogen to plasmin.

In patients with acute PE, the thrombolytic agent should be given via a peripheral intravenous line. If a central line is required, it should be placed in a compressible site such as the internal jugular or femoral vein under ultrasound guidance. Comparisons of different thrombolytic regimens in patients with acute PE have not yielded conclusive findings. Short infusion times (≤ 2 hours) are recommended since they achieve more rapid thrombolysis and are probably associated with less bleeding. No single agent or dosing regimen has proven superior over another in the treatment of patients with massive and submassive PE.[18] The Urokinase–Streptokinase Pulmonary Embolism Trial (USPET) documented equal efficacy of urokinase and streptokinase infused over a period of 12 to 24 hours.[19] The infusion of 100 mg of rtPA over two hours led to faster angiographic and hemodynamic improvement compared to urokinase infused over 12 to 24 hours at the rate of 4400 IU/kg·h; there were no differences in the mortality rates. The two-hour infusion of rtPA appeared to be superior to a 12-hour streptokinase infusion (at 100,000 IU/h), but no difference was observed when the same streptokinase dose was given over two hours. Trials that compared the two-hour, 100-mg rtPA regimen with a short infusion (over 15 min) of 0.6 mg/kg rtPA reported non-significant trends toward both slightly faster improvements and slightly higher bleeding rates.[20] Case reports and cases series have demonstrated good results with the administration of a single dose of tenecteplase (TNK) for the treatment of massive PE.[21] Despite its favorable profile, TNK is not yet licensed by the FDA for use in patients with PE. It is administered as a single dose based on the patient's weight, which may prove very attractive. Heparin should be administered as an 80-IU/kg bolus, followed by an 18-IU/kg·h continuous infusion, titrated to maintain an aPTT of twice the control value. Heparin should be stopped as soon as the decision is made to administer the thrombolytic agent, and aPTT should be measured. Heparin should not be infused concurrently with a thrombolytic agent because of the increased risk of serious bleeding.

Dosing regimens

Alteplase

The FDA-approved regimen for alteplase in patients with PE is 100 mg as an infusion over two hours. Administer a 15-mg bolus followed by 85 mg over a two-hour period. Heparin must be discontinued during the infusion. An accelerated 90-minute regimen that appears to be faster acting, safer, and more efficacious than the two-hour infusion is used at some centers. For patients weighing less than 67 kg, the drug is administered as a 15-mg IV bolus, followed by 0.75 mg/kg infused over the next 30 minutes (maximum, 50 mg) and then 0.50 mg/kg over the next 60 minutes (maximum, 35 mg). For patients weighing more than 67 kg, 100 mg is administered as a 15-mg IV bolus, followed by 50 mg infused over the next 30 minutes and then 35 mg over the next 60 minutes.[15,18]

Urokinase

The FDA-approved regimen for urokinase is 4400 IU/kg as a loading dose given at a rate of 90 mL/h over a period of 10 minutes, followed by a continuous infusion of 4400 IU/kg·h at a rate of 15 mL/h for 12 to 24 hours. In the accelerated regimen, 3×10^6 IU are infused over two hours.

Streptokinase

The FDA-approved regimen for the use of streptokinase in patients with PE is 250,000 IU as a loading dose over 30 minutes, followed by 100,000 IU/h over 12 to 24 hours. In the accelerated regimen, 1.5×10^6 IU are infused over two hours.

Potential benefits and harm

When considering thrombolytic therapy for a patient with PE, just as in the treatment of patients with ST-segment elevation myocardial infarction (STEMI) or acute cerebral ischemia, one must conduct a risk–benefit assessment.[1–3] Potential benefits include rapid resolution of symptoms, stabilization of respiratory and cardiovascular function without need for mechanical ventilation or vasopressor support, reduction of RV damage, improved exercise tolerance, prevention of PE recurrence, and increased probability of survival.[13] Potential harm includes hemorrhage. Whether a life-threatening result such as ICH or a minor hemorrhage occurs, such a complication prolongs hospitalization, heightens the need for blood product replacement, and increases the monetary cost. Presumably, patients at higher risk of death from PE have greater potential for benefit from thrombolytic therapy. Data from the International Cooperative Pulmonary Embolism Registry revealed the three-month mortality rate from PE to be 17.4%.[22] Factors associated with a higher mortality rate from PE include age > 70 years, congestive heart failure, chronic obstructive lung disease, the presence of only one lung, cancer, hypotension, tachypnea, hypoxia, tachycardia, altered mental status, RV hypokinesis, syncope, chronic renal failure, previous cerebral vascular accident, elevated troponin level, elevated BNP level, and right heart thrombus.[1,21,22] Factors that are associated with an increased risk of bleeding are age > 65 years, uncontrolled hypertension, recent stroke or surgery, and bleeding diathesis.[15] Among thrombolytic-treated patients, intracranial bleeding occurred in about 3% and major bleeding in as many as 21.7%.[22] As a result of the increased rates of major bleeding and ICH, thrombolytic therapy is not recommended in the treatment of PE in patients who are hemodynamically stable and have normal RV function. To minimize the risk of harm, patients should be screened carefully for contraindications to thrombolysis (Table 22.2). The thrombolytic dose should be adjusted in patients who weigh < 70 kg, and the increased risk for ICH in patients > 65 years of age should be factored heavily.

Non-medical and embolectomy options

The practical application and delivery of interventional therapy is beyond the scope of most emergency physicians and is not applicable in a low-resource center. This treatment is best performed by a multidisciplinary team, including an interventional radiologist and a cardiothoracic surgeon. Techniques include percutaneous embolectomy, catheter-directed thrombolysis, percutaneous fragmentation, and surgical embolectomy in centers in which cardiothoracic surgery is available. Most studies reported to date have

Table 22.2 Contraindications to fibrinolysis[1,2,3]

Cardiac arrest resulting from PE is *not* a contraindication

Absolute contraindications

- Any previous intracranial hemorrhage.
- Known structural intracranial cerebrovascular disease (e.g., arteriovenous malformation).
- Known malignant intracranial neoplasm.
- Ischemic stroke within three months.
- Suspected aortic dissection.
- Active bleeding or bleeding diathesis.
- Recent surgery encroaching on the spinal canal or brain.
- Recent significant closed-head or facial trauma with radiographic evidence of bony fracture or brain injury.

Relative contraindications

- Age > 75 years.
- Current use of anticoagulation.
- Pregnancy.
- Non-compressible vascular punctures.
- Traumatic or prolonged cardiopulmonary resuscitation (> 10 minutes).
- Recent internal bleeding (within two to four weeks).
- History of chronic, severe, and poorly controlled hypertension.
- Severe uncontrolled hypertension on presentation (systolic blood pressure > 180 mmHg or diastolic blood pressure > 110 mmHg).
- Dementia.
- Remote (> 3 months) ischemic stroke.
- Major surgery within three weeks.

not shown that catheter-based delivery of lytics is safer than systemically administered lytics.

Possible indications for this approach include hemodynamic instability with contraindications to systemic thrombolysis and patients with massive PE who, despite undergoing thrombolysis, are still hemodynamically unstable.[3]

Thrombolysis and deep venous thrombosis (DVT)

The mainstay of treatment of DVT is anticoagulation. Thrombolytic therapy may be associated with rapid and complete lysis of DVT, as well as a decrease in the incidence and severity of post-thrombotic syndrome. The clinical relevance of earlier clearance of a venous obstruction is uncertain, bearing in mind that thrombolytic therapy does increase the risk of major bleeding. In this section, the discussion is limited to indications for thrombolysis and thrombolytic regimens.

DVT-induced phlegmasia cerula dolens is the most widely accepted indication for thrombolysis,[3,23] because, if untreated, it can result in loss of limb.[23] The decision to initiate thrombolytic therapy should be made on a case-by-case basis, after the risks and benefits are discussed with the patient. The thrombolytic agent should be administered via catheter, and the intervention should be discussed with an interventional radiologist or vascular surgeon.[24] In environments with limited resource, if no such service is readily available, administration of a thrombolytic agent should be considered, provided there are no contraindications. Anticoagulant therapy should be discontinued during thrombolytic infusion.

Systemic thrombolytic regimens for thrombolysis in deep vein thrombosis are presented below[3]:

- rtPA – administer 100 mg intravenously over two hours.
- Streptokinase – administer 250,000 IU intravenously over 30 minutes, then 100,000 IU/h for 24 to 72 hours.
- Urokinase – administer 4400 IU/kg intravenously over the initial 10 minutes, then 2200 IU/kg·h for 12 hours.

When the infusion of the thrombolytic agent is complete, heparin therapy can be resumed, depending on the aPTT.

Conclusion

The use of thrombolytics in patients with PE is a controversial topic that leaves many clinicians with clinical uncertainties. Pulmonary embolism with hypotension and acute RV dysfunction mandates rapid evaluation and management. There is a clear benefit versus risk of harm for thrombolytic therapy in a patient who presents in cardiac arrest from PE and in those who are hemodynamically unstable. Heparinization and thrombolytic therapy are essential in this subgroup of patients. Patients who are diagnosed with PE but have stable hemodynamics and no evidence of RV strain should not receive thrombolytics. Emergency physicians who are armed with a structured, rational approach to the assessment and treatment of a patient with a massive PE are in the best position to limit patient morbidity and mortality.

Critical actions

- Consider early thrombolytic therapy in the hemodynamically unstable patient with suspected massive PE.

- Stop the administration of heparin during the infusion of thrombolytic therapy and resume it when the infusion is completed.
- Alteplase is the recommended thrombolytic because of its short infusion time.

Pearls and pitfalls

- Cardiac arrest caused by pulmonary embolism is not an absolute contraindication to thrombolysis.
- The administration of thrombolytic therapy for acute PE is within the scope of emergency medicine.
- Thrombolytics are *not indicated* for clinically stable patients without evidence of RV strain.
- The treating physician is in the best position to judge the relative merits of thrombolysis on a case-by-case basis.

References

1. American College of Emergency Physicians. Critical issues in the evaluation and management of adult patients presenting to the emergency department with suspected pulmonary embolism. *Ann Emerg Med* 2011; 57: 628–52.

2. Tapson V. Acute pulmonary embolism. *N Engl J Med* 2008; 358: 1037–52.

3. Jaff MR, McMurtry MS, Archer SL, *et al.* Management of massive and submassive pulmonary embolism, ileofemoral deep vein thrombosis, and chronic thromboembolic pulmonary hypertension: a scientific statement from the American Heart Association. *Circulation* 2011; 123(16): 1788–830.

4. Jerjes-Sanchez C, Ramirez-Rivera A, de Lourdes Garcia M, *et al.* Streptokinase and heparin versus heparin alone in massive pulmonary embolism: a randomized controlled trial. *J Thromb Thrombolysis* 1995; 2(3): 227–9.

5. Fengler BT, Brady WJ. Fibrinolytic therapy in pulmonary embolism: an evidence-based treatment algorithm. *Am J Emerg Med* 2009; 27: 84–95.

6. British Thoracic Society Standards of Care Committee Pulmonary Embolism Guideline Development Group. British Thoracic Society guidelines for the management of suspected acute pulmonary embolism. *Thorax* 2003; 58: 470–84.

7. Janata K, Holzer M, Kürkciyan I, *et al.* Major bleeding complications in cardiopulmonary resuscitation: the place of thrombolytic therapy in cardiac arrest due to massive pulmonary embolism. *Resuscitation* 2003; 57: 49–55.

8. Scholz KH, Tebbe U, Herrmann C, *et al.* Frequency of complications of cardiopulmonary resuscitation after thrombolysis during acute myocardial infarction. *Am J Cardiol* 1992; 69: 724–8.

9. Wan S, Quinlan DJ, Agnelli G, *et al.* Thrombolysis compared with heparin for the initial treatment of pulmonary embolism: a meta-analysis of the randomized controlled trials. *Circulation* 2004; 110: 744–9.

10. Goldhaber SZ. Echocardiography in the management of pulmonary embolism. *Ann Intern Med* 2002; 136: 691–700.

11. Casazza F, Bongarzoni A, Capozi A, Agostoni O. Regional right ventricular dysfunction in acute pulmonary embolism and right ventricular infarction. *Eur J Echocardiography* 2005; 6(1): 11–14.

12. Ribeiro A, Lindmarker P, Johnsson H, *et al.* Pulmonary embolism: one-year follow-up with echocardiography Doppler and five-year survival analysis. *Circulation* 1999; 99: 1325–30.

13. Loebinger MR, Bradley JC. Thrombolysis in pulmonary embolism: are we under-using it? *Q J Med* 2004; 97: 361–4.

14. Torbicki A, Perrier A, Konstantinides S, *et al.* Guidelines on the diagnosis and management of acute pulmonary embolism: the Task Force for the Diagnosis and Management of Acute Pulmonary Embolism of the European Society of Cardiology (ESC). *Eur Heart J* 2008; 29(18): 2276–315.

15. Rivera-Bou WL, Cabanas JG, Villanueva SE, *et al.* Thrombolytic therapy in emergency medicine. Last updated May 3, 2012. Available at http://emedicine.medscape.com/article/811234-overview. Accessed on September 26, 2012.

16. Bailen MR, Cuadra JA, Aguayo De Hoyos E. Thrombolysis during cardiopulmonary resuscitation in fulminant pulmonary embolism: a review. *Crit Care Med* 2001; 29(11): 2211–19.

17. Capstick T, Henry MT. Efficacy of thrombolytic agents in the treatment of pulmonary embolism. *Eur Respir J* 2005; 26: 864–74.

18. Goldhaber SZ. Advanced treatment strategies for acute pulmonary embolism, including thrombolysis and embolectomy. *J Thromb Haemost* 2009; 7(suppl 1): 322–7.

19. Urokinase-streptokinase embolism trial. Phase 2 results. A cooperative study. *JAMA* 1974; 229: 1606–13.

20. Meneveau N, Schiele F, Metz D, *et al.* Comparative efficacy of a two-hour regimen of streptokinase versus alteplase in acute massive pulmonary embolism: immediate clinical and hemodynamic outcome and one-year follow-up. *J Am Coll Cardiol* 1998; 31: 1057–63.

21. Kline J, Hernandez-Nino J, Jones AE. Tenecteplase to treat pulmonary embolism in the emergency department. *Thromb Haemost* 2010; 103(5): 877–83.

22. Goldhaber SZ, Visani L, De Rosa M. Acute pulmonary embolism: clinical outcomes in the International Cooperative Pulmonary Embolism Registry (ICOPER). *Lancet* 1999; 353: 1386–9.

23. Wicky ST. Acute deep vein thrombosis and thrombolysis. *Tech Vasc Interv Radiol* 2009; 12(2): 148–53.

24. Enden T, Sandvik L, Kløw NE, *et al.* Catheter-directed Venous Thrombolysis in acute ileofemoral vein thrombosis–the CaVenT study: rationale and design of a multicenter, randomized, controlled, clinical trial. *Am Heart J* 2007; 154(5): 808–14.

Chapter

23

Ultrasound-guided central venous access

Sarah K. Sommerkamp and Alisa Gibson

Central venous access has developed into an essential procedure in emergency care since its introduction in the 1950s. Traditionally, the landmark technique has been used for placement of all central venous lines. The introduction of ultrasound into emergency departments has led to a novel approach to central venous access. Ultrasound guidance for central-line placement is quickly gaining favor as physicians become more comfortable with the machine and experienced with line placement. The use of ultrasound to guide line placement has many benefits, including improved accuracy and a decreased number of attempts, both of which improve complication rates and safety.[1–5]

Central lines are frequently required in the critically ill and can facilitate life-saving interventions. However, their placement is far from risk free. Complications occur in more than 15% of patients who receive a central venous catheter via the traditional landmark technique. Infectious complications occur in 5 to 26%, thrombotic complications in 2 to 26%, and mechanical complications in 5 to 19%.[6] Mechanical complications include hematoma, arterial puncture, and pneumothorax. Overall, the highest rates of mechanical complications occur with femoral access, although the frequency of serious mechanical complications is equivalent to the frequency of such complications when subclavian access is used.[7,8]

Complications from central venous access not only cause harm to patients, but also add considerably to the cost of health care. The excess healthcare cost of a single central-line–associated blood stream infection (CLABSI) is estimated at $16,550.[9] Iatrogenic pneumothorax is associated with four to seven excess days in hospital, 1 to 14% in excess mortality, and $17,000 to $45,000 in excess charges.[10] There is also a large cost in terms of malpractice claims paid because

of these complications. In 1999 dollars, the median payout ranged from $40,000 to $185,000 (depending on the type of complication).[11]

The impetus to reduce complications is obvious. Many hospitals have implemented quality improvement initiatives to reduce the incidence of CLABSI, which have proven to be quite effective.[12] Another means of decreasing the frequency of complications is the use of ultrasound guidance. A meta-analysis of eight studies showed that this technique is associated with significantly fewer mechanical complications than the standard landmark placement technique.[13] In addition, the use of ultrasound decreases the time from needle to skin to flashback,[14] the number of catheter-placement failures, the time required for insertion,[6] and the frequency of bloodstream infection.[15] The data available for subclavian and femoral veins are limited but promising.[12] They are clear enough (level 1b evidence) that the Centers for Disease Control now recommends the use of ultrasound guidance to place central lines whenever possible.[16]

The National Institute for Health and Clinical Excellence (NICE) has also become a strong supporter of ultrasound-guided central-line placement, recommending its use since 2002. In an economic evaluation, NICE investigators acknowledged that the major impediment to ultrasound guidance for central access is the initial cost of the ultrasound machine. Taking into account the sizable upfront costs, their cost–benefit analysis still favored the use of ultrasound, showing savings of £2 per line. This was largely related to the decreased cost stemming from complications.[17] Another British economic model, developed by Calvert and colleagues for the National Health Service, yielded similar findings.[18]

Despite the promising messages of the studies mentioned above, the cost of ultrasound machines continues to be an impediment to their regular use. The ever-increasing variety of machines, at multiple price points, is reducing that impediment. Many models are being targeted specifically to the demands of an emergency department. The micronization of technology is also decreasing the cost and improving the portability of ultrasound machines. The cost of a portable ultrasound machine can range from $20,000 to $60,000, with each probe adding an additional few thousand dollars. The expected life span of an ultrasound machine in the ED is four to seven years.

Indications/contraindications/anatomy

Central venous access is needed in the ED for a variety of reasons. Indications range from inability to obtain a peripheral intravenous (IV) line in a code situation to sepsis requiring vasoactive agents. Specific disease conditions that tend to require access include vascular emergencies, trauma, sepsis, and renal failure. Central access may be required in other disease conditions when dependable access, frequent blood sampling, administration of vasoconstricting and sclerosing medications, or hemodialysis is needed. Subclavian and internal jugular veins can be used for hemodynamic monitoring, transvenous pacing, and monitoring response to therapeutic interventions.

Multiple considerations come into the choice of a site for central venous access. In a code or other true emergency situation, the fastest and easiest central line to place is in the femoral vein. Benefits associated with the femoral line include the ability to use it immediately after placement without a confirmatory radiograph, the lack of potential to cause a pneumothorax, and its compressibility in the event of arterial puncture. In a code situation in which multiple care providers are crowded around the torso, practitioners can more easily position themselves to place a femoral line. Ultrasound can be used to make placement even easier. However, the significantly higher risks of infection[16] and thrombosis[19] make a code essentially the only situation in which femoral access should be used.

Emergency practitioners should consider intraosseous access or placement of an ultrasound-guided peripheral IV line as an alternative to a central line. Subclavian lines have the lowest infectious complications.[20] The subclavian vein is not compressible, so it should not be used in a patient with coagulopathy, because bleeding may go unrecognized and cannot be controlled with direct pressure. The internal jugular vein is compressible and is thought to pose less risk of infection than femoral access. While this continues to be true for patients with body mass index over 28.4 kg/m^2, for non-obese patients, there seems to be minimal improvement in infection rate.[21] The right internal jugular vein has the lowest rate of catheter malposition[22] and is the preferred choice for transvenous pacing (the left subclavian vein is second best).

If time permits, laboratory tests to check for coagulopathy should be obtained. These include a platelet count and coagulation factors (PT/INR and PTT). No absolute numbers prohibit placement of a central line. However, a platelet count of less than 50,000/μL is associated with a higher risk of bleeding, more so than a prolonged clotting time.[23] Platelet transfusions and/or FFP can be administered if time allows, though there is no compelling evidence to support their use.[24]

No specific imaging needs to be done before placement of a central line. However, ultrasound can be used to evaluate both sides of the patient's anatomy to avoid thrombosis and evaluate the distance between the artery and vein and thus determine the ideal location for the central line. Ultrasound can (and should) be used to provide real-time guidance. A post-procedure chest film is mandatory after placement of a subclavian or internal jugular line.

Another consideration when choosing an access site is the number of times that the site has been used previously. The presence of extensive scarring from some other cause could also be a factor. Finally, if long-term hemodialysis is anticipated, it may be best to leave an extremity free for a fistula or graft.

Management of central-line placement

Once the need for a central line has been determined, and all contraindications have been reviewed, several critical actions must be performed. Informed consent should be obtained whenever possible. Time-out documentation or other hospital-specific policies may be required. It is crucial to have the proper armamentarium in the room before beginning the procedure.

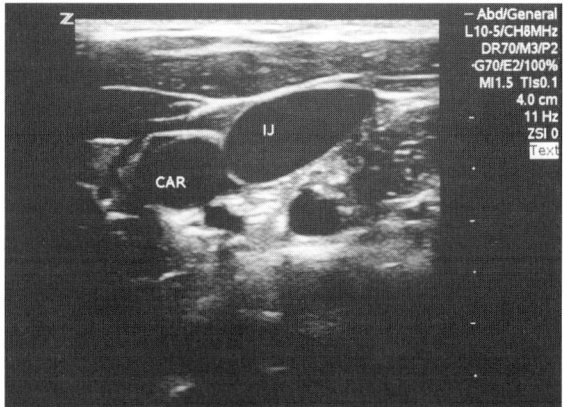

Figure 23.1 The internal jugular vein (IJ) and carotid artery (CAR) are shown on ultrasound. The vein is larger and has thinner walls compared to the artery.

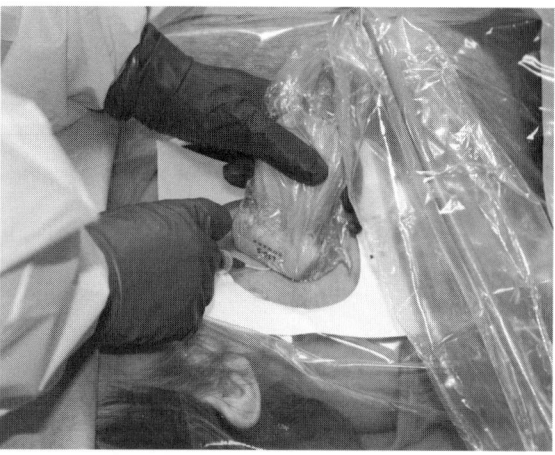

Figure 23.2 Patient positioning and probe placement for internal jugular vein access.

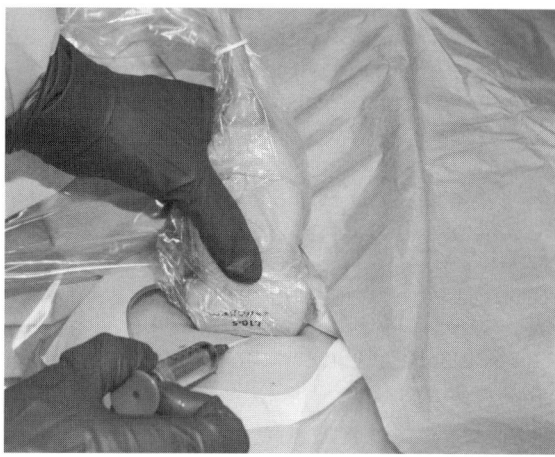

Figure 23.3 Patient positioning and probe placement for femoral vein access.

This includes a commercially available central-line kit as well as saline, caps, antiseptic supplies, and sterile drapes and gowns, depending on the kit your hospital uses. Anesthesia must also be used, and in some cases procedural sedation may be appropriate. Ultrasound-specific supplies include the machine itself (ideally with a linear array transducer with frequency of 7.5 to 10 MHz), a sterile probe cover, and sterile acoustic gel.

Before creating a sterile field, use ultrasound to compare the desired vessel on the left and right and optimize the patient's positioning (Figure 23.1). For internal jugular venous access, place the patient in Trendelenburg position. This decreases the risk of air embolism and maximizes the size of the vein. Twenty-five degrees of tilt is optimal, although as little as ten degrees is effective.[25] Turning the patient's head only partially to the side puts the vein more lateral to the carotid artery, which minimizes the risk of arterial puncture.[26] Either the left or right internal jugular may be used, based on the indications/contraindications reviewed above or simply based on which vein appears larger or easier to access. The operator stands behind the patient's head. Orient the probe marker toward the patient's left (Figure 23.2).

For subclavian venous access, place the patient in Trendelenburg position. A shoulder roll may be helpful. Pulling the patient's ipsilateral arm toward the feet (requires an assistant) may facilitate venous access and threading of the catheter. In theory, the anatomy of the right subclavian vein decreases the risk of pneumothorax because of the lower pleural apex and absence of the thoracic duct. However, use of the right sub-clavian vein is associated with higher rates of catheter malposition and vessel trauma.[27] Ultrasound guidance for subclavian access is generally difficult to accomplish because the clavicle creates a shadow, obscuring the operator's view of the vein in all but the most lateral approach. Alternate approaches such as axillary or supraclavicular vein cannulation are not yet standard; they are discussed below, in the Future directions section. For femoral venous access, the optimal position of the hip is abducted and externally rotated. This increases the mean diameter of the vein and prevents it from being directly posterior to the artery.[28] The operator stands on the same side as the target vessel, with the probe marker toward the patient's right (Figure 23.3).

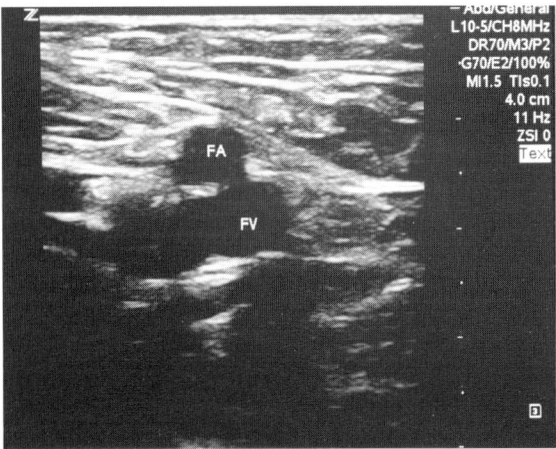

Figure 23.4 The femoral vein (FV) and artery (FA) are shown on ultrasound. The vein is larger and has thinner walls compared with the artery. Note that the vein is deep in relation to the artery. External rotation of the patient's leg decreases the FA–FV overlap and the FV depth.

After the patient is positioned satisfactorily and the desired vein has been located, prepare and drape the patient. Place the ultrasound probe into the probe cover, being sure to use copious amounts of acoustic gel inside the cover and avoiding air bubbles. Sterile sleeves that are very easy to use are commercially available. A sterile glove can be used as well, with the aid of an assistant. Once the operator is sterile, he or she should hold the sleeve. Apply the acoustic gel into the sleeve, then have the assistant place the probe into it. To maintain sterility, only the interior portion of the sleeve can be touched with the probe. Apply sterile gel to the patient or the outside of the probe cover. Acoustic ultrasound gel is preferred to sterile lubricating gel because of its acoustic properties and therefore its sound transmission. Acoustic gel improves the image quality, but sterile lubricating gel will work. Use the probe to identify the exact location of the vein. Distinguishing the vein from the artery is generally straightforward. Vessels are hypoechoic (black) structures. When using a transverse approach, the vein is typically the larger structure and should be easily compressible. The diameter of the internal jugular and subclavian veins increases with the Valsalva maneuver and Trendelenburg position. Vein walls are thinner than those of arteries. The artery is usually smaller and visibly pulsates. Images of the internal jugular and femoral veins are shown in Figures 23.1 and 23.4. The femoral vein is always medial to the artery (remember

the mnemonic "NAVEL": nerve, artery, vein, endothelial, lymphatics).

When in doubt, use color Doppler to clearly distinguish vein from artery. The artery shows pulsations in the color pattern, while the vein has a more stable flow. Do not be misled; the red and blue colors do NOT indicate which vessel is which. The color indicates flow toward or away from the transducer, not the heart. If the transducer is 90° from the direction of flow, color Doppler will not be visible.

The choice to use the longitudinal or transverse approach depends on a number of factors, including the patient's anatomy and the operator's experience and comfort. In the longitudinal approach, the vein and artery cannot be seen in the same view, but they can be distinguished by compressibility versus pulsation. Find the vessels in the transverse orientation, and then rotate the probe 90° to view them longitudinally. The needle tip is much more difficult to visualize entering the vein in the transverse view, but the entire length of the needle can be watched using the longitudinal orientation.[29] The two approaches can be combined as well. Some operators prefer to enter the skin while viewing the vessels transversely and then switch to a longitudinal view to visualize the needle as it enters the vein. An alternative to real-time ultrasound guidance is a static technique. Simply find the vein with ultrasound, mark its position on the skin, and then use that mark to facilitate the landmark technique. The drawback of this approach is that you are not able to watch the needle enter the specific vessel. The benefit is that you are able to use both hands to place the line.

Local anesthetics are usually instilled using the transverse view. Keep the vein in view to facilitate administration of the anesthetic, both subcutaneously and along the anticipated needle path. Use as much local anesthesia as necessary to achieve patient comfort, but avoid overzealous subcutaneous infiltration as well as introduction of air, both of which may distort anatomy and impair visualization with ultrasound.

After adequate analgesia is obtained, the next step is to align the needle with the vein. Be sure to use a needle that is at least 1.5 times as long as the measured depth of the vessel. Initial alignment is accomplished by centering the vein along the probe. Survey the vein along its course; gaining access and placing the catheter are much easier if done in a long, straight section of the vessel. Once a site has been selected, use a blunt object to push down on the skin at the site of anticipated puncture. Use the movement of the tissue

Table 23.1 Troubleshooting

Problem	Solution
It looks like the needle is in the vein, but there is no blood flow.	The vessel may be tented at the site of the needle. Slight advancement of the needle may be required to pierce the vessel wall. The needle may have gone through the other side of the vein. Try withdrawing the syringe slightly while aspirating.
I can't see the needle on the ultrasound monitor.	Gently move the needle up and down, and look for tissue motion on the screen. Do not move the needle from side to side, as this is more likely to lacerate the vessel and surrounding tissue. Keep the needle in one spot and sweep the transducer up and down, looking for the echogenic (white) spot.

seen on the ultrasound image to confirm that site is in the middle of the screen. Alternatively, place the needle on top of the skin under the ultrasound probe and align the "ring down" artifact (a white shadow) that it produces with the vein to ensure correct placement. Pierce the skin with the needle. You should see a hyperechoic (white) spot on the screen. Move the transducer forward, keeping the needle in one place until the needle is no longer visible. Advance the needle until it comes into view again. Align the needle tip with the middle of the vein, and proceed in a step-wise fashion until the needle can be seen in the vessel and there is good blood return. Although this may seem like a technically difficult, multistep procedure, with practice it becomes a simple, fluid motion. If difficulty is encountered with the procedure, review the common problems and solutions in Table 23.1.

Adjunct techniques that may be helpful

Some operators find it helpful to have an ultrasound-savvy assistant hold the ultrasound probe, so that they have both their hands free for the procedure. Another adjunct technique is to use a needle guide. These are commercial products that attach to the ultrasound probe and ensure that the needle is inserted along its midline. Specialized needles with echogenic tips are available and make visualization with ultrasound much simpler. The guidewire is echogenic and can be visualized in the vessel if there is any doubt about placement.

Post-procedure care is the same for a central line established based on anatomy or aided by ultrasound guidance. After the line is sutured in place, apply a sterile dressing and an antibiotic-coated disc (Biopatch). Order a chest film for an internal jugular or subclavian line to confirm appropriate positioning and exclude pneumothorax. Document the procedure in accordance with hospital policy. If a patient will be discharged to a long-term care facility (as opposed to being admitted to a hospital bed), a peripherally inserted central catheter (PICC) is probably a safer alternative.

Future directions

As the technology surrounding ultrasound continues to advance, its uses related to central venous access are expanding. One of the most exciting areas of research is ultrasound access to the subclavian vein. Two methods have been proposed. The first is use of the axillary vein, the lateral extension of the subclavian vein. The line is placed transpectorally. Initial results are promising, but larger studies are needed.[30] The second method is the supraclavicular approach. The endocavitary probe is placed into the supraclavicular fossa and the subclavian vein is identified and cannulated dynamically.[31]

A number of products have been developed to facilitate ultrasound-guided central access, including needle-tracking systems. These devices can improve needle visibility and project needle pathways.[32,33] Handheld ultrasound devices are already on the market and may prove beneficial for line placement. Limitations include their small screen size (which makes dynamic imaging more challenging with a single operator) and maintaining a sterile barrier for this smaller device. Handheld devices are also limited, at the time of this writing, by probe choice. A single probe is offered and is not a high-frequency linear transducer, which is generally the preferred probe for procedural guidance for central access.

Clinical approach when resources are limited

Healthcare providers with limited resources have some lower-cost alternatives. No ultrasound machine can be considered "cheap," but a small machine such as a Site-Rite is less expensive than a full capability machine. If a linear probe is not available, a curvilinear probe, though not ideal, can be used to assist in gaining vascular access. If a commercial sheath is not available,

Table 23.2 Critical actions

Before procedure	During procedure	After procedure
Obtain consent.	Maintain sterile field, including the probe.	Apply appropriate dressing.
Perform a time out.	Induce effective anesthesia.	Obtain a chest film.
Gather equipment.	Localize the vessel with ultrasound.	
Position patient and ultrasound machine.	Visualize entry of the needle/guidewire into the vessel.	

a sterile glove can be used to cover the ultrasound probe. Obviously, the traditional landmark techniques for central-line placement can be used if ultrasound is not available.

Conclusion

Ultrasound guidance for central access continues to gain popularity. It makes catheter placement easier and safer and should be used whenever possible. The choice of location depends on many factors; an upper site is preferred. The use of sterile probe covers and acoustic gel facilitates maintenance of the crucial sterile field. A dynamic imaging technique allows the use of adjunctive tools and is optimal. As technology and care providers' experience continue to improve, ultrasound might be used for placement of subclavian lines as well. Ultrasound is no longer just a "back up" method to be employed when the landmark technique fails, or a sophisticated technology accessible only at academic centers. It is not the future; it is the present.

Pearls and pitfalls

Pearls

- Use sedation if necessary to ensure the patient is calm and comfortable and remains still during the procedure.
- Use ultrasound guidance to improve accuracy and decrease the procedure length and complications.
- Find a long, straight section of the vessel to access to improve ease of placement.
- Use the transverse approach to find the vein.
- Use the longitudinal approach to visualize the needle along its path.
- Use copious amounts of gel both inside and outside the probe cover.
- Advance the needle slightly if no flash is obtained despite the appearance of the catheter in the vein.

The needle might be just above the tenting of the vessel.
- Watch movement of the tissue displaced by the needle to assist with needle localization.

Pitfalls

- Overzealous subcutaneous infiltration or introduction of air distorts anatomy and impairs visualization with ultrasound.
- Failing to gather all needed supplies before beginning the procedure.
- Failure to use ultrasound to locate the desired vessel *before* prepping and draping the patient.
- Using the red and blue colors on Doppler to distinguish artery from vein (they do NOT indicate which vessel is which).
- Posterior penetration of the vessel wall is common; use the step-wise method of keeping the needle tip in view.

Critical actions

See Table 23.2.

References

1. Hudson PA, Rose JS. Real-time ultrasound guided internal jugular vein catheterization in the emergency department. *Am J Emerg Med* 1997; 15: 79–82.
2. Slama M, Novara A, Safavian A, *et al.* Improvement of internal jugular vein cannulation using an ultrasound-guided technique. *Intensive Care Med* 1997; 23: 916–19.
3. Teichgräber UK, Benter T, Gebel M, *et al.* A sonographically guided technique for central venous access. *AJR* 1997; 169: 731–3.
4. Denys BG, Uretsky BF, Reddy PS. Ultrasound-assisted cannulation of the internal jugular vein: a prospective comparison to the external landmark-guided technique. *Circulation* 1993; 87: 1557–62.

5. Keyes LE, Frazee BW, Snoey ER, *et al.* Ultrasound-guided brachial and basilic vein cannulation in emergency department patients with difficult intravenous access. *Ann Emerg Med* 1993; 34: 711–14.

6. McGee DC, Gould MK. Preventing complications of central venous catheterization. *N Engl J Med* 2003; 348:1123–33.

7. Merrer J, De Jonghe B, Golliot F, *et al.* Complications of femoral and subclavian venous catheterization in critically ill patients: a randomized controlled trial. *JAMA* 2001; 286: 700–7.

8. Sznajder JI, Zveibil FR, Bitterman H, *et al.* Central vein catheterization: failure and complication rates by three percutaneous approaches. *Arch Intern Med* 1986; 146: 259–61.

9. Centers for Disease Control and Prevention (CDC). Vital signs: central line–associated blood stream infections – United States, 2001, 2008, and 2009. *MMWR Morb Mortal Wkly Rep* 2011; 60(8): 243–8.

10. Zhan C, Smith M, Stryer D. Incidences, outcomes and factors associated with iatrogenic pneumothorax in hospitalized patients. In *Academy Health 2004 Annual Research Meeting: Abstracts. Quality & Patient Safety.* Washington DC: Academy Health; 2004: 54. Available at http://www.academyhealth.org/files/2004/abstracts/quality.pdf. Accessed on October 11, 2012.

11. Domino KB, Bowdle TA, Posner KL, *et al.* Injuries and liability related to central vascular catheters: a closed claims analysis. *Anesthesiology* 2004; 100: 1411–18.

12. Frasca D, Dahyot-Fizelier C, Mimoz O. Prevention of central venous catheter-related infection in the intensive care unit. *Crit Care* 2010; 14: 212.

13. Randolph AG, Cook DJ, Gonzales CA, *et al.* Ultrasound guidance for placement of central venous catheters: a meta-analysis of the literature. *Crit Care Med* 1996; 24: 2053–8.

14. Miller AH, Roth BA. Ultrasound guidance versus the landmark technique for the placement of central venous catheters in the emergency department. *Acad Emerg Med* 2002; 9: 800–5.

15. Karakitsos D, Labropoulos N, De Groot E, *et al.* Real-time ultrasound-guided catheterisation of the internal jugular vein: a prospective comparison with the landmark technique in critical care patients. *Crit Care* 2006; 10: R162.

16. O'Grady NP, Alexander A, Burns LA, *et al. Guidelines for the Prevention of Intravascular Catheter-Related Infections, 2011.* Atlanta, GA: Centers for Disease Control; 2011. Available at www.cdc.gov/hicpac/pdf/guidelines/bsi-guidelines-2011.pdf. Accessed on March 28, 2012.

17. Atkinson P, Boyle A, Robinson S, *et al.* Should ultrasound guidance be used for central venous catheterisation in the emergency department? *Emerg Med J* 2005; 22: 158–64.

18. Calvert N, Hind D, McWilliams RG, *et al.* The effectiveness and cost-effectiveness of ultrasound locating devices for central venous access: a systematic review and economic evaluation. *Health Technol Assess* 2003; 7(12): 1–84.

19. Joynt GM, Kew J, Gomersall CD, *et al.* Deep venous thrombosis caused by femoral venous catheters in critically ill adult patients. *Chest* 2000; 117: 178–83.

20. Trottier SJ, Veremakis C, O'Brien J, *et al.* Femoral deep vein thrombosis associated with central venous catheterization: results from a prospective, randomized trial. *Crit Care Med* 1995; 23: 52–9.

21. Parienti JJ, Thirion M, Mégarbane B, *et al.* Femoral vs jugular venous catheterization and risk of nosocomial events in adults requiring acute renal replacement therapy: a randomized controlled trial. *JAMA* 2008; 299: 2413–22.

22. Ruesch S, Walder B, Tramèr MR. Complications of central venous catheters: internal jugular versus subclavian access – a systematic review. *Crit Care Med* 2002; 30: 454–60.

23. Polderman KH, Girbes AJ. Central venous catheter use. Part 1: mechanical complications. *Intensive Care Med* 2002; 28: 1–17.

24. Segal JB, Dzik WH, Transfusion Medicine/Hemostasis Clinical Trials Network. Paucity of studies to support that abnormal coagulation test results predict bleeding in the setting of invasive procedures: an evidence-based review. *Transfusion* 2005; 45: 1413–25.

25. Clenaghan S, McLaughlin RE, Martyn C, *et al.* Relationship between Trendelenburg tilt and internal jugular vein diameter. *Emerg Med J* 2005; 22: 867–8.

26. Geria R, Hoffmann B. Ultrasound guide for emergency physicians 2008: Ultrasound guided vascular access. Available at www.sonoguide.com/line_placement.html. Accessed on March 28, 2012.

27. American Association of Clinical Anatomists, Educational Affairs Committee. The clinical anatomy of several invasive procedures. *AUSO Clin Anat* 1999; 12(1): 43.

28. Werner SL, Jones RA, Emerman CL. Effect of hip abduction and external rotation on femoral vein exposure for possible cannulation. *J Emerg Med* 2008; 35: 73–5.

29. Stone MB, Moon C, Sutijono D, *et al.* Needle tip visualization during ultrasound-guided vascular access: short-axis vs long-axis approach. *Am J Emerg Med* 2010; 28: 343–7.

30. Sandhu NS. Transpectoral ultrasound-guided catheterization of the axillary vein: an alternative to standard catheterization of the subclavian vein. *Anesth Analg* 2004; 99: 183–7.

31. Mallin M, Lewis H. A novel technique for ultrasound-guided supraclavicular subclavian cannulation. *Am J Emerg Med* 2010; 28: 966–9.

32. MedicalPhysicsWeb. SonoSite software offers enhanced needle visualization. Newsfeed, July 14, 2010. Available at http://medicalphysicsweb.org/cws/article/newsfeed/43176. Accessed on March 28, 2012.

33. Medical Health Imaging. GE Healthcare launches its new ultrasound needle technology. March 15, 2010. Available at www.healthimaginghub.com/126-medical-imaging/450-ge-healthcare-launches-its-new-ultrasound-needle-technology.html. Accessed on March 28, 2012.

Chapter

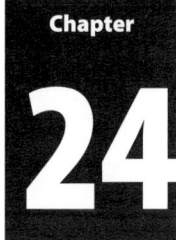

24

Use of ultrasound to assess the patient with hypotension and shock

Leah Bright and Beatrice Hoffmann

Point-of-care sonography in the emergency department (ED), also called "emergency ultrasound," is now a commonly used diagnostic tool in the acute care setting. Although it is operator dependent, it is also fast and portable, has a growing number of diagnostic indications, and has been found to be reliable in several clinical studies.[1–3] One of the developing applications for point-of-care sonography is its use in patients presenting with undifferentiated hypotension and shock.[1–3]

Hypotensive patients are frequently more ill than normotensive patients,[1] mainly because hypotension may signify the presence of decompensated shock. Circulatory shock is a common endpoint of many medical and surgical conditions and can be divided into four types: hypovolemic shock, cardiogenic shock, obstructive shock, and distributive shock. Quick diagnosis and goal-directed management for each type of shock are of utmost importance for critical care and emergency physicians. Important clinical data may not be readily available because the patient's ability to participate in history taking and the physical examination may be compromised by severe illness. In this situation, ultrasound may help distinguish between types of shock and even identify the underlying cause. Thus, it has the potential to improve the management and outcome of patients in shock.

When using bedside ultrasound, a focused, goal-directed approach to hypotension and shock is important.[3] Protocols for the use of sonography to assess patients with undifferentiated hypotension have been developed. These standardized protocols recommend a goal-directed approach, which includes abdominal, cardiac, and thoracic ultrasound views.[3] Each of these views addresses the differential diagnosis of medical problems that can cause hypotension.

Diagnosis

Circulatory shock can be defined as a medical emergency in which tissues do not receive sufficient perfusion, leading to inadequate tissue oxygenation. It can have a variable presentation, depending on the patient's age and medical problems. Some patients have only minimal symptoms, such as a minor change in mental status and generalized weakness; others present with profound hypotension, renal failure, tachypnea, and tachycardia. Although tachycardia is common in patients in shock, patients on β-blockers can have a normal or slow heart rate. Specific subtypes of shock are associated with additional symptoms. On examination, the patient can be diaphoretic with cool and clammy skin, have a weak pulse, and exhibit changes in mental status as cranial perfusion decreases. Depending on the cause of shock, other physical examination findings may be notable, including ecchymosis in trauma patients, a warm torso or limbs in septic patients with fever, or profound dyspnea in patients with pneumothorax or pulmonary embolism.

Laboratory tests obtained in the ED to help evaluate for shock include a complete blood count, a comprehensive metabolic panel, coagulation panel, as well as urinalysis. Routine blood tests can reveal acidosis through decreased carbon dioxide levels, but specific testing for increased anaerobic metabolism can be performed by measuring lactic acid levels and central venous oxygen saturation ($ScvO_2$). Central venous oxygen saturation obtained from a central venous catheter usually correlates well with mixed venous oxygen saturation ($SmvO_2$) obtained from a pulmonary artery catheter.

Imaging the hypotensive patient may yield helpful additional information but is often limited to bedside

Vascular Emergencies, ed. Robert L. Rogers, Thomas Scalea, Lee Wallis, and Heike Geduld. Published by Cambridge University Press. © Cambridge University Press 2013.

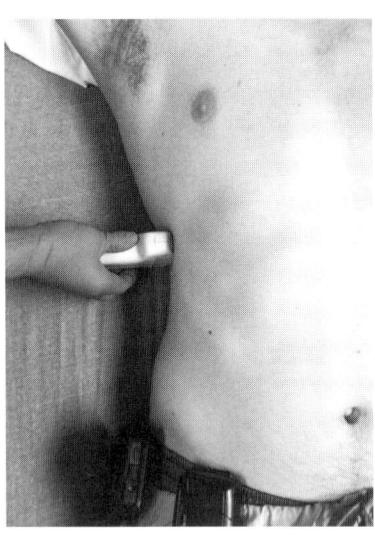

Figure 24.1 Right upper quadrant view of the FAST examination.

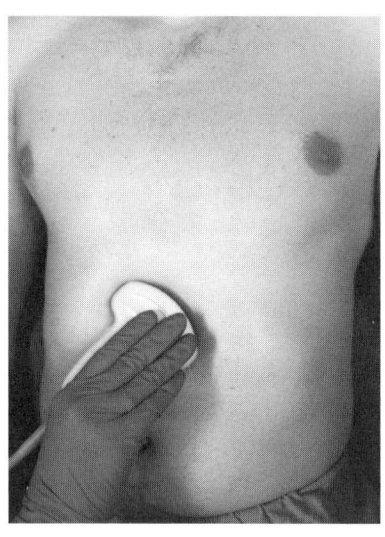

Figure 24.2 Subxyphoid cardiac view of the FAST examination.

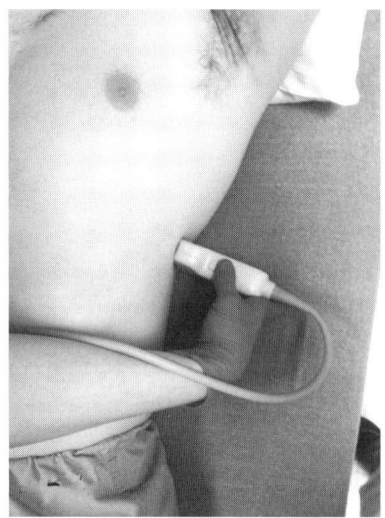

Figure 24.3 Left upper quadrant view of the FAST examination.

diagnostics. The patient is usually too ill to leave the ED, so a portable X-ray machine and emergency ultrasound equipment should be employed as necessary. If resuscitation is underway, it can be continued in the ED while bedside imaging is in progress.

The goals of initial ED management are twofold: identification of the underlying cause of the shock state, and resuscitation of the patient. Initial resuscitative actions include airway management to maximize oxygen delivery with nasal cannula, non-breather mask, or intubation with assisted ventilation if necessary, and aggressive fluid resuscitation.

Urine output should reach more than 0.5 ml/kg·h, with a central venous pressure goal of 8 to 12 mmHg and a mean arterial pressure (MAP) goal of 60 to 65 mmHg. Other specific therapies can be initiated once the cause of the hypotension and shock is identified. Bedside ultrasound can be used to rapidly identify reversible causes and ensure definitive treatment is initiated as soon as possible.

Hypovolemic shock

Hypovolemic shock can be caused by absolute hypovolemia (loss of blood or fluid through bleeding or profound diarrhea) and relative hypovolemia (vasomotor dysfunction). Ultrasound can identify intraperitoneal bleeding and hemothorax in trauma patients and free abdominal fluid in patients with a ruptured abdominal aneurysm or a ruptured ectopic pregnancy.

The FAST examination (focused assessment with sonography for trauma) can be employed to rule out intra-abdominal or intrathoracic bleeding in trauma patients.[4] It can also be used to assess for bleeding in the non-trauma patient. The FAST examination accurately detects bleeding in both normotensive[5] and hypotensive trauma patients and has high specificity with variable sensitivity.[2] The conventional FAST examination uses four views to detect free intra-abdominal or pericardial fluid: the right upper quadrant (RUQ) (Figure 24.1), the subcostal cardiac (Figure 24.2), the left upper quadrant (LUQ) (Figure 24.3), and the pelvic (Figure 24.4). The extended FAST examination (eFAST) evaluates the anterior chest for pneumothorax and the spaces above the diaphragm for intrathoracic bleeding (Figure 24.5).

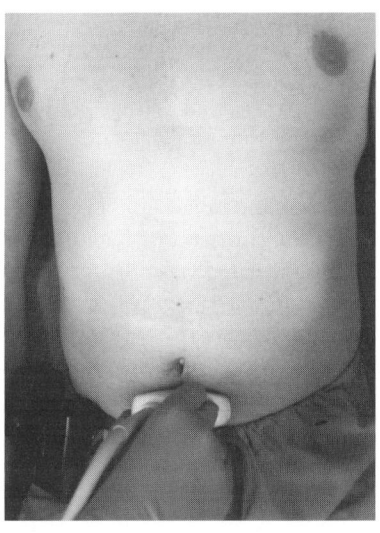

Figure 24.4 Pelvic view of the FAST examination.

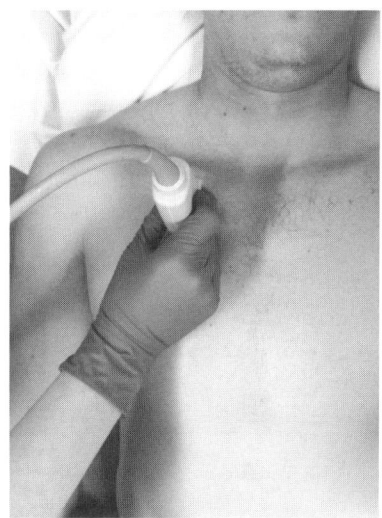

Figure 24.5 Anterior chest view of the extended FAST examination.

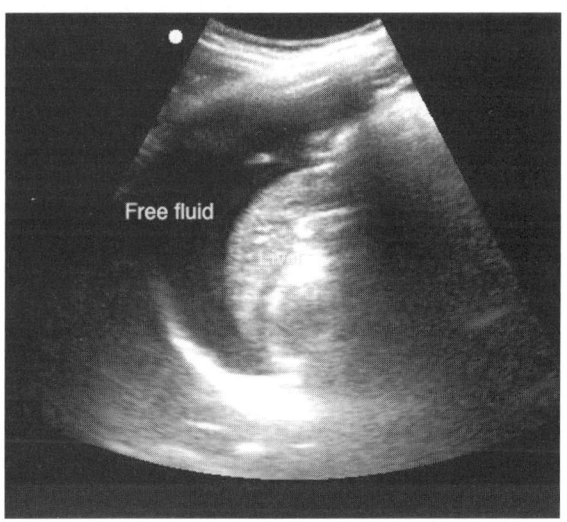

Free fluid

Figure 24.6 RUQ view showing free fluid.

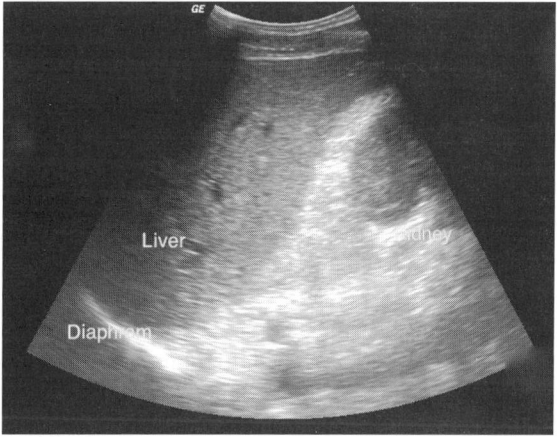

Liver

Diaphragm

Figure 24.7 Normal ight upper quadrant view obtained during the FAST examination.

The RUQ view is believed to be the most useful for diagnosing intra-abdominal fluid. It focuses on Morrison's pouch, the potential space between the liver and the right kidney (Figure 24.1). Free intra-abdominal fluid tends to collect here first and appears on ultrasound as a dark black (hypoechoic) space, separating the kidney from the liver. The minimum amount of fluid needed for detection is approximately 250 ml. Free fluid can also be located between the diaphragm and the liver and around the tip of the liver. All three areas can be visualized easily with the RUQ view, and all should be assessed properly to rule out free fluid (Figures 24.6 and 24.7).

The cardiac view is part of the original FAST examination and is discussed below in the section on obstructive and cardiogenic shock. It is used to evaluate the patient for traumatic pericardial effusion.

For the LUQ view of the FAST examination, the probe should be placed in the posterior axillary line. Because of the smaller size of the spleen, it is often necessary to angle the probe more posteriorly and position it more cephalad than for the RUQ view to obtain an adequate view. An ideal image includes the spleen, the diaphragm, and the left kidney (Figure 24.8).

The pelvic view evaluates the perivesicular spaces and is optimized with the urine-filled bladder acting as

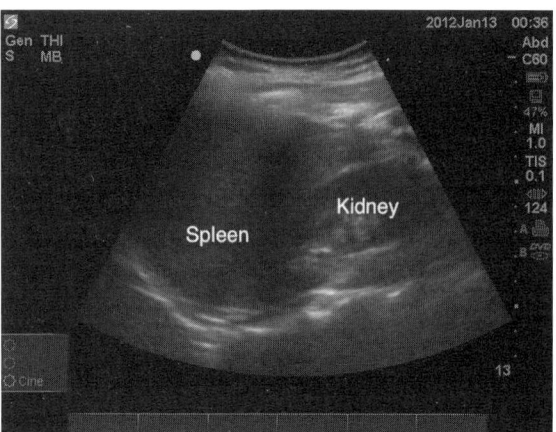

Figure 24.8 Normal left upper quadrant view of the FAST examination, capturing the spleen, diaphragm, and left kidney.

a sonographic window. The probe is placed at the mid-suprapubic area in transverse and longitudinal orientations. It is imperative to use both views, as the longitudinal view is sensitive for a smaller amount of fluid. Free fluid usually collects in the vesicouterine or vesicorectal area. In female patients, potential amounts of free fluid should be correlated with the clinical presentation.

The RUQ and LUQ views can also be used to evaluate a patient for hemothorax. A hemothorax occurs when blood accumulates in the thoracic cavity (pleural space), between the lung and the chest wall. This usually occurs after trauma, both blunt and penetrating. Accumulation of blood can cause hypotension and dyspnea as the lung has difficulty inflating against increasing volume. This can be diagnosed during the extended FAST examination views by identifying fluid above the diaphragm.

A patient with a ruptured abdominal aortic aneurysm can also present in hypovolemic shock. Emergency ultrasound is frequently used to identify the aortic aneurysm itself or, if the aneurysm has ruptured, to accurately locate free intra-abdominal fluid using the RUQ view of the FAST examination.[6] Several sonographic views are obtained to assess the integrity of the upper and lower aspects of the abdominal aorta. One can begin the examination with the probe in transverse orientation, placed just distal to the xiphoid process. The left lobe of the liver can be used as a sonographic window into the deeper retroperitoneum. Normal aortic diameter is less than 3 cm. The sonographic measurement is made from outer wall to outer wall, to avoid a false-negative diagnosis in patients with a significant intraluminal thrombus. The aortic diameter should also decrease from cephalad to caudal. An increase of over 50% in size from proximal to distal aorta should raise concern for an abdominal aortic aneurysm.

Usually, both transverse and longitudinal views are obtained, if feasible, for the entire aortic length, from upper aorta to bifurcation. Patients with a ruptured aortic abdominal aneurysm have a grave prognosis, so timely management is critical. The treating physician should have a high degree of suspicion and a low threshold to perform this ultrasound examination, as it can be completed quickly and accurately at the bedside.[7]

Females who are of child-bearing age and in hypotensive shock should be evaluated immediately for ectopic pregnancy. Free fluid can be identified with the RUQ or pelvic view of the FAST examination.[8,9]

Ultrasound allows assessment of the filling and collapsibility of the inferior vena cava (IVC), indicating fluid status in hypotensive patients, but it is best used in conjunction with cardiac ultrasound.[10,11] The IVC can be evaluated at the level of the hepatic vein influx. The patient is considered hypovolemic if the walls of the IVC collapse more than 50% throughout the respiratory cycle. If the walls of the IVC do not collapse significantly and have little variation with respiration, the patient is considered hypervolemic. Measurements in between can be considered euvolemic.[12] These measurements are reliable in the setting of normal cardiac function in non-ventilated patients.[13] An IVC collapse of 30% is considered a sign of euvolemia in patients who have undergone endotracheal intubation and are receiving positive-pressure ventilation.

Obstructive shock

Obstructive shock can be caused by extrinsic and intrinsic factors, and hypotension is a common finding. Causes include cardiac tamponade, pulmonary embolism, tension pneumothorax, and proximal aortic dissection.[14]

Cardiac tamponade can be challenging to diagnose in the acute setting. Trauma and medical conditions such as lupus, rheumatoid arthritis, end-stage renal disease with uremia, and cancer can cause cardiac effusions that lead to tamponade physiology. All echocardiographic views are able to diagnose tamponade; parasternal long- and short-axis views, the

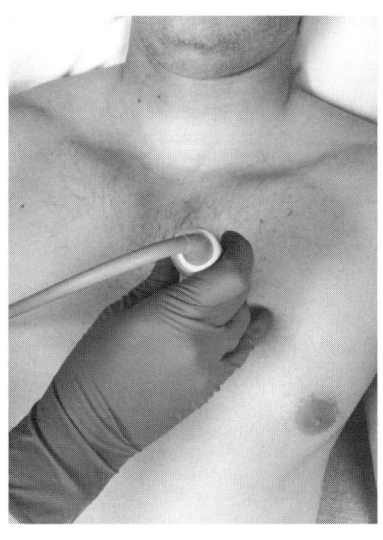

Figure 24.9 Parasternal long-axis cardiac view, with probe pointing toward the patient's right shoulder.

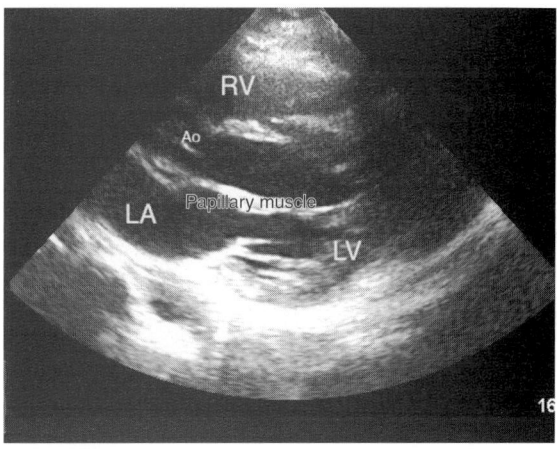

Figure 24.10 Normal cardiac parasternal long-axis view. LA, left atrium; Ao, aorta.

subxyphoid view, and apical four-chamber views are used frequently by emergency physicians.[14,15] The cardiac views are obtained using the low-frequency cardiac probe due to its smaller footprint, which assists the user in visualizing between ribs. The parasternal long view is obtained by placing the probe directly to the left of the sternum, at approximately the fourth intercostal space. The marker should point toward the patient's right shoulder (Figure 24.9). This view reveals the long axis of the heart, including the left (LV) and right (RV) ventricles, the mitral valve, and the aortic valve. The descending aorta can also be visualized. This view offers the most information; it can be used for evaluation of an effusion, right heart strain, and left ventricular failure (Figure 24.10).

The effusion will be a hypoechoic, black area around the heart. Although many diagnostic criteria exist, tamponade is usually characterized by collapse of the right ventricle during diastole and a decrease in left ventricle size (Figure 24.11).

Tension pneumothorax can be a cause of obstructive shock. Bedside ultrasound has been shown to be more accurate and efficient than portable radiography in the detection of pneumothorax, making it a valuable alternative to conventional imaging.[16,17] In patients with suspected pneumothorax, sonography is used to evaluate if the interface of visceral and parietal pleura is intact. In normal inflated lung, the movement of the visceral pleura along the inner wall of the thoracic cavity can be observed as a motion of sonographic artifacts distal to the chest wall. The intact

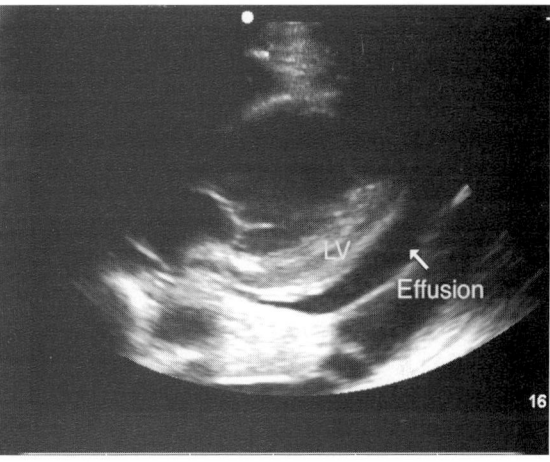

Figure 24.11 Cardiac parasternal long view indicating effusion.

pleural interface also generates small comet-tail artifacts, which move with respirations. In pneumothorax, both of these artifacts are lost. M-mode sonography can be used to document either motion of the pleura or the lack of it, and B-mode sonography can be used to depict the presence or absence of small comet-tail artifacts. The M-mode sonogram across the sliding pleura will have two images, commonly known as "beach" and "waves" (Figure 24.12). With a pneumothorax, the image becomes only the "waves," also known as the "barcode sign" (Figure 24.13). In a complete pneumothorax, all areas of the hemithorax lack pleural movement and comet-tail artifacts. In a partial pneumothorax, the leading edge of the partially inflated

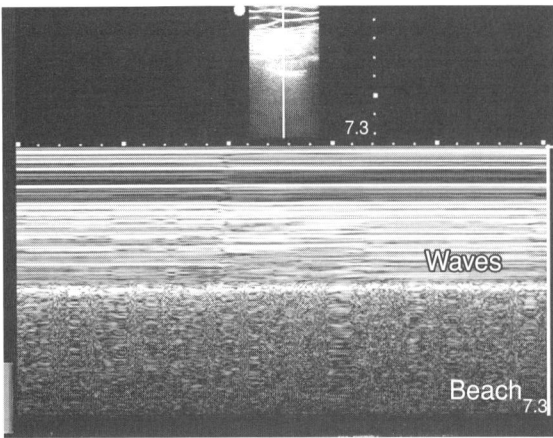

Figure 24.12 Normal M-mode lung ultrasound findings: waves and beach.

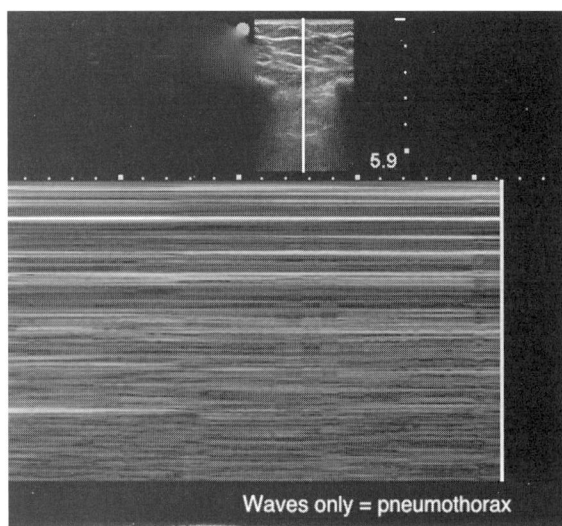

Figure 24.13 Abnormal M-mode lung ultrasound: waves only.

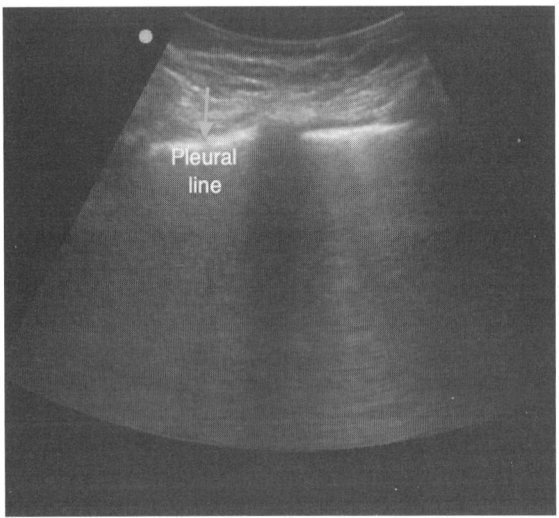

Figure 24.14 Normal pleural line shown on lung ultrasound image.

lung can be observed with respirations, marking the border between an inflated lung and a chest cavity filled with air.[16]

Lung ultrasound can be performed in minutes and can answer challenging clinical questions rapidly.[17] The patient must be supine, with the high-frequency transducer placed on the anterior chest wall at the third intercostal space. The pleural sliding can be identified as a hyperechoic line between rib shadows (Figures 24.5 and 24.14).

Obstructive shock can also be caused by right ventricle failure resulting from pulmonary embolism.

Pulmonary embolism is difficult to diagnose, and the current gold standard is computed tomography (CT). However, patients in obstructive shock can be too unstable to leave the acute treatment area for comprehensive imaging that will secure the diagnosis. In this scenario, ultrasound can be used to support difficult treatment decisions such as administration of thrombolytics. Evaluation of the right ventricle in an unstable patient suspected of having pulmonary embolism can assist in making this diagnosis.[18] The right ventricle can be viewed in the cardiac parasternal long- and short-axis views and the apical four-chamber view. The parasternal long-axis view is used to identify McConnell's sign in an enlarged right ventricle to differentiate between acute failure and chronic dilatation.[19] McConnell's sign is a paradoxic movement, in which the right ventricular wall aspect of the apex contracts while the rest of the right ventricle does not. The movement can also be evaluated in the apical four-chamber view. McConnell's sign is believed to be highly specific for acute pulmonary embolism. In a patient with massive pulmonary embolism, the right ventricle can be enlarged significantly, due to high pressures, and the septum may bow into the left ventricle during systole, its pressures overwhelming its usually stronger partner (Figure 24.15). However, the right ventricle can be enlarged for other reasons, including chronic pulmonary hypertension. In these conditions, however, the left ventricle should not be affected. This

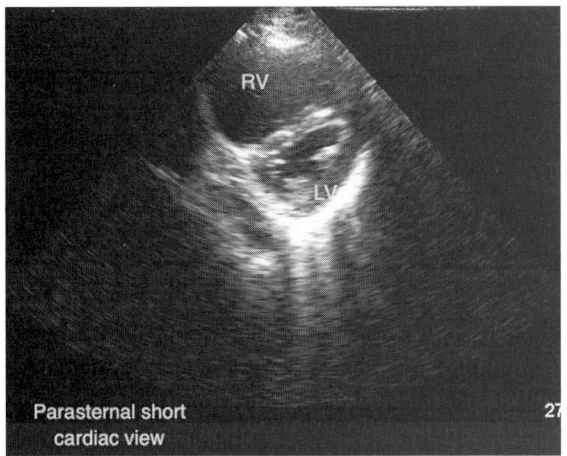

Figure 24.15 Enlarged right ventricle.

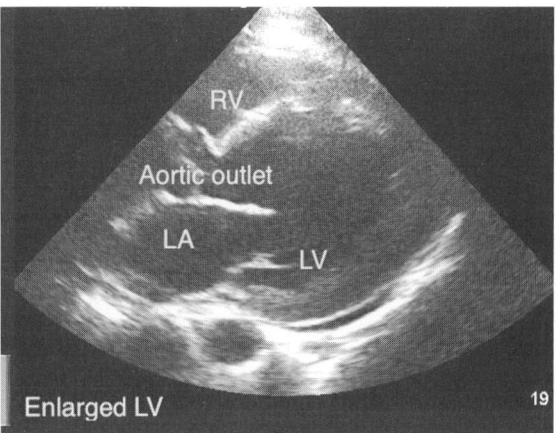

Figure 24.16 Cardiac parasternal long view revealing left ventricle enlargement. LA, left atrium.

differentiation in presentation can lead to the diagnosis of massive pulmonary embolism.

Several studies by European investigators suggest that transthoracic ultrasound of the lungs can detect embolic changes in lung tissue. Case reports have described the diagnosis of pulmonary embolism, confirmed by CT, by the identification of wedge-shaped hypodense lung parenchyma with ultrasound and of the loss of perfusion identified with Doppler ultrasound. This technique was found to be feasible in the emergency medicine setting and could prove useful for patients being evaluated in austere settings where CT is not available.[20] More studies are needed to determine the utility of this ultrasound use.

Cardiogenic shock

Cardiogenic shock often arises from left or right ventricular failure (also a form of obstructive shock.) Studies have demonstrated that a physician trained in bedside echocardiography can accurately determine left ventricular ejection fraction.[21,22] Echocardiography can evaluate for acute myocardial infarction with associated wall-motion abnormalities, reduced left ventricular function in a patient with congestive heart disease, and valvular abnormalities such as acute valvular insufficiencies. Administration of intravenous fluids can put the patient at risk for acute pulmonary edema if the left ventricle is failing. Experience in visualizing the left ventricle is important for the emergency physician, as a failing left ventricle will have poor inotropy (Figure 24.16).

Valvular abnormalities can cause acute heart failure. Echocardiography can assess the mitral valve in patients in whom chordae tendinae rupture and acute mitral insufficiency are suspected. The parasternal long-axis view and apical four-chamber view also can be used to visualize the mitral valve.

Distributive shock

Distributive shock also presents as symptomatic hypotension. Examples of distributive shock include sepsis and anaphylaxis. Low systemic vascular resistance caused by peripheral vasodilation with concurrent high cardiac output and tachycardia can be detected with echocardiography and IVC ultrasound; these conditions are found in patients with sepsis or anaphylaxis. Point-of-care ultrasound can help guide treatment. In a septic patient, the heart beats rapidly, a state often described as "hyperdynamic," and the IVC may show signs of hypovolemia. Neurogenic shock may manifest as bradycardia with IVC collapse; the mechanism of injury can help confirm the diagnosis.

Pearls and pitfalls

- Ultrasound is an operator-dependent diagnostic tool, making training and practice of utmost importance to reach acceptable accuracy.
- Body habitus, bowel gas, and emphysema can cause sonographic barriers and impede sonographic visualization of key structures.
- Findings from point-of-care sonographic evaluations should be considered within the

context of the patient's clinical presentation. Chronic medical problems may be mistaken for acute presentations. Examples are chronic ascites leading to false-positive results in trauma, false-positive sonographic findings for pneumothorax in patients with severe emphysema and peripheral bullous lung changes, and physiologic fluid in the pelvis of a woman with abdominal pain and in an early stage of pregnancy.

- The interpretation of a sonographic image of the inferior vena cava can be problematic if echocardiography results are not taken into account. Chronic right-sided heart failure or tricuspid insufficiency may cause the IVC to appear to be "full" and distended, even if the patient is acutely septic. In some patients with left-sided heart failure, the IVC can appear to be collapsed, but the echocardiogram shows that the patient would benefit from inotropic support. Thus, it is important that all aspects of the patient's presentation are taken into consideration and that ultrasound is not used as an isolated tool. A bolus of intravenous fluid can worsen heart failure and cause pulmonary edema and respiratory failure if the left heart cannot manage the extra fluid. These scenarios must be investigated to ensure safe medical decision-making.

Clinical approach when resources are limited

Ultrasound is a viable imaging tool for patients in rural or hostile environments. Many of the hand-carried ultrasound machines are robust, portable, and inexpensive in comparison with other advanced imaging modalities, such as CT. The portability of the ultrasound machine allows the physician to come to the patient instead of transporting the patient to the physician. If maintenance is required, the machine can be brought or shipped to the appropriate service center. This is a clear advantage over equipment that cannot be moved and requires repair services to reach its location. However, portable ultrasound equipment is not indestructible. Adequate precautions can avoid equipment failure.[23]

Conclusion

Emergency ultrasound is a useful tool for patients with hypotension and shock. With training and experience,

the emergency physician can become adept with the evaluation, requiring only minutes to solve diagnostic questions and guide patient care decisions during the most critical minutes. Training and experience are of utmost importance for the safe and appropriate use of this technology.

Critical actions for undifferentiated hypotension

1. Place two large-bore IV lines, cardiac monitor, supplemental oxygen, take rectal temperature, and pulse oximetry.
2. IV infusion of 2 L of normal saline.
3. If ventilation or oxygenation is not adequate, the patient should be intubated.
4. If blood pressure remains low after administration of 1 to 2 L normal saline, vasopressors should be started.
5. Emergent causes of hypotension must be evaluated and treated: tension pneumothorax, cardiac tamponade, massive pulmonary embolism.
6. Treat cardiac arrhythmias according to standard ACLS (Advanced Cardiovascular Life Support) guidelines.
7. If septic shock is suspected, administer empiric antibiotics within an hour of presentation.

References

1. Jones AE, Stiell IG, Nesbit LP, *et al*. Non-traumatic out of hospital hypotension predicts in hospital mortality. *Ann Emerg Med* 2004; 43(1): 106–13.

2. Jones AE, Tayal VS, Sullivan DM, *et al*. Randomized, controlled trial of immediate versus delayed goal-directed ultrasound to identify the cause of nontraumatic hypotension in emergency department patients. *Crit Care Med* 2004; 32(8): 1703–8.

3. Rose JS, Blair AE, Mandaria E, *et al*. The UHP Ultrasound Protocol: a novel ultrasound approach to the empiric evaluation of the undifferentiated hypotensive patient. *Am J Emerg Med* 2001; 19(4): 299–302.

4. Helling TS, Wilson J, Augustosky K. The utility of focused abdominal ultrasound in blunt abdominal trauma: a reappraisal. *Am J Surg* 2007; 194(6): 728–32.

5. Moylan M, Newgard CD, Ma OJ, *et al*. Association between a positive emergency department FAST examination and therapeutic laparotomy in

normotensive blunt trauma patients. *J Emerg Med* 2007; 33(3): L65–71.

6. Tayal VS, Graf CD, Gibbs MA, *et al.* Prospective study of accuracy and outcome of emergency ultrasound for abdominal aortic aneurysm over two years. *Acad Emerg Med* 2003; 10(8): 867–71.

7. Constantino TG, Bruno EC, Handly N, *et al.* Accuracy of emergency medicine ultrasound in the evaluation of abdominal aortic aneurysm. *J Emerg Med* 2005; 29(4): 455–60.

8. Adhikari S, Blaivis M, Lyon M. Diagnosis and management of ectopic pregnancy using bedside ultrasound in the emergency department: a 2-year experience. *Am J Emerg Med* 2007; 25(6): 591–6.

9. Moore C, Todd WM, O'Brien E, *et al.* Free fluid in Morrison's pouch on bedside ultrasound predicts the need for operative intervention in suspected ectopic pregnancy. *Acad Emerg Med* 2007; 14(8): 755–8.

10. Carr BG, Dean AJ, Everett WW, *et al.* Intensivist bedside ultrasound (INBU) for volume assessment in the intensive care unit: a pilot study. *J Trauma* 2007; 63(3): 495–500.

11. Blehar DJ, Dickman E, Gaspari R. Identification of congestive heart failure via respiratory variation of inferior vena cava diameter. *Am J Emerg Med* 2009; 27: 71–5.

12. Wong SP, Otto CM. Echocardiographic findings in acute and chronic pulmonary disease. In Otto CM, ed. *Textbook of Clinical Echocardiography*, 2nd edition. Philadelphia: Saunders; 2000: 747.

13. Gullace G, Savola MT. Echocardiographic assessment of the inferior vena cava wall motion for studies of right heart dynamics and function. *Clin Cardiol* 1984; 7(7): 393–404.

14. Mandavia DP, Hoffner RJ, Mahaney K, *et al.* Bedside echocardiography by emergency physicians. *Ann Emerg Med* 2001; 38(4): 377–82.

15. Blaivias M. Incidence of pericardial effusion in patients presenting to the emergency department with unexplained dyspnea. *Acad Emerg Med* 2001; 8(12): 1143–6.

16. Alrajhl K, Woo MY, Vaillancourt C. Test characteristics of ultrasonography for the detection of pneumothorax; a systematic review and meta-analysis. *Chest* 2011; 141: 703–8.

17. Volpicelli G. Sonographic diagnosis of pneumothorax. *Intensive Care Med* 2011; 37(2): 224–32.

18. Goldhaber SZ. Echocardiography in the management of pulmonary embolism. *Ann Intern Med* 2002; 136(9): 691–700.

19. McConnell MV, Solomon SD, Rayan ME, *et al.* Regional right ventricle dysfunction detected by echocardiography in acute pulmonary embolism. *Am J Cardiol* 1996; 78: 469–73.

20. Hoffmann B, Gullet JP. Bedside transthoracic sonography in suspected pulmonary embolism: a new tool for emergency physicians. *Acad Emerg Med* 2010; 17(9): e88–93.

21. Moore CL, Rose GA, Tayal VS, *et al.* Determination of left ventricular function by emergency physician echocardiography of hypotensive patients. *Acad Emerg Med* 2002; 9(3): 186–93.

22. Randazzo MR, Snoey ER, Levitt MA, *et al.* Accuracy of emergency physician assessment of left ventricular ejection fraction and central venous pressure using echocardiography. *Acad Emerg Med* 2003; 10(9): 973–7.

23. Brooks A, Connolly T, Chan O. *Ultrasound in Emergency Care.* Malden, MA: Blackwell Publishing Ltd; 2004.

Use of ultrasound to assess abdominal vascular emergencies

Sam Hsu

Ultrasound is an ideal modality for the assessment of abdominal vascular emergencies. It can be performed rapidly, accurately, and at the bedside. Ultrasound is a reliable and portable technology. Once the initial cost of obtaining the equipment is surmounted, ultrasound machines require very little maintenance or recurrent cost. This makes ultrasound highly suitable for practice environments with limited resources.

Evaluation for abdominal aortic aneurysm (AAA) is the most common indication for ultrasound of the aorta. The technique is easily mastered, and the interpretation is straightforward. This chapter focuses on abdominal aortic aneurysms and briefly discusses aortic dissection, aortic occlusion, and mesenteric ischemia.

Most of the applications can be accomplished with B-mode imaging, the default mode that produces the familiar black-and-white images. All ultrasound machines have B-mode imaging, so these examinations can be performed with even the most basic machines. A working knowledge of B-mode ultrasound imaging is assumed in this chapter. Doppler mode imaging is used to detect and quantify vascular flow. It is not available on basic or older ultrasound machines. Performing Doppler examinations is significantly more complex and difficult than B-mode imaging. Doppler findings will be described where applicable, but Doppler theory and technique are beyond the scope of this chapter. Users interested in learning Doppler imaging should seek other instructional material and/or bedside instruction from an experienced operator. Fortunately, Doppler is not necessary for any of the applications in this chapter, except mesenteric ischemia.

General technique for imaging the aorta

To evaluate the aorta, a 3- to 6-mHz curvilinear or phased-array probe is used. To begin, the probe is placed in transverse orientation, with the probe indicator toward the patient's right. The epigastrium is the best starting point, as the liver provides a large acoustic window, creating the easiest area in which to obtain a view of the aorta. If there is any uncertainty about the location of the aorta, increasing the depth of view to allow identification of the long shadow of the spine provides an easily recognizable landmark. The aorta and inferior vena cava can be found immediately superficial to the spine. The aorta will be on the image right (the patient's left) and the inferior vena cava (IVC) will be on the image left (the patient's right) (Figure 25.1). Occasionally, the IVC is collapsed because of low intravascular volume and therefore is difficult to identify. In such cases, the single vessel superficial to the spine will be the aorta. It is common for the IVC to pulsate due to right atrial contractions, so the presence of pulsations does not reliably differentiate the aorta from the IVC. If Doppler is available, it can help identify the aorta. With color Doppler, the aorta will show pulsatile flow, while the IVC will show a subtly varying continuous flow. Spectral Doppler illustrates the differences in flow. Doppler will not be necessary to find the aorta in most cases. Once the aorta is identified, the depth of view can be decreased so that the aorta is in the center of the screen. Occasionally, bowel gas will cast a deep shadow, simulating the spine. The peristalsis of bowel will differentiate it from the spine. The aorta is surveyed by sliding the probe caudally, until the aortic bifurcation is reached,

Vascular Emergencies, ed. Robert L. Rogers, Thomas Scalea, Lee Wallis, and Heike Geduld. Published by Cambridge University Press. © Cambridge University Press 2013.

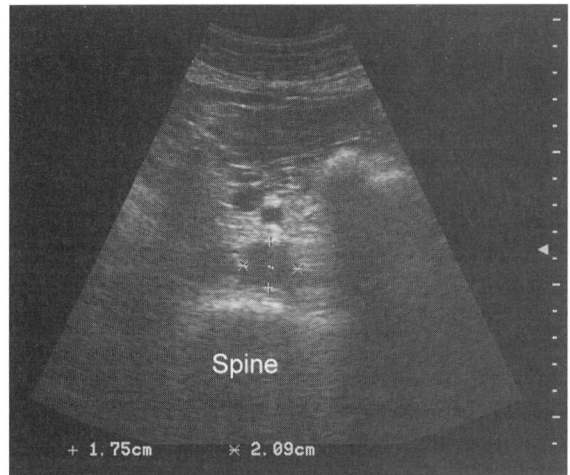

Figure 25.1 Normal transverse appearance of the aorta. The left side of the image represents the patient's right. The aorta is superficial to the spine and is shown with normal measurements. The inferior vena cava is to the left (the patient's right) of the aorta.

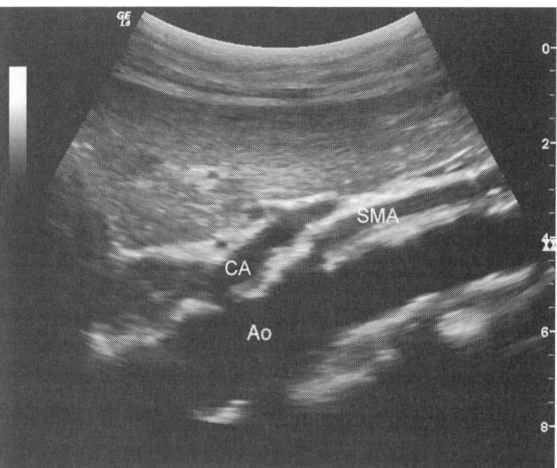

Figure 25.2 Normal longitudinal appearance of the aorta (Ao), celiac artery (CA), and superior mesenteric artery (SMA).

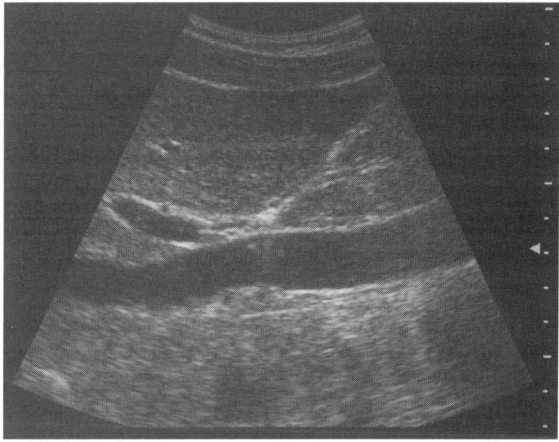

Figure 25.3 Longitudinal view of the inferior vena cava. Compared with the aorta, the IVC has thinner walls and an irregular lumen.

typically at the level of the umbilicus. The aorta becomes more superficial as it progresses caudally due to lumbar lordosis; the depth of view can be adjusted as needed.

Bowel gas frequently obscures the view. Applying graded pressure with the probe can displace the bowel and clarify the view. Do not apply pressure while sliding the probe, since this is painful to the patient and tiring to perform. Instead, apply pressure to obtain a view, and then release the pressure before sliding further. If pressure does not displace the bowel, positioning the probe off center can provide a window. Positioning the probe far on the patient's right, over the liver, may be necessary to obtain a view. If these measures fail, rescanning after a few minutes might allow time for bowel gas to move out of the way. It is reasonable to skip over 1–2 cm of the aorta that prove impossible to image, since it is not likely that significant pathology will be present exclusively in such a short segment.

A longitudinal image of the aorta is obtained by turning the probe so that the indicator is pointed cephalad. The aorta can be distinguished from the IVC by the presence of the celiac and superior mesenteric arteries branching from the aorta (Figure 25.2). The aorta has thicker walls and a more constant caliber compared to the IVC (Figure 25.3). The longitudinal view is used to measure the length of any abnormalities and to evaluate flow through the aorta and its branches.

Evaluation for abdominal aortic aneurysm

Ultrasound is 94 to 100% sensitive for detection of AAA.[1,2] Missed diagnoses are largely due to technical difficulties in obtaining an image of the aorta rather than inherent inaccuracies of ultrasound technology. Ultrasound is much less reliable for detecting a ruptured AAA, with sensitivity for retroperitoneal rupture of only 4%.[3] An intraperitoneal rupture can

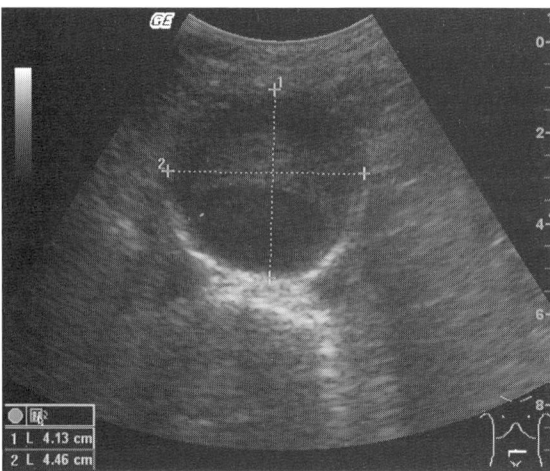

Figure 25.4 Transverse view of an abdominal aortic aneurysm. Note the mural thrombus along the superficial wall. The aortic diameter is measured from outside wall to outside wall. Measuring the inner lumen would underestimate the aortic diameter. The aorta is the same size as the spine – a rapid method for recognizing an aneurysm.

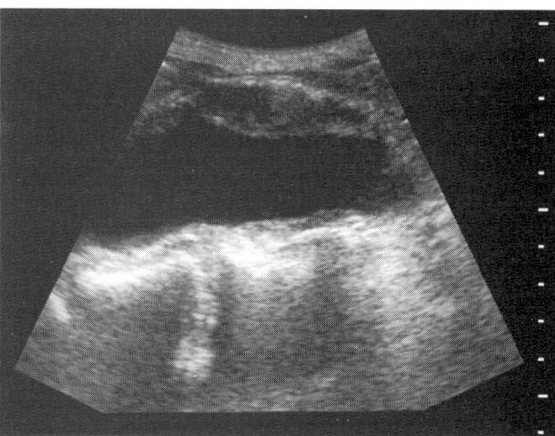

Figure 25.5 Longitudinal view of a fusiform aneurysm. The ends of the aneurysm taper. An anterior mural thrombus is present.

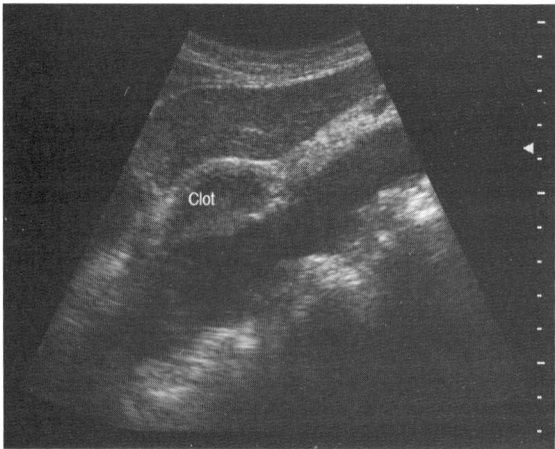

Figure 25.6 Longitudinal view of a saccular aneurysm. The boundaries of the aneurysm are well defined compared to a fusiform aneurysm.

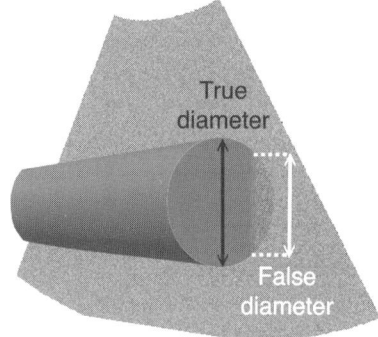

Figure 25.7 A pitfall in measuring the aortic diameter while imaging in the longitudinal plane. If the beam is not aligned with the center of the aorta, the measurement will be falsely small. The aortic diameter is best measured in the transverse plane.

lumen can underestimate the diameter of an AAA due to the frequent presence of a mural thrombus. An AAA is present if the diameter exceeds 3 cm; although clinically significant AAAs typically exceed 5 cm. When the aorta approaches or exceeds the size of the spine, an AAA can be recognized rapidly even before making a measurement (Figure 25.4). Document at least three images in the transverse plane, typically at the proximal and distal ends of the aorta and another in between. More images might be needed to fully document any abnormalities.

The longitudinal image is helpful in distinguishing a fusiform from a saccular aneurysm, since in transverse they appear similar (Figures 25.5 and 25.6). The aortic diameter should not be measured on the longitudinal plane since this can underestimate the diameter of the aorta if the ultrasound beam is not aligned with the center of the aorta (Figure 25.7).

be seen with a *focused assessment with sonography for trauma* (FAST) examination, but patients with this disruption do not often survive to presentation. Rupture should be presumed in a hemodynamically unstable patient when an AAA is present on ultrasound.

While surveying the aorta in transverse orientation, note any areas of enlargement. Measure the aortic diameter in two planes – depth and width. The measurement must be taken from the outside wall to the opposing outside wall of the aorta. Measuring only the

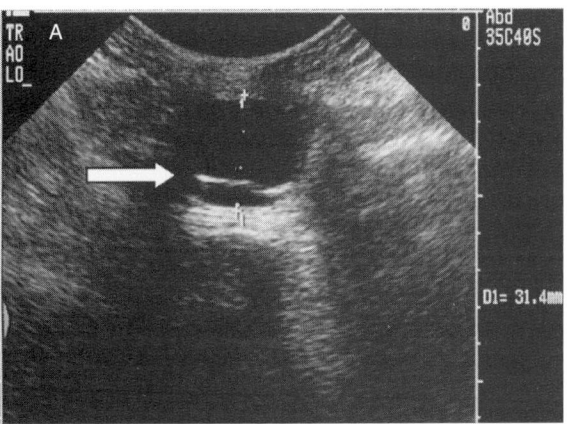 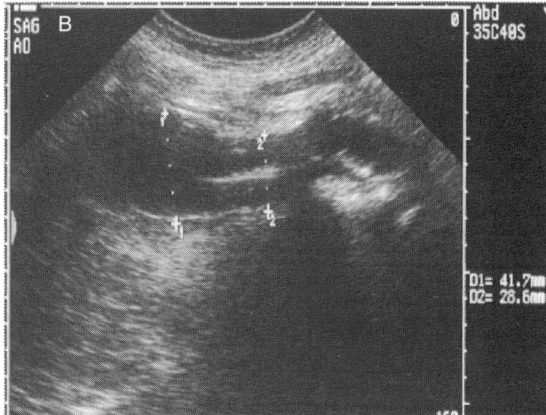

Figure 25.8 Aortic dissection. Transverse view (A) and longitudinal view (B). The intimal flap flutters with cardiac contractions. (Reprinted from Fojtik et al.,[4] with permission from Elsevier.)

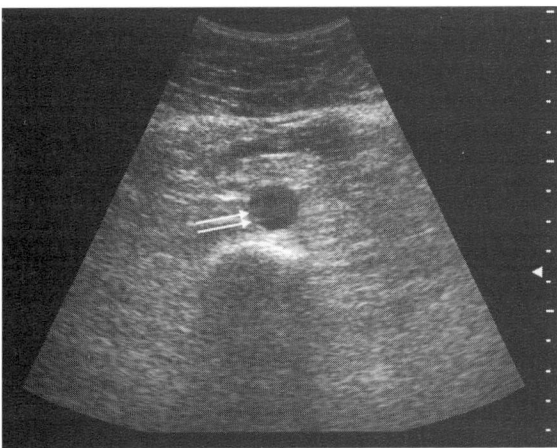

Figure 25.9 Reverberation artifacts (arrows) can simulate dissection. Artifacts vary with probe position and not with cardiac contractions. Reverberations also appear as multiple parallel lines, whereas a dissection appears as a single line.

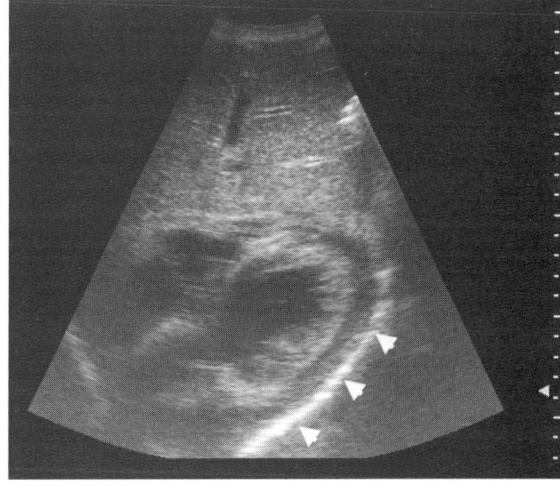

Figure 25.10 A pericardial effusion appears as an anechoic stripe between the pericardium (arrowheads) and the myocardium. If a pericardial effusion is present in conjunction with an aortic dissection, a Type A dissection must be suspected.

Evaluation for aortic dissection

Aortic dissections can extend into the abdominal aorta, where they can be detected on ultrasound. The dissection will appear as a tissue plane within the lumen of the aorta, which flutters with the patient's pulse (Figure 25.8). A reverberation artifact can mimic a dissection but will consist of characteristic parallel lines that do not move in time with the patient's pulse (Figure 25.9). Doppler may not show flow in the false lumen if a thrombus is present. The detection of a mobile flap within the lumen has a specificity of 99 to 100% for dissection, but because not all dissections extend into the abdomen, the sensitivity is poor.[4] If a dissection is noted, examination of the pericardium for effusion or tamponade is warranted. If present, this suggests a Type A dissection that has ruptured into the pericardium. An ultrasound image of the pericardium can be obtained by placing the probe transversely in the epigastrium and directing the beam cephalad toward the heart. This will produce the subxyphoid view of the heart. An effusion will appear as an anechoic stripe between the echogenic pericardium and the myocardium (Figure 25.10).

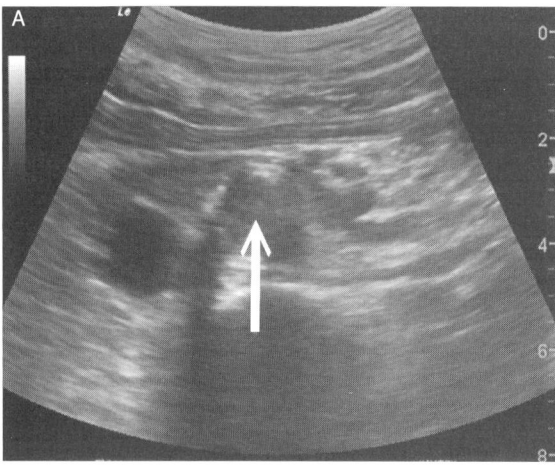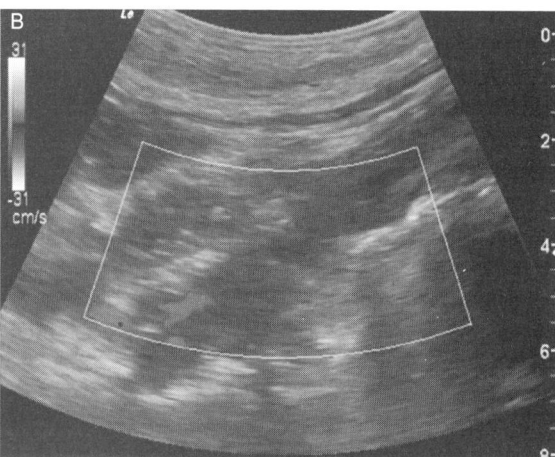

Figure 25.11 Aortic occlusion. (A) In transverse view, the thrombus appears in the aortic lumen (arrow). The IVC is to the left of the aorta. (B) In longitudinal, there is an absence of color flow. See plate section for color version of panel B. (Reprinted from Roxas *et al.*,[5] with permission from Elsevier.)

Evaluation for aortic obstruction

Acute aortic obstruction is an unusual and catastrophic clinical entity. Ultrasound will reveal a thrombus in the aortic lumen and a lack of Doppler flow (Figure 25.11).[5] Recognizing an aortic occlusion requires a high degree of suspicion, since artifacts frequently appear in the aortic lumen and can simulate a thrombus. Artifacts typically change in appearance with alterations in probe placement or angle; thrombus will not. Clinical clues will also help, since aortic occlusion will be associated with severe ischemia of the mesentery and/or lower extremities.

Evaluation for mesenteric ischemia

Mesenteric ischemia is a notoriously difficult diagnosis to confirm in the emergency department. Unfortunately, ultrasound does not provide a straightforward dichotomous answer. Published reports are based on stable patients with chronic arterial mesenteric ischemia, not on patients with acute undifferentiated abdominal pain. The ultrasound criteria for arterial stenosis are not necessarily diagnostic of mesenteric ischemia, since severe stenosis can be present without ischemia due to collateral circulation. The clinical history and additional imaging, e.g., invasive or CT arteriography, are needed to confirm the diagnosis. Of note, there are no established ultrasound criteria for venous mesenteric ischemia.

Performing an ultrasound examination of the mesenteric arteries is difficult and time consuming. It requires a working knowledge of duplex and spectral Doppler. The study should be performed only by operators with experience in vascular ultrasound. This is not a study that novice ultrasound users should perform.

Ultrasound examination of the mesenteric blood supply focuses on the celiac artery (CA) and superior mesenteric artery (SMA). The proximal aorta is imaged in the longitudinal plane and duplex Doppler is activated (Figure 25.12). Complete arterial occlusion is present when there is no color flow through the CA or SMA. Celiac artery occlusion can also be inferred when there is retrograde flow through the common hepatic artery, which is seen as the right branch of the CA in the transverse plane (Figure 25.13).[6]

If flow is present on duplex scanning, spectral Doppler is used to quantify the flow. The peak systolic velocity and end diastolic velocity through the CA and SMA are measured (Figure 25.14). As blood flow is restricted by stenosis, the flow rate increases to maintain perfusion. The criteria for critical stenosis are shown in Table 25.1.[6,7] There are no criteria for the inferior mesenteric artery since it is difficult to image and not usually the singular cause of mesenteric ischemia.

In summary, ultrasound is highly accurate for detecting complete occlusion of the CA and SMA but not conclusive for subtotal occlusion. Ultrasound is reported to have negative predictive values of 91 to 99%, depending on the specific criteria referenced, so it can be useful to exclude chronic arterial

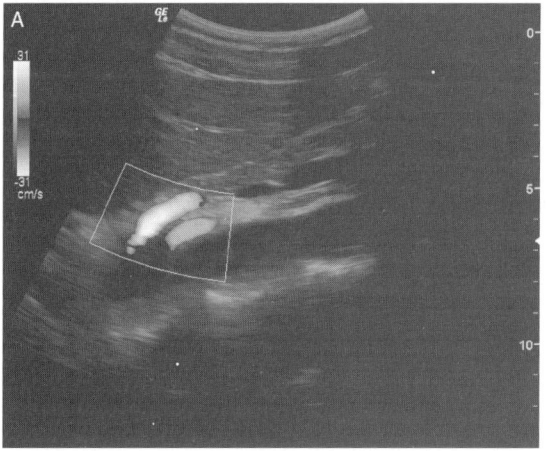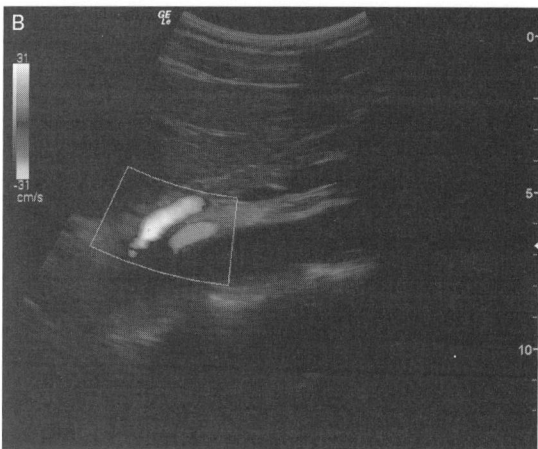

Figure 25.12 Duplex Doppler of celiac and superior mesenteric arteries. Normal flow is present. Complete occlusion of either vessel would appear as an absence of color in the vessel. See plate section for color version of panel B.

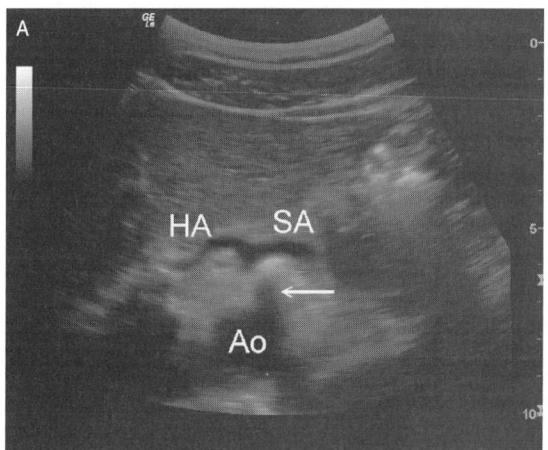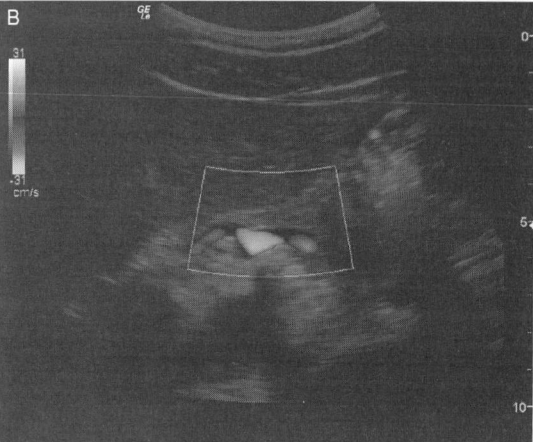

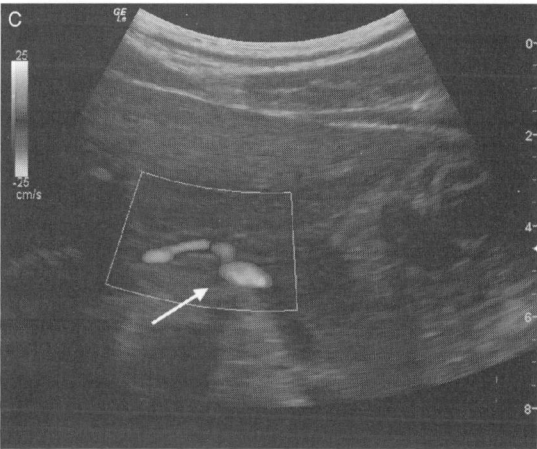

Figure 25.13 Branches of the celiac artery. (A) The "seagull" appearance consists of the hepatic artery (HA) and the splenic artery (SA). The third branch of the celiac artery, the left gastric artery, is not shown. Aorta (Ao) and branch point of the superior mesenteric artery are indicated (arrow). (B) Normal color Doppler flow through the celiac branches. Flow toward the ultrasound probe (upward on screen) is colored red, and flow away (downward on screen) is colored blue. Blood flows anteriorly through the celiac artery, then posteriorly through the HA and SA. Note that the wingtips of the "seagull" are the same color. (C) Retrograde flow through the hepatic artery. The HA is red due to flow from posterior to anterior, toward the celiac artery (arrow). Note that the wingtips of the "seagull" are different colors. See plate section for color version of panels B and C.

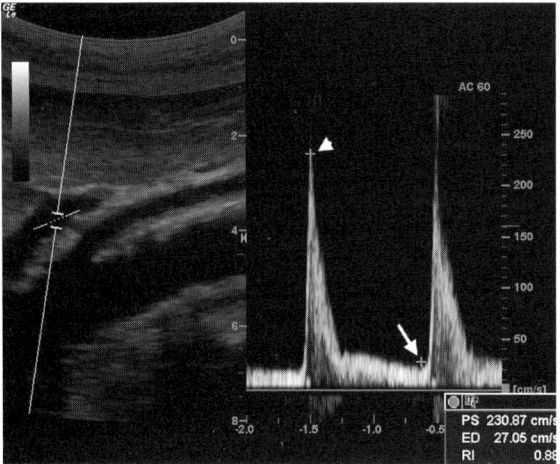

Figure 25.14 Spectral Doppler signal of celiac stenosis. The peak systolic velocity (PS, arrowhead) of 230 cm/s exceeds the cutoff of 200 cm/s, indicating > 70% stenosis. The end diastolic velocity (ED, arrow) does not meet the criteria for stenosis.

Table 25.1 Flow criteria for mesenteric stenosis

	Celiac artery	Superior mesenteric artery	Degree of stenosis
Peak systolic velocity (cm/sec)	> 200 or 0	> 275 or 0	> 70% stenosis[7]
End diastolic velocity (cm/sec)	> 55 or 0	> 45 or 0	> 50% stenosis[6]

4. Survey the entire aorta from epigastrium to bifurcation.
5. Measure the outside-to-outside diameter of the aorta in transverse.
6. Look for luminal objects that could be indicators of dissection or thrombus.
7. If more than 2–3 cm of the aorta cannot be imaged, another imaging modality is needed.

Pearls and pitfalls

1. If the aorta is difficult to find, increase the depth and look for the spine shadow. The aorta will always be immediately superficial and slightly to the right (on the monitor).
2. Make sure the probe is oriented to the patient's right. If not, the position of the aorta and IVC will be reversed on the monitor and could cause misidentification of the aorta.
3. Do not use pulsations to differentiate between the aorta and IVC. Pulsations can be present in either, both, or neither.
4. If the aorta is obscured by bowel gas, graded pressure with the probe or placing the probe off-midline can obtain the view. Rescanning in a few minutes to allow gas to move away can also improve the view.
5. If the aorta is as large as or larger than the spine shadow, it is abnormal.
6. Ultrasound is not sensitive for aortic rupture. If the aorta is large and the patient is hemodynamically unstable, assume rupture has occurred.
7. If an aortic dissection is present, image the heart to look for a pericardial effusion. If present, a Type A dissection is suggested and tamponade must be considered.
8. If an aortic thrombus appears to be present, consider whether the patient's clinical presentation is consistent with a thrombus and

mesenteric ischemia.[8] Positive studies for subtotal occlusion require further definitive imaging.

Clinical actions when resources are limited

The use of ultrasound is ideal for resource-limited situations. Although CT, aortography, and MRI might provide higher sensitivity and better surgical detail than ultrasound, they are expensive and not always available. Ultrasound provides an alternative imaging modality that is relatively inexpensive, is easy to maintain, and provides high accuracy for AAA, the most common abdominal vascular emergency. The cost of an ultrasound system can be as low as US$10,000 to $30,000 for handheld models and older models with a single probe. The latest models with several probes range from US$40,000 to $60,000. The cost of operating an ultrasound consists simply of the price of ultrasonic gel and electricity. No technician salary is needed since the study is performed by the clinician.

Critical actions

1. Orient the probe indicator to the patient's right when scanning in transverse.
2. Confidently identify the aorta. It should appear immediately superficial to the spine shadow.
3. Adjust the depth and gain to optimize the image.

widespread ischemia. Improper gain settings or misuse/misunderstanding of Doppler can create the illusion of a luminal thrombus.

9. Leave the use of ultrasound for mesenteric ischemia to experienced vascular operators. Consider another imaging modality, since ultrasound is time consuming and not necessarily conclusive.

References

1. Costantino TG, Bruno EC, Handly N, Dean AJ. Accuracy of emergency medicine ultrasound in the evaluation of abdominal aortic aneurysm. *J Emerg Med* 2005; 29(4): 455–60.

2. Tayal VS, Graf CD, Gibbs MA. Prospective study of accuracy and outcome of emergency ultrasound for abdominal aortic aneurysm over two years. *Acad Emerg Med* 2003; 10(8): 867–71.

3. Shuman WP, Hastrup W Jr, Kohler TR, *et al.* Suspected leaking abdominal aortic aneurysm: use of sonography in the emergency room. *Radiology* 1988; 168: 117–19.

4. Fojtik JP, Costantino TG, Dean AJ. The diagnosis of aortic dissection by emergency medicine ultrasound. *J Emerg Med* 2007; 32(2): 191–6.

5. Roxas R, Gallegos L, Bailitz J. Rapid detection of aortic occlusion with emergency ultrasound. *Ann Emerg Med* 2011; 58(1): 21–3.

6. Zwolak RM, Fillinger MF, Walsh DB, *et al.* Mesenteric and celiac duplex scanning: a validation study. *J Vasc Surg* 1998; 27(6): 1078–88.

7. Moneta GL, Lee RW, Yeager RA, *et al.* Mesenteric duplex scanning: a blinded prospective study. *J Vasc Surg* 1993; 17(1): 79–86.

8. Mitchell EL, Moneta GL. Mesenteric duplex scanning. *Perspect Vasc Surg Endovasc Ther* 2006; 18(2): 175–83.

Hemodialysis access emergencies

Eugene J. Schweitzer

Introduction

Most emergency department complaints from patients with end-stage renal disease (ESRD) relate to infection, dyspnea, chest pain, dysrhythmia, cardiac tamponade, and electrolyte or gastrointestinal disturbances. About 15% relate to complications of hemodialysis AV (arteriovenous) access.[1–5] These complications embody a wide range of severity and urgency (Table 26.1).[6,7] Life-threatening bleeding and limb-threatening ischemia must be recognized and treated immediately, while other complications can be managed in more relaxed timeframes. This chapter outlines the recognition and treatment of these complications with a focus on those that are true emergencies.

Bleeding

Overview

External bleeding from an AV access can range from a slow but persistent trickle from a dialysis needle puncture site to massive hemorrhage that could lead to exsanguination in minutes. Massive hemorrhage can occur with a ruptured aneurysm, pseudoaneurysm, or buttonhole. Management depends upon the etiology, location, and severity of the bleeding, but in all cases should include direct pressure to the bleeding site and correction of coagulopathies.

Diagnosis

Pseudoaneurysm of AV graft. A pseudoaneurysm is a pulsatile hematoma between the access and the skin. It forms after multiple dialysis needle sticks disrupt the integrity of the access wall such that blood flows in and out of a subcutaneous space with each cardiac cycle (Figure 26.1). Like a true

aneurysm, it feels like a pulsatile mass. It is called a "pseudoaneurysm" because, in contrast to a true aneurysm, its wall does not contain the histologic layers of a blood vessel. It is much more common with an AV graft than a fistula (see Is it a fistula or a graft?).

True aneurysm of AV fistula. A true aneurysm forms in an AV fistula as an undesirable progression of the normal maturation process (Figure 26.2). It consists of dilation of a segment of the vein that was used to construct the fistula as it is exposed to pulsatile arterial pressure. Ideally the vein would stop growing once it "matures" to a size that will support dialysis (diameter of 1 cm, flow of 300 mL/min), but often parts of it will continue to expand beyond that. Fistula aneurysms can attain diameters of 5 cm or more and usually have flow rates over 1000 mL/min.[8] It is called a "true" aneurysm because its wall contains all the histologic layers of a blood vessel.

Anastomotic pseudoaneurysm of AV graft. A pseudoaneurysm can form after an AV graft is placed if the suture line between the graft and the artery becomes partially or totally disrupted. This usually occurs where a prosthetic conduit like a PTFE graft is sutured to an artery. It is rarely seen at a vein-to-artery or graft-to-vein anastomosis. An anastomosis can become disrupted because of technical errors caused by suture purchases on the artery that are too small, especially if the artery is diseased from atherosclerosis, or if the sutures do not encompass some adventitia. Infection in the area with certain organisms like *Staphylococcus aureus* or *Pseudomonas aeruginosa* can also cause anastomotic disruption. Blood leaking out of the anastomosis can pool and swirl in a pocket under

Vascular Emergencies, ed. Robert L. Rogers, Thomas Scalea, Lee Wallis, and Heike Geduld. Published by Cambridge University Press. © Cambridge University Press 2013.

Table 26.1 Presentation and differential diagnosis of acute hemodialysis access complications

Presentation	Differential diagnosis for:	
	Graft	**Fistula**
Bleeding, massive	Ruptured pseudoaneurysm Ruptured anastomotic pseudoaneurysm	Ruptured true aneurysm Ruptured buttonhole
Bleeding, slow but persistent	Needle puncture site bleeding Impending pseudoaneurysm rupture	Needle puncture site bleeding Impending aneurysm rupture
Mass, pulsatile	Pseudoaneurysm Anastomotic pseudoaneurysm	True aneurysm
Mass, non-pulsatile	Hematoma Thrombosed pseudoaneurysm Abscess Lymphocele	Hematoma Thrombosed aneurysm
Hand or foot ischemia	Arterial steal Surgical technical error	
Purulent drainage from needle puncture site or surgical incision	Abscess Peri-graft infection	Infected hematoma
Painful, possibly erythematous, AV access	Infection, cellulitis	Thrombosed AV fistula
Absence of thrill, pulse, bruit in access	Thrombosis, outflow stenosis	Thrombosis, inflow or mid-fistula stenosis
Marked edema of extremity containing the access	Central venous stenosis	

the skin, creating a pseudoaneurysm similar to that formed when a graft is damaged by repeated needle sticks.

Buttonhole of AV fistula. The buttonhole technique is a method for access cannulation that involves creating a track through the skin with sharp dialysis needles applied at the same angle and direction over a two-to-four-week period.[9] Once the track develops, blunt needles are used. Some practitioners reported better hemostasis and less cannulation pain with the technique,[10] while others have found buttonholes are prone to infection.[11]

Ruptured pseudoaneurysm, true aneurysm, or buttonhole. The skin over a pseudoaneurysm or aneurysm is the strong barrier that contains it and keeps it from rupturing. Rupture occurs when the skin breaks down. It can become weakened by repeated needle sticks in the same area; so dialysis needles should not be placed through pseudoaneurysms. Unfortunately, dialysis technicians often find the large bulge too tempting to resist. A favorite "sweet spot" over a pseudoaneurysm where the needles are often introduced becomes traumatized until its integrity is compromised. The overlying skin is also weakened by ischemia as pressure from an

expanding pseudoaneurysm compresses skin blood flow, similar to how decubiti develop from prolonged bed rest. Skin necrosis with pseudoaneurysm rupture is heralded by epithelial sloughing which gives the impending rupture site a moist appearance, an ominous sign (Figure 26.1). The track of a buttonhole can open up spontaneously and bleed profusely (Figure 26.3).

Emergency department management

First 15 minutes: direct pressure. First aid for external bleeding of any kind, including that from an AV access, includes direct pressure. To be maximally effective, the bleeding point should be directly observed so that the size of the defect can be appreciated and pressure can be accurately applied. This involves having the emergency physician or vascular surgeon remove the field dressing to quickly assess the bleeding point. If it is a dialysis needle hole, a fingertip or adhesive bandage holding a 4″ by 4″ (10 × 10 cm) gauze pad folded in quarters over the spot is appropriate. If bleeding is from a ruptured pseudoaneurysm or aneurysm with a large open defect, then a compressive force over a wider area than a fingertip should be used, perhaps the heel of a gloved hand. This point pressure over large defects should be

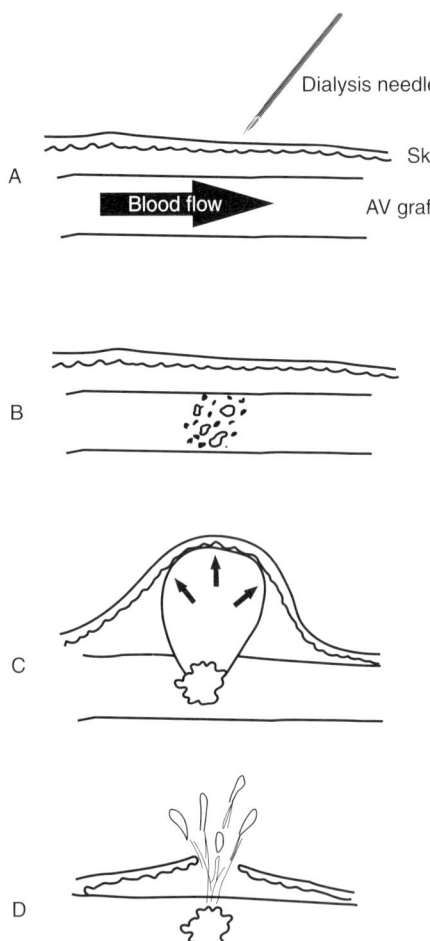

Figure 26.1 Mechanism of *pseudoaneurysm* formation and rupture. (A) Dialysis needles penetrate the skin and wall of the graft twice per treatment, two treatments per week. (B) If puncture sites are not rotated because the technician continuously uses the same "sweet spot" that gives good flow, graft structure breaks down. (C) Eventually a hole forms, allowing blood to pulsate in and out of a subcutaneous pseudoaneurysm cavity with each heartbeat. (D) As the pseudoaneurysm grows it exerts pressure against the under surface of the overlying skin, causing ischemic necrosis and eventual rupture.

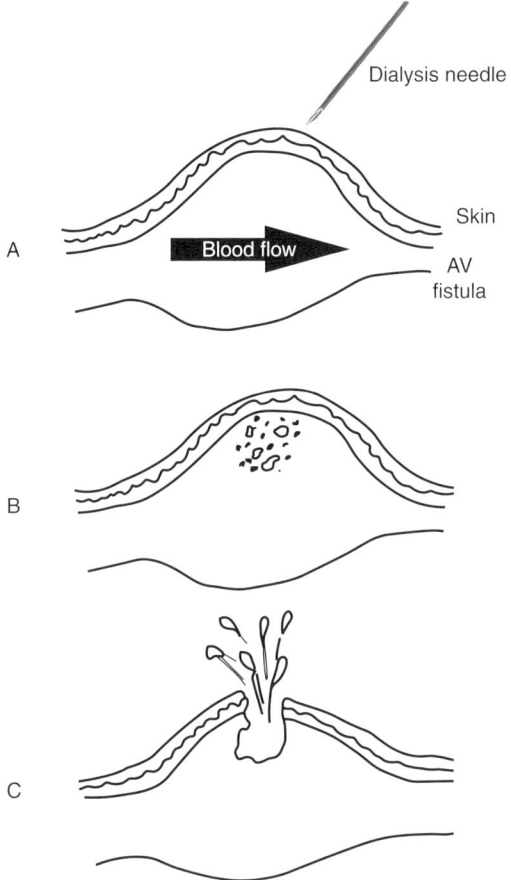

Figure 26.2 Mechanism of *true* aneurysm formation and rupture. (A) AV fistulas form true aneurysms, where the pulsatile mass represents dilation of the fistula, an area of over-exuberant maturation. (B) Repeated needle puncture of the aneurysm because it presents an easy target damages both the fistula wall and overlying skin. (C) If the fistula and skin are damaged enough that they break down, rupture can occur, especially if pressure from aneurysm expansion causes ischemic necrosis of the skin.

maintained continuously as the patient is taken to the operating room and prepared for surgery.

Indirect pressure. Besides direct pressure over the bleeding site, one can firmly compresses the access proximally and distally with a finger or palm of the hand (Figure 26.4). This prevents blood from getting to the bleeding area.

Tourniquet. Anastomotic pseudoaneurysm can cause massive bleeding, especially if it occurs in the immediate postoperative period, before the surgical incision over the anastomosis has healed. This bleeding can be difficult to control for several reasons. Blood is entering the disrupted anastomosis from three directions: proximal artery, distal artery, and venous back bleeding from the AV graft. Direct pressure on the bleeding point at the skin level may not be effective if the wound is fresh, with tissue planes that are still open from the surgery. In rare instances it may be necessary to apply a pneumatic tourniquet such as a manual blood-pressure cuff above the bleeding point. The cuff pressure must be higher than systolic arterial pressure to stop blood flow. Tourniquets are not often used because direct and indirect pressure

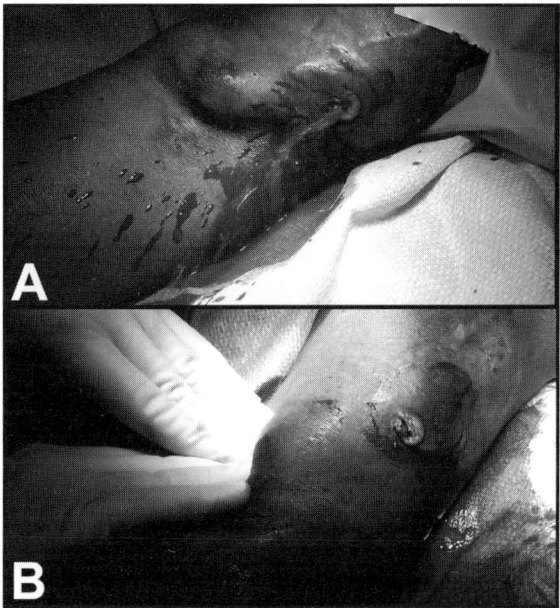

Figure 26.3 (A) Vigorous bleeding from a brachial-cephalic AV fistula buttonhole that spontaneously broke open. (B) Technique of hemorrhage control by digital compression of arterial end of fistula. See plate section for color version.

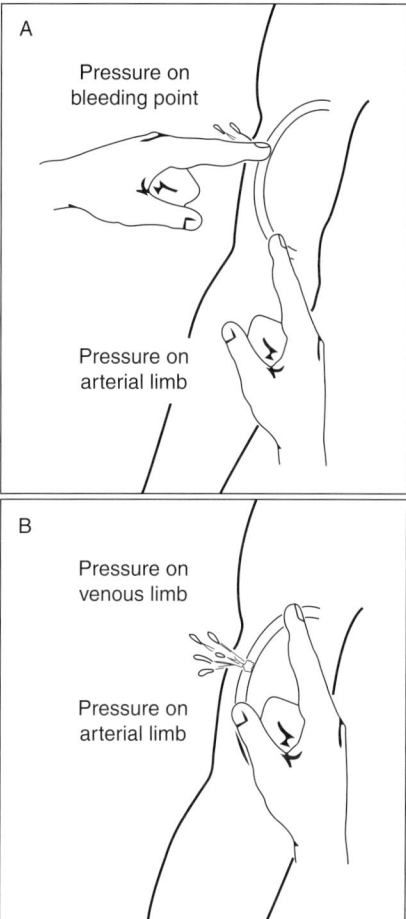

Figure 26.4 First aid for ruptured AV access. (A) Direct pressure on the bleeding point using a fingertip or folded piece of gauze will usually stop the bleeding. This can be improved if necessary by digitally occluding the arterial limb of the access. (B) If the bleeding point needs to be inspected, firm simultaneous pressure over both the arterial and venous limbs of the access will often stop or markedly slow the bleeding.

methods are usually effective while not imposing a risk of distal ischemia.

First few hours: correction of hemostasis. Many patients with ESRD have coagulopathy. The pathophysiology is multifactorial, but is mainly attributable to platelet dysfunction. It manifests as gastrointestinal bleeding, post-surgical bleeding, and excessive bleeding from AV access sites. Vasopressin (DDAVP) is useful for improving hemostasis in patients with uremia by releasing endogenous von Willebrand factor (vWF) from storage sites. It can be given intravenously (0.3 μg/kg in a 50-mL bolus of saline over 30 minutes), subcutaneously (0.3 μg/kg), or intranasally (2 μg/kg).[12,13] Conjugated estrogens have also been useful for treatment of uremic bleeding, but the effect is not detectable until six hours after the first infusion.[14] Transfusion of packed red blood cells to a hematocrit over 30% has the benefits of not only correcting the acute anemia and hypovolemia resulting from hemorrhage, but also reducing bleeding time through a rheologic effect.[7,15] A hemodialysis treatment without heparin in the circuit might be useful in some cases where acute uremia is thought to be contributing to

inadequate hemostasis. Other blood products such as platelet transfusions, fresh frozen plasma, and cryoprecipitate[16] may also be beneficial, especially when an elevated bleeding time or other coagulation defects are demonstrated.

Dialysis needle bleeding. Depending on the size of the defect, a figure-of-eight suture with nylon or silk may help reduce the size of the skin defect and assist the intrinsic hemostatic mechanisms by slowing the bleeding rate and tamponading the defect in the access. This will fail if the defect in the access wall beneath the skin opening is too large.

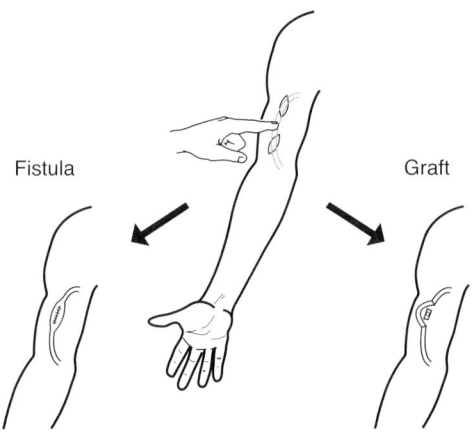

Figure 26.5 Surgery for ruptured fistula aneurysm and graft pseudoaneurysm. In all cases the patient is brought to the operating room with an assistant holding continuous digital pressure on the bleeding point. After the area is prepared and draped, an incision is made on either side of the bleeding point, and the access is controlled with vascular clamps or vessel loops. Digital pressure can then be released. **Fistula**: if the access is a fistula, the two incisions can be joined across the top of the ruptured area. An elliptical area of the aneurysm encompassing the rupture can be excised, then closed to reduce the diameter of the aneurysm. The fistula can then be repositioned more laterally into a subcutaneous pocket so it is away from the surgical scar. The skin is then debrided and closed primarily. **Graft**: if the access is a graft, a fresh piece of PTFE can be tunneled around the area of rupture, and anastomosed to the arterial and venous ends of the graft to restore continuity. The two surgical incisions are closed primarily, and the area of rupture packed open after the shredded PTFE at the base is debrided out.

Definitive treatment

Ruptured pseudoaneurysm. While stent placement may be applicable to some pseudoaneurysms that are enlarging or at risk for rupture,[17] once rupture occurs the best option is surgery. After the surgeon is scrubbed and gloved, he can take over applying direct pressure in a sterile surgical field. Incisions are made over the graft proximal and distal to the rupture, through which the graft can be isolated and clamped. At this point direct pressure over the rupture can be released. The graft and overlying necrotic skin is debrided. Healthy skin can be approximated over the area, or more often the area can be packed to heal by secondary intention. An interposition graft of PTFE can then be sewn to the proximal and distal graft to bypass the involved area and re-establish graft flow (Figure 26.5). Uninvolved areas of the graft can be used for dialysis needle access immediately after the reconstruction, and the new bypass segment can be used after three weeks.

Ruptured true aneurysm. In the case of ruptured aneurysm, the surgical reconstruction often does not require a bypass (Figure 26.5). The damaged aneurysm wall and overlying necrotic skin can be debrided and closed after proximal and distal control have been achieved in the operating room. As with repair of pseudoaneurysm, the uninvolved areas of the fistula can be used for dialysis access immediately.

Anastomotic pseudoaneurysm. During repair of ruptured anastomotic pseudoaneurysm it can be difficult to identify structures depending on the timing after the original surgery, and degree of inflammation, especially if infection was the cause of the anastomotic breakdown. A pneumatic tourniquet on the arm above the anastomosis may be required for a brief period of time to arrest bleeding while vascular structures are identified and controlled. Repair of a ruptured anastomotic pseudoaneurysm usually entails removal of the AV graft and repair of the artery with a vein or bovine pericardium patch, or bypass with saphenous vein.

Inpatient care

Depending on the amount of blood loss, hemodynamic instability, and fluids administered during resuscitation, a short hospitalization may be needed after definitive treatment. The patient may need a temporary dialysis catheter if the bleeding access is no longer usable, and a dialysis treatment to correct volume overload. The patient can be discharged after the hematocrit, electrolytes, and fluid balance are restored to stable, acceptable levels.

Critical actions

- Direct pressure to bleeding point.
- Indirect pressure to inflow and outflow ends of access if direct pressure is not sufficient.
- Fluid resuscitation.
- Correction of coagulopathy.
- Vascular surgical repair in some cases.

Hand and foot ischemia

Overview

Placement of an AV access can impair distal arterial perfusion and lead to ischemic symptoms, gangrene, and limb loss. In every case of AV fistula or graft place-ment it is accepted that the access will cause some drop in arterial pressure at the level of the anastomosis, but this will be sufficient to cause symptoms in only about 10% of patients.[18,19]

Diagnosis

Signs and symptoms of ischemia can develop immedi-ately after AV access placement, or appear slowly over time. They include diminished pulse, cyanosis, pares-thesias, cold feeling, weakness, pain, paralysis, ulcer-ation, cellulitis, and gangrene. The type and number of symptoms can suggest the degree of ischemia, but it is easy to underestimate the severity and urgency of the problem. The difficulty of trying to decide whether the symptoms warrant aggressive treatment arises from the fact that spontaneous resolution can occur over several weeks, suggesting a period of obser-vation. On the other hand, even if tissue necrosis has not occurred, periods of ischemia can result in a long-standing or permanent neuropathy that persists after the steal has been treated, suggesting prompt attention.

The safest approach is to presume that any new symptoms in the ipsilateral hand or foot following AV access placement represent ischemia until proven otherwise. Initial workup of possible ischemia should include blood pressures of both the affected and con-tralateral side, usually performed in a vascular non-invasive laboratory.[20] The test is simple to perform, and measurements are made with several different sized blood-pressure cuffs and a Doppler probe. Typ-ical pressure measurements include bilateral wrist pressures with a forearm cuff, several digital pres-sures with a finger cuff, and a contralateral brachial artery pressure with an upper arm cuff. Ipsilateral pressures can be obtained with and without tempo-rary compression and occlusion of the AV access. The ratio of the ipsilateral digital to contralateral brachial pressure of less than 0.4–0.6 (digital-brachial index), or an absolute digital pressure < 60 mmHg, is strongly suggestive that ischemia is the cause of symptoms.[21,22] The change in digital pressure with compression of the access may be useful in pre-dicting which patients will benefit from an inter-vention that targets the access.[22] If digital pres-sure does not improve with compression of the access, one should consider other diagnoses, such as arterial stricture at the anastomosis, atherosclerotic occlusive disease somewhere between the aortic arch

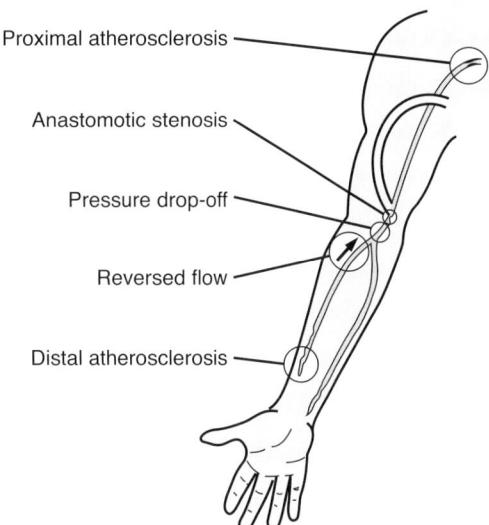

Figure 26.6 Potential contributors to distal ischemia in an extremity containing an AV access.

and the hand, or perhaps an unrecognized arterial thrombus or embolus that occurred during the AV access surgery (Figure 26.6). Digital-brachial index > 0.6, or pressure > 60 mmHg, suggest tissue loss from ischemia is not imminent, and that symptoms may be due to surgical nerve damage, or a problem unrelated to the access such as ischemic monomelic neur-opathy,[23] arthritis, or carpal tunnel syndrome.

If non-invasive testing suggests that the hand is ischemic, then an arteriogram should be performed. Arterial steal is confirmed if contrast is seen beyond the arterial anastomosis with the AV access temporar-ily occluded, but not when it is open. An arteri-ogram is needed for preoperative planning if a DRIL bypass (distal revascularization and interval ligation, Table 26.2) is planned to treat steal. The arteriogram defines the vascular anatomy to help plan the sites of anastomosis for the bypass, and identifies other problems that might need to be addressed, such as a proximal atherosclerotic stenosis that could be angio-plastied, an anastomotic stricture that could be cor-rected, or an arterial thrombus or embolus that could be extracted.

Emergency department management

It is critical that distal ischemia from a dialysis access be suspected in patients with ipsilateral pain in the hand or foot. A delay in diagnosis and treatment can quickly progress to irreversible tissue necrosis or a

Table 26.2 Procedures to treat arterial steal

Procedure	Advantages	Disadvantages
Ligation	Quickest, easiest, most reliable means of eliminating arterial steal by the access	Access is lost
Distal Revascularization Interval Ligation	High likelihood of improving ischemic symptoms while preserving the access	Major surgery that includes ligation of the main blood supply to the extremity
Banding	Simple procedure compared to DRIL. Has the potential to resolve ischemic symptoms while preserving access	Disappointing results, including high probability of access thrombosis

chronic painful neuropathy, which is tragic insofar as it can cause a lifelong disability and is often preventable. All patients with symptoms possibly due to vascular steal should have, at minimum, an early evaluation by a surgeon experienced with dialysis access.

Definitive treatment

A DRIL bypass for vascular steal carries an 80 to 90% likelihood of resolving the ischemic symptoms without sacrificing the AV access. Its principal disadvantage is that it is a major vascular surgical procedure that further alters extremity anatomy by ligating a major artery. It may not be appropriate if there are other problems with the AV access such as pseudoaneurysms or outflow stenosis, where tissue loss has already occurred, or where ischemia is progressing rapidly. In these cases a simple surgical ligation of the AV access is a quick, reliable way to arrest progression of ischemic damage. Banding the access to limit flow and reduce steal is intuitively appealing, but experience with it is associated with a high thrombosis rate, so it is considered a suboptimal technique (Table 26.2).

Inpatient care

Inpatient care of a patient with vascular steal depends on its severity. As described above, it can range from a decision to observe mild symptoms, to access ligation with possible amputation, to a bypass operation.

Critical actions

- Hand or foot symptoms in an extremity with a dialysis access is due to ischemia from vascular steal until proven otherwise.
- Do not discharge the patient for a remote clinic appointment without consultation with a vascular surgeon. Delay in diagnosis and treatment can lead to progression of ischemia, tissue loss, and chronic neuropathic pain.

Hematoma

Overview

A hematoma between the AV access and skin presents as a non-pulsatile mass which may or may not be painful. It usually occurs just after a dialysis needle is withdrawn, resulting from failure of the needle puncture to seal, allowing blood to leak out under arterial pressure into the subcutaneous tissues. Such hematomas can impair the dialysis technician's ability to palpate and cannulate the AV access. They can also compress the access, causing diminished flow or thrombosis. Some hematomas expand so rapidly under such pressure that they cause ulceration and necrosis of the overlying skin.

Diagnosis

Diagnosis of a hematoma around a dialysis access is made on history and physical examination. They commonly present as a non-pulsatile mass occurring shortly after removal of a dialysis needle. An ultrasound examination may be helpful in differentiating a pseudoaneurysm in some cases.

Emergency department management

Soft hematomas that are minimally symptomatic will resolve slowly with observation. No emergency treatment is needed. Referral to a vascular surgeon should be made for those that are painful, tense, ulcerated, expanding, or compressing the access.

Definitive treatment

Symptomatic hematomas may require surgical exploration with drainage, and suture of the puncture in the access. The incision should be placed to the side of the hematoma so that the resultant surgical scar does not overlie the access. During hematoma evacuation the offending puncture hole is usually obvious at the base of the wound and can be approximated with a figure-of-eight suture. Treatment with angiographic stenting may control the bleeding, but does not resolve any mass effect from the hematoma.

Critical actions

- Discharge for follow-up at the dialysis unit if the hematoma is soft and asymptomatic.
- Refer for surgical repair if it is painful, tense, ulcerated, expanding, or compressing the access.

Infection

Overview

As with thrombosis, AV access infections occur more frequently with grafts than fistulas.[24] Staphylococcal and streptococcal species are responsible for 70 to 80% of dialysis access infections.[25,26]

Diagnosis

An access infection can present as cellulitis, induration, fluctuant mass, purulent drainage, and exposure of the access if infection erodes the overlying skin.[26] However, a graft infection can be also insidious, with no local signs at all, just systemic manifestations such as fever, leukocytosis, and bacteremia. This pattern is observed when the graft's surrounding reactive fibrous capsule keeps the infection from spreading into the surrounding subcutaneous tissues. Ultrasound imaging to look for fluid collections,[27] or indium-111-labeled white-blood cell scanning, may be helpful in such cases.[28] Before an investigation for an insidious access infection is undertaken, any central venous catheters should be removed, since they are the source of the majority of bacteremias in the ESRD population.[29]

Emergency department management

Patients with suspected access infection should have blood cultures drawn. Purulent drainage from surgical wounds, dialysis needle puncture sites, or exposed graft material should also be cultured. Empiric antibiotic therapy should cover both Gram-positive and

Gram-negative bacteria like *Pseudomonas*, which is relatively common in this setting, and is a virulent organism capable of disrupting native arteries, vein grafts, and anastomoses.[30]

Definitive treatment

Antibiotics alone are a reasonable choice as initial therapy for a localized cellulitis without abscess around a native fistula (see Is it a fistula or a graft?). Most AV graft infections also require surgery. Total or subtotal access excision is indicated when the infection is causing septicemia, the access is occluded, infection is due to aggressive bacteria like *S. aureus* or *Pseudomonas* spp., or the majority of the access is involved. A limited segmental excision with a PTFE jump graft bypass around the involved area and preservation of the access can be performed when the infection is confined to a focal area of the access.[7]

Critical actions

- Draw blood cultures.
- Culture purulent drainage from around the access.
- Start empiric antibiotics.
- Refer to vascular surgeon.

Thrombosis

Overview

Arteriovenous access thrombosis is a frequent complication. Thrombosis within the first 30 days after access placement usually results from either a surgical technical problem, or selection of an access site where the vessels are too small or diseased to support it. After this early time period, thrombosis usually results from one or more stenoses in the access circuit.

Diagnosis

With AV grafts there is turbulent flow at the outflow anastomosis, which causes inflammation of the vein. This inflammation leads to a neointimal hyperplasia which progressively narrows the lumen, reducing flow and eventually leading to thrombosis. While an AV fistula is not susceptible to outflow stenosis (there is no venous anastomosis at the outflow), it can thrombose after stenoses occur at needle stick sites. The thrombosis rate is much lower than with grafts, which is one of the reasons fistulas are preferred. Thrombosis of an AV graft is often asymptomatic, coming to light when the

dialysis technician is unable to feel a pulse or thrill. In contrast, thrombosis of a fistula can cause symptoms similar to a superficial phlebitis, presenting with pain, tenderness, and possibly erythema. This presentation can appear to be a cellulitis, so it is important to try to determine if the access is a fistula or a graft (see Is it a fistula or a graft?).

Emergency department management

When patients present to an emergency department because of a thrombosed access, they should be referred to a vascular surgeon or interventional radiologist (depending on local practice) for thrombectomy, thrombolysis, and possible angioplasty. Patients should be treated as early as possible (ideally within 24 hours) for an AV fistula, since thrombus in the valves of the fistula is difficult to remove once it becomes organized.

Definitive treatment

There are multiple treatment options available for declotting an AV access. Early thromboses require either correction of the technical problem or a decision to move on to another site. The surgeon who placed the access should be in the best position to decide.[31] With later thromboses, percutaneous pharmacologic thrombolysis and/or mechanical thrombectomy is often the approach utilized at the initial episode, because it can restore flow without surgery. It also gives a radiographic depiction of the anatomy which can guide decision-making for subsequent thromboses. For example, if the graft has a focal outflow stenosis that responds well to angioplasty and stays patent for several months, it may be reasonable to try angioplasty again. On the other hand, if there are multiple or long-segment stenoses that do not dilate nicely, it may be more appropriate to attempt surgical thrombectomy and revision. Sometimes the access is in such bad shape, with multiple aneurysms, pseudoaneurysms, stenoses, angioplasties, and revisions, that it is best to abandon it and plan a new site.

Critical actions

- Refer the patient to a vascular surgeon or interventional radiologist (depending on local practice) for thrombectomy, thrombolysis, and possible angioplasty.

- Patients should be treated as early as possible (ideally within 24 hours) for an AV fistula, since thrombus in the valves of the fistula is difficult to remove once it becomes organized.

Swelling

Overview

Swelling in an extremity with an AV access is usually caused by high flow in the access combined with a stenosis somewhere in the venous circuit back to the heart. The resulting venous hypertension leads to edema, which can be quite painful to the patient, and which can obscure the location of the access to the point where it is useless for dialysis. Edema can involve the chest wall, breast, and head if the stenosis is in the innominate vein or superior vena cava.

Diagnosis

Swelling often presents within days of a new access placement, when the altered hemodynamics uncover a central stenosis that was previously subclinical. Central stenoses and thromboses are often due to prior central venous catheters,[32] or indwelling pacemaker/defibrillator wires. Beyond swelling, venous stenoses can also cause excessive needle-hole bleeding, recirculation, loss of the extremity for future dialysis access, thrombosis of the access, airway obstruction, and central nervous system symptoms.[33]

Venography or fistulography should be performed to identify the location and degree of the venous stenoses. Venography is preferred for swelling early after access placement, since fistulography could damage a small, immature fistula vein, or dissect a hematoma around a poorly incorporated AV graft. After a fistula is sufficiently large, or a graft is well incorporated (three weeks after placement), fistulography is preferred since it shows both the access and venous outflow anatomy.

Emergency department management

When patients present to an emergency department because of swelling of an extremity with a dialysis access, they should be referred to a vascular surgeon or interventional radiologist (depending on local practice) for venography or fistulography to look for central venous stenosis, and angioplasty or stenting if one is found.

Definitive treatment

Central venous stenoses are best treated with endovascular angioplasty, with stent placement for lesions that recoil or recur.[34] Subclavian stenoses can be problematic because stents are usually not an option since they become damaged by scissoring between the clavicle and first rib. When endovascular techniques fail, a number of surgical options are available, some of which are rather aggressive and invasive.[35] If relief of the venous obstruction is not possible or does not resolve the swelling, ligation of the access usually does.

Critical actions

- Refer the patient to a vascular surgeon or interventional radiologist (depending on local practice) for venography or fistulography to look for central venous stenosis, and angioplasty or stenting if one is found.

Is it a fistula or a graft?

"Dialysis access" is a non-specific term that can refer to either an arteriovenous (AV) "fistula" or "graft." For patients with a suitable vein,[36] the National Kidney Foundation recommends an "AV fistula" as the preferred conduit because of higher patency, lower cost, and reduced mortality.[37] It is constructed by suturing a patient's artery to a vein without the use of exogenous materials. In the absence of a suitable vein for a fistula, an alternative is a prosthetic conduit such as polytetrafluoroethylene (PTFE) sewn between an artery and vein, commonly referred to as an "AV graft." Management of some complications (especially bleeding, aneurysm, and infection) is affected by whether the access is a fistula or graft. For example a bleeding or aneurysmal site is often managed by direct repair for a fistula, but would be bypassed for a graft. Pain and erythema around a graft is often due to infection, but would more likely be an acute thrombosis or infiltration for a fistula. In the absence of a surgical procedure note, an educated guess about whether it's a fistula or graft can be made on clinical grounds. Grafts usually feel harder and narrower than fistulas. The number and location of the surgical scars is also helpful, as shown in Table 26.3. If the configuration is a loop, or if there is a surgical scar on both ends of the access, it is often a graft.

Table 26.3

Configuration	Surgical scars	It's probably a …
Loop, in the volar forearm	One scar in the antecubital fossa	Forearm loop GRAFT (brachial artery to basilic, cephalic, or brachial vein)
Straight, in the volar forearm	Two scars, one at the distal and one at the proximal end of the access	Forearm straight GRAFT (radial artery to basilic, cephalic, or brachial vein)
Curve, antero-lateral upper arm	Two scars, one at the distal and one at the proximal end of the access	Upper arm GRAFT (brachial artery to axillary vein)
Loop, in the antero-lateral upper arm	One scar near the axilla	Upper arm loop GRAFT (axillary artery to axillary vein)
Straight, along the lateral forearm	One scar at the distal end of the access	Forearm FISTULA (radial artery to cephalic vein)

Table 26.3 (*cont.*)

Configuration		Surgical scars		It's probably a ...
	Curve, in the antero-lateral upper arm		One scar at the distal end of the access	Upper arm FISTULA (brachial artery to cephalic vein)
	Curve, in the antero-lateral upper arm		One long, or multiple small scars along the medial upper arm	Upper arm FISTULA (brachial artery to transposed basilic vein)
	Loop, in the upper thigh		One scar near the groin crease	Thigh loop GRAFT(femoral artery to femoral vein)

References

1. Cloonan CC, Gatrell CB, Cushner HM. Emergencies in continuous dialysis patients: diagnosis and management. *Am J Emerg Med* 1990; 8(2): 134–48.

2. Loran MJ, McErlean M, Eisele G, Raccio-Robak N, Verdile VP. The emergency department care of hemodialysis patients. *Clin Nephrol* 2002; 57(6): 439–43.

3. McAllister CJ, Gibson R. Emergencies in dialysis patients. *JACEP* 1978; 7(3): 96–8.

4. Wolfson AB, Singer I. Hemodialysis-related emergencies – Part 1. *J Emerg Med* 1987; 5(6): 533–43.

5. Wolfson AB, Singer I. Hemodialysis-related emergencies – Part II. *J Emerg Med* 1988; 6(1): 61–70.

6. Anton NS. Arteriovenous hemodialysis access: the Society for Vascular Surgery practice guidelines. *J Vasc Surg* 2008; 48(5 suppl): S1.

7. Padberg FT Jr, Calligaro KD, Sidawy AN. Complications of arteriovenous hemodialysis access: recognition and management. *J Vasc Surg* 2008; 48(5 suppl): 55S–80S.

8. Begin V, Ethier J, Dumont M, Leblanc M. Prospective evaluation of the intra-access flow of recently created native arteriovenous fistulae. *Am J Kidney Dis* 2002; 40(6): 1277–82.

9. Verhallen AM, Kooistra MP, van Jaarsveld BC. Cannulating in haemodialysis: rope-ladder or buttonhole technique? *Nephrol Dial Transplant* 2007; 22(9): 2601–4.

10. Pergolotti A, Rich E, Lock K. The effect of the buttonhole method vs. the traditional method of AV fistula cannulation on hemostasis, needle stick pain, pre-needle stick anxiety, and presence of aneurysms in ambulatory patients on hemodialysis. *Nephrol Nurs J* 2011; 38(4): 333–6.

11. Labriola L, Crott R, Desmet C, Andre G, Jadoul M. Infectious complications following conversion to

buttonhole cannulation of native arteriovenous fistulas: a quality improvement report. *Am J Kidney Dis* 2011; 57(3): 442–8.

12. Mannucci PM, Remuzzi G, Pusineri F, *et al.* Deamino-8-D-arginine vasopressin shortens the bleeding time in uremia. *N Engl J Med* 1983; 308(1): 8–12.

13. Vigano GL, Mannucci PM, Lattuada A, Harris A, Remuzzi G. Subcutaneous desmopressin (DDAVP) shortens the bleeding time in uremia. *Am J Hematol* 1989; 31(1): 32–5.

14. Livio M, Mannucci PM, Vigano G, *et al.* Conjugated estrogens for the management of bleeding associated with renal failure. *N Engl J Med* 1986; 315(12): 731–5.

15. Livio M, Gotti E, Marchesi D, *et al.* Uraemic bleeding: role of anaemia and beneficial effect of red cell transfusions. *Lancet* 1982; 2(8306): 1013–15.

16. Janson PA, Jubelirer SJ, Weinstein MJ, Deykin D. Treatment of the bleeding tendency in uremia with cryoprecipitate. *N Engl J Med* 1980; 303(23): 1318–22.

17. Vesely TM. Use of stent grafts to repair hemodialysis graft-related pseudoaneurysms. *J Vasc Interv Radiol* 2005; 16(10): 1301–7.

18. Rutherford RB, ed. *Rutherford's Vascular Surgery*, 6th edition. Philadelphia: Elsevier Saunders; 2005.

19. Morsy AH, Kulbaski M, Chen C, Isiklar H, Lumsden AB. Incidence and characteristics of patients with hand ischemia after a hemodialysis access procedure. *J Surg Res* 1998; 74(1): 8–10.

20. Wixon CL, Hughes JD, Mills JL. Understanding strategies for the treatment of ischemic steal syndrome after hemodialysis access. *J Am Coll Surg* 2000; 191(3): 301–10.

21. Goff CD, Sato DT, Bloch PH, *et al.* Steal syndrome complicating hemodialysis access procedures: can it be predicted? *Ann Vasc Surg* 2000; 14(2): 138–44.

22. Schanzer A, Nguyen LL, Owens CD, Schanzer H. Use of digital pressure measurements for the diagnosis of AV access-induced hand ischemia. *Vasc Med* 2006; 11(4): 227–31.

23. Miles AM. Upper limb ischemia after vascular access surgery: differential diagnosis and management. *Semin Dial* 2000; 13(5): 312–15.

24. Butterly DW, Schwab SJ. Dialysis access infections. *Curr Opin Nephrol Hypertens* 2000; 9(6): 631–5.

25. Tokars JI, Miller ER, Stein G. New national surveillance system for hemodialysis-associated infections: initial results. *Am J Infect Control* 2002; 30(5): 288–95.

26. Ryan SV, Calligaro KD, Scharff J, Dougherty MJ. Management of infected prosthetic dialysis arteriovenous grafts. *J Vasc Surg* 2004; 39(1): 73–8.

27. Rutherford RB. The value of noninvasive testing before and after hemodialysis access in the prevention and management of complications. *Semin Vasc Surg* 1997; 10(3): 157–61.

28. Williamson MR, Boyd CM, Read RC, *et al.* 111 In-labeled leukocytes in the detection of prosthetic vascular graft infections. *AJR Am J Roentgenol* 1986; 147(1): 173–6.

29. Klevens RM, Tokars JI, Andrus M. Electronic reporting of infections associated with hemodialysis. *Nephrol News Issues* 2005; 19(7): 37–8, 43.

30. Geary KJ, Tomkiewicz ZM, Harrison HN, *et al.* Differential effects of a Gram-negative and a Gram-positive infection on autogenous and prosthetic grafts. *J Vasc Surg* 1990; 11(2): 339–45; discussion 46–7.

31. Sidawy AN, Spergel LM, Besarab A, *et al.* The Society for Vascular Surgery: clinical practice guidelines for the surgical placement and maintenance of arteriovenous hemodialysis access. *J Vasc Surg* 2008; 48(5 suppl): 2S–25S.

32. Joffe HV, Kucher N, Tapson VF, Goldhaber SZ. Upper-extremity deep vein thrombosis: a prospective registry of 592 patients. *Circulation* 2004; 110(12): 1605–11.

33. Cuadra SA, Padberg FT, Turbin RE, Farkas J, Frohman LP. Cerebral venous hypertension and blindness: a reversible complication. *J Vasc Surg* 2005; 42(4): 792–5.

34. Anaya-Ayala JE, Smolock CJ, Colvard BD, *et al.* Efficacy of covered stent placement for central venous occlusive disease in hemodialysis patients. *J Vasc Surg* 2011; 54(3): 754–9.

35. El-Sabrout RA, Duncan JM. Right atrial bypass grafting for central venous obstruction associated with dialysis access: another treatment option. *J Vasc Surg* 1999; 29(3): 472–8.

36. Allon M, Lok CE. Dialysis fistula or graft: the role for randomized clinical trials. *Clin J Am Soc Nephrol* 2010; 5(12): 2348–54.

37. Murad MH, Elamin MB, Sidawy AN, *et al.* Autogenous versus prosthetic vascular access for hemodialysis: a systematic review and meta-analysis. *J Vasc Surg* 2008; 48(5 suppl):S34–47.

Complications of central venous catheterization

Ronald Tesoriero

Introduction

Central venous access has become ubiquitous in both its utilization and necessity in the care of the acutely and chronically ill patient. Over five million central venous catheters (CVCs) are inserted each year in the United States.[1,2] Complications from their placement can have a profound impact on patient morbidity, mortality, and the cost of providing health care.[3] While the majority of complications that will be faced by the acute care physician will occur secondary to the insertion of CVC lines, it is important to recognize the potential complications related to indwelling, and extraction of these catheters.

Epidemiology

Unfortunately, complications of central venous access are commonplace, affecting more than 15% of patients.[1,2] Mechanical complications occur in 5 to 19%,[2] and thrombotic complications occur in 2 to 59% of patients.[1,2,4] Infectious complications occur in 5 to 26% of patients, with a significant increase in their incidence in patients who experience a mechanical complication during their placement of CVCs.[3,5] Femoral catheters are associated with an increased incidence of both thrombotic (21.5% vs. 1.9%) and major infectious (4.4% vs. 1.5%) complications when compared to subclavian catheters, though the rate of mechanical complications are similar.[4]

Risk factors for mechanical complications are listed in Table 27.1. Additionally, there are patient factors that may make significant complications more likely if a mechanical complication occurs; for instance, moderate to severe atherosclerosis may make thromboembolic phenomenon more likely if inadvertent fine gauge needle arterial puncture occurs.[3]

Table 27.1 Risk factors for the development of mechanical complications

1. Inexperience of the practitioner or supervisor ($<$ 50 CVC insertions). [1,3]
2. Number of attempts; three or more is associated with a sixfold increase in mechanical complications. [1,2,6]
3. Emergency situations. [3]
4. Significant hypovolemia. [1]
5. Significant obesity; BMI $>$ 30.
6. Low body weight; BMI $<$ 20. [1]
7. Previous catheterizations or vascular thrombosis.
8. Previous operative therapy, injury, or radiation in or near the area of proposed venous cannulation (e.g., median sternotomy, clavicular fracture). [2,3]
9. Presence of thrombocytopenia or coagulopathy. [3]

BMI, body mass index.

Though many of these factors are non-modifiable, care should be taken to correct factors that can be modified (thrombocytopenia, coagulopathy, hypovolemia), avoid high-risk sites of cannulation if able (sites that have been previously accessed, have a known thrombosis, or are within prior surgical or radiation fields), and ensure that inexperienced providers are supervised appropriately. If available, ultrasound guidance should be utilized to assist placement of CVCs, as its use appears to significantly reduce the number of mechanical complications associated with central venous access.[6,7,8]

Complications of central venous catheterization, and their management

Complications of central venous catheterization can be divided into those that occur during insertion, those

Vascular Emergencies, ed. Robert L. Rogers, Thomas Scalea, Lee Wallis, and Heike Geduld. Published by Cambridge University Press. © Cambridge University Press 2013.

Table 27.2 Complications of central venous access

Complications of insertion

Pneumothorax

Arterial puncture/laceration/catheterization

Hemothorax

Air embolization

Cardiac tamponade

Dysrhythmias

Pseudoaneurysm, AV fistula, vertebral artery injury

Guidewire loss/fracture/embolization

Cerebrovascular accident

Brachial plexus injuries

Thoracic duct injury/chylothorax

Esophageal injury and mediastinitis

Tracheal injury

Complications of indwelling

Vascular erosion and perforation

Catheter fracture and embolization

Thrombosis

Infection

Vascular stenosis

Extravasation injury

Complications of extraction

Air embolization

Catheter fracture and embolization

Hemothorax

that are related to indwelling, and those that occur secondary to catheter extraction (Table 27.2). The majority of events that are encountered by the acute care/emergency physician are those that occur during catheter insertion. However, as patients increase in complexity there will invariably be more patients that present to the emergency department in transfer from rehabilitation and subacute care facilities where they are being managed with chronic indwelling venous catheters. Thus it is important to recognize and understand the initial treatment for complications that occur due to indwelling catheters and their removal.

Pneumothorax

Pneumothorax (PTX) represents the most common complication that will be encountered and treated by emergency care providers. It accounts for up to 30% of all mechanical complications with an incidence

that ranges from 0.2 to 6.6%,[2,3] with a 0.2 to 1.5% incidence being the most common reported range. Pneumothorax occurs more commonly after subclavian vein CVC attempts (0.5–2%) than with internal jugular vein CVC attempts (0.2–0.5%).[2,3,9] Pneumothorax may present in a delayed fashion, with the majority of patients developing symptoms within six hours, though delays of up to 72 hours have been reported.[2,3]

Diagnosis

History and physical examination

Clinicians should suspect pneumothorax should any of the following findings occur during or after placement of CVCs:[10]

- Aspiration of air into the syringe during needle localization of the central vein.
- Absence or decrease in breath sounds (usually on the ipsilateral side of the cannulation attempt, though contralateral PTX has been described).
- Hyper-resonance on percussion of the thorax.
- Decreased chest movement.
- Hyper-inflation of the affected hemithorax.
- Tracheal deviation away from the side of PTX.
- Pleuritic chest pain and shortness of breath.
- Tachycardia.
- Hypotension.

It may be particularly difficult to diagnose PTX in patients who are critically ill and receiving mechanical ventilation. Factors that should increase clinical suspicion include:[10]

- increasing ventilatory or oxygen requirements
- increased peak and plateau airway pressures
- metabolic acidosis/hyperlactemia
- decreased urine output.

Laboratory assessment

There is no laboratory profile that is pathognomonic for PTX. In patients who develop an unexplained fall in PaO_2 on ABG (arterial blood gas), or an increasing lactate, re-evaluation for the presence of PTX is warranted.

Imaging

Chest X-ray (CXR). Chest X-ray is the most commonly used imaging study to detect the presence of pneumothorax. Upright

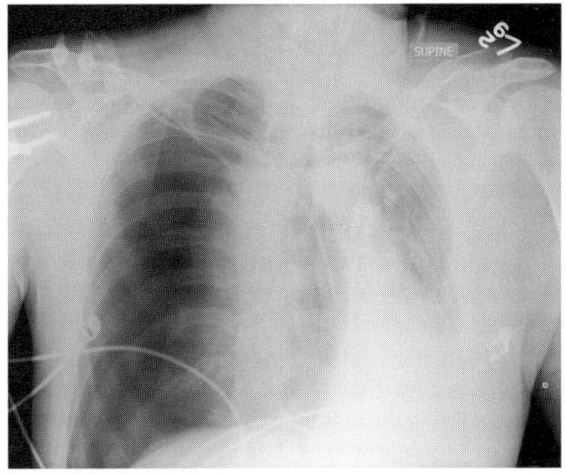

Figure 27.1 Right-sided tension pneumothorax after insertion of a right subclavian CVC.

posteroanterior is the most sensitive CXR technique to detect the presence of PTX and should be used preferentially. However, as most patients are critically ill, these films tend to be done with a supine or semi-upright anteroposterior technique. In these cases up to 500 mL of gas must be introduced into the pleura to definitively diagnose PTX, and many may be missed.[10,11]

Ultrasound (US). Ultrasound has been shown to be more sensitive than bedside CXR for the detection of pneumothorax.[10,12,13,14] In the correct clinical context it will allow early diagnosis and placement of a pleural drainage catheter. However, it is operator dependent, and the optimal management of the occult pneumothorax (pneumothorax seen only on US or CT) remains unclear.[10,12]

Computed tomography (CT). Computed tomography scan is the most sensitive and specific test for the detection of pneumothorax and may be utilized in stable patients who have unexplained hypoxia or evidence of decreased cardiac output after CVC placement.

Emergency department management

Tension pneumothorax

See Figure 27.1.

- Perform initial needle decompression with a 45 mm, 14-gauge angiocatheter over the rib in the second intercostal space at the mid-clavicular line on the affected side.
- Follow with chest tube thoracostomy with a 20-French or larger tube in the fifth intercostal space at the anterior axillary line.

Symptomatic pneumothorax

Treat with a pleural drain (standard chest tube thoracostomy or percutaneously placed drain larger than 7 French[10,15,16]) when:

- 15% PTX (1–2 cm air rim on anteroposterior (AP) CXR);
- 15% PTX (by CXR) if the patient is on mechanical ventilation.

There is evidence that percutaneously placed drains are adequate to treat PTX, and tube thoracostomy is not needed.[10,15,16] However, if the PTX is causing hemodynamic instability or significant clinical deterioration, preference should be given to placing a chest tube thoracostomy of larger than 20-French size.

Asymptomatic pneumothorax

Aspiration or observation may be considered when the PTX is:

- < 15% on CXR;
- only seen with US or on CT.

The optimal treatment of non-mechanically ventilated asymptomatic patients with PTX of less than 15% or patients with PTX seen only on US or CT (ventilated or not) is debatable. Available evidence suggests these may be managed with observation or aspiration, though data are derived from literature on spontaneous pneumothorax and occult traumatic pneumothorax.[10,17,18,19]

Definitive treatment and inpatient care

When required, pleural drainage is the definitive management for nearly all cases of CVC-related pneumothorax. Most patients can be managed on a non-monitored floor, after appropriate placement of a pleural drain is confirmed. In rare instances, where an unresolving air leak is present or patients develop complications related to tube thoracostomy or pleural drainage (hemothorax, empyema), video-assisted thorascopic surgery (VATS) or thoracostomy may be necessary.

Arterial puncture/laceration/catheterization

The most commonly accessed central veins lie in close proximity to major arteries, and their accidental puncture and catheterization is an unfortunately common complication of CVC access. Arterial puncture may occur as frequently as 5%, with accidental catheterization occurring in 0.1 to 1% of attempts.[2,20,21,22] Inadvertent arterial catheterizations cause subsequent complications in up to 47% of patients.[20] When symptomatic (up to 30%), they carry an associated mortality of 20 to 40%.[2,20] The most commonly affected arteries are the carotid, subclavian, and femoral; however smaller arteries and side branches such as the vertebral, thyrocervical trunk, and internal mammary may also be injured.

The consequences of arterial injury and catheterization include hematoma, hemothorax, arterial dissection and occlusion, limb ischemia, pseudoaneurysm, arteriovenous (AV) fistula, and cerebrovascular accident (CVA). Though uncommonly reported, embolic stroke has occurred after simple carotid puncture. It is most often seen in the setting of significant carotid atherosclerotic disease, and may present in a delayed fashion, generally within 48 hours.[21,23,24]

Diagnosis

Arterial puncture is generally immediately recognizable due to the return of high-pressure pulsatile, bright red blood through the finder or introducer needle or into the syringe. Arterial catheterization may still occur, as these signs are not always present, especially in the hypoxic, hypovolemic, or hypotensive patient.

History and physical examination

The inserter should be observant for bright red, pulsatile, high-pressure blood at the time of needle puncture. If there is uncertainty, a wire may be placed via the introducer needle and the included single-lumen, 18-gauge angiocatheter may be placed into the vessel. This should then be connected to a 50-cm extension set of IV tubing or the included manometry tubing. Blood is then aspirated into the length of the tubing using a syringe. The syringe is then disconnected as the tubing is elevated and a slowly descending column of blood should be observed.[25] Alternatively, manometry can be performed via the introducer needle without placing a catheter.

If there continues to be uncertainty, an arterial pressure transducer should be connected and the waveform observed. The same procedure should be performed through the most distal port site of a catheter that is already in place if there is concern for arterial cannulation.

Arterial punctures and catheterizations that are missed at the time of CVC insertion may present in a myriad of ways depending on the type of complication that develops. A pseudoaneurysm may present as a pulsatile or non-pulsatile mass. A thrill or bruit at an attempted or successful cannulation site may indicate an arteriovenous fistula. Distal ischemia may result due to arterial dissection or thrombosis. A hemothorax or retroperitoneal hematoma may develop, with their associated signs and symptoms. A stroke may be the first sign of an incorrectly placed internal jugular catheter.

Laboratory assessment

When there is concern for arterial catheterization, blood gas assessment to determine oxygen saturation should be performed on sampled blood from the catheter.

Imaging

CXR. All post-CVC chest X-rays should be closely reviewed for any aberrant CVC path that may indicate an arterial cannulation. Examples include catheters that follow the path of the descending aorta (Figure 27.2). However, given the anatomic similarities in the paths of the major arteries and veins, CXR may miss many cases of arterial catheterization. Other concerning findings that suggest an arterial injury has occurred include a widened mediastinum and apical cap.[26]

Ultrasound. Ultrasonography may be used to confirm wire or catheter placement within the vein near the site of cannulation. Advanced operators may be able to confirm placement in the distal SVC of certain patients.

Computed tomography. CT shows excellent anatomic detail and may be obtained to confirm catheter position or define arterial injury in difficult to interpret cases.

Angiography. Angiographic studies will definitively diagnose arterially placed CVCs, and can be helpful in managing complications related to their placement.

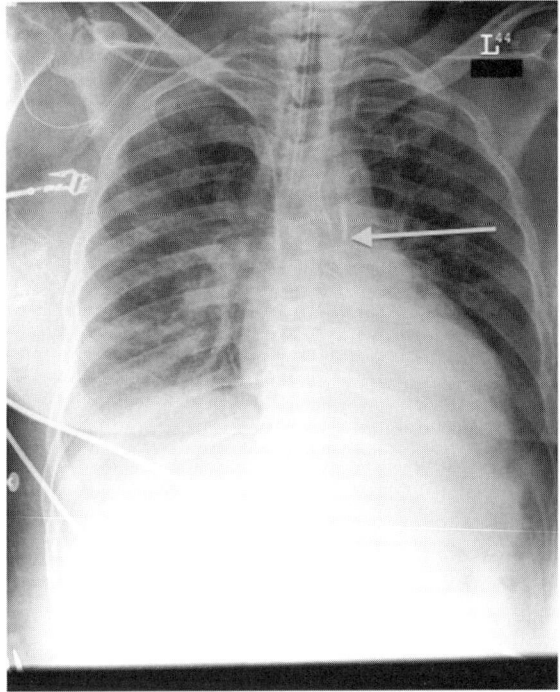

Figure 27.2 Catheterization of the left carotid artery with dialysis catheter. The tip of the catheter is seen overlying the aortic knob (arrow). Arterial placement was confirmed with manometry and blood gas assessment. Surgical extraction was required.

Emergency department management

Arterial puncture with finder or introducer needle

- **Withdraw the needle immediately** and hold gentle pressure for at least five minutes.[22]
- Perform a thorough neurologic (carotid) or distal arterial examination (subclavian or femoral).
- Control hypertension.[20]
- Record the arterial puncture in procedure notes and inform the admitting team so that delayed presentation of neurologic sequelae or other complications can be closely monitored.
- If hematoma develops:
  - obtain prompt duplex ultrasound evaluation to evaluate for pseudoaneurysm or dissection;
  - correct coagulopathy or thrombocytopenia;
  - monitor closely for airway compromise.

- If neurologic change/CVA develop:
  - obtain emergent CT of the head to evaluate for hemorrhagic stroke;

- obtain emergent duplex ultrasound to evaluate for dissection, pseudoaneurysm, or thrombosis/occlusion of the vessel; CTA of the neck at the time of the head CT may also be considered;
  - obtain emergent vascular surgery consultation;
  - if indicated by protocol, tPA may be considered if:
    - no other contraindications exist
    - there is no evidence of hematoma or pseudoaneurysm at the puncture site
    - the arterial puncture occurred at a compressible site
    - the decision is discussed and made in conjunction with the vascular surgery service.

- If distal extremity ischemia occurs:
  - obtain emergent vascular surgery consultation;
  - obtain emergent duplex ultrasound;
  - administer an intravenous fluid bolus of 500–1000 mL;
  - consider anticoagulation with unfractionated heparin with a goal PTT of 50–70 if:
    - there is no evidence of hematoma, enlarging pseudoaneurysm, hemothorax, or pericardial tamponade on physical or duplex ultrasound examination;
    - the injury occurred at a compressible site.

In select cases, anticoagulation may be administered even when the injury occurred at a non-compressible site, but the decision to do so should be made in consultation with the vascular surgery service.

Arterial catheterization

If arterial catheterization occurs with a catheter less than 7 French:

- **Remove the catheter** and follow the steps as above.
- If there is no immediate complication obtain interval duplex evaluation of the vessel in 24 to 48 hours.

The risk of complication for catheters less than 7 French appears to be similar to that of arterial puncture.[20] If the catheterized vessel is non-compressible due to anatomic location (subclavian), vascular surgery consultation should occur prior to catheter removal.

If arterial catheterization occurs with a catheter that is 7 French or larger:

- **Do not remove catheter** as it may be partially occluding an injury.
- Obtain immediate vascular/cardiothoracic surgery consultation.
- If immediate treatment is not available, and there are no associated complications, consider anticoagulation while awaiting transfer/intervention.

Large-bore arterial catheterization treated by the pull/pressure technique has a complication rate of over 50%, with a stroke risk of 5.9% (for carotid catheterization) and associated mortality of 12.5%.[2,20] Surgical exploration or angiographic assessment and treatment should be utilized, as the complication rate with a directed approach is nearly 0%.[20,21]

It is often safe to remove catheters up to 9 French in size from the femoral artery and control with manual pressure; however, these decisions should be made in conjunction with the vascular surgery service.

Definitive treatment and inpatient care

Arterial puncture and cannulation with catheters of less than 7 French caliber are generally associated with a low complication rate. After their removal, patients should be observed as inpatients for 12–24 hours in a non-ICU setting for delayed sequelae. The liberal use of duplex will allow most complications to be diagnosed and treated at an early stage.

Due to the high complication rate, carotid arterial cannulation with catheters of greater than 7 French should be managed with immediate open exploration, catheter removal, and arterial repair. In subclavian vessels cannulated with catheters of greater than 7 French, immediate arteriography should be performed and arterial injury may be treated with stenting, coil embolization, or with percutaneous closure devices. If there is delay in intervention, patients should be monitored in an ICU-level setting with frequent neurologic checks until definitive repair. When treated with open surgical or angiographic means the significant complication rate approaches 0%.[20,21]

Due to its high compressibility and tolerance to microembolism, femoral artery cannulations up to 9 French can be selectively managed with pull and pressure techniques in consultation with the

vascular surgery service. Any anticoagulation should be fully reversed and pressure should be held for a minimum of 25 minutes. Catheterization with catheters of greater than 9 French should be treated with percutaneous closure devices or open exploration and direct repair.

Hemothorax/pleural effusion

Hemothorax may occur at the time of CVC insertion and is most commonly a result of an arterial injury during attempts at subclavian access.[2] It may also occur as a result of venous injury, of delayed perforation/erosion related to a poorly positioned central venous catheter, or to direct placement of the catheter into the pleural space. Delayed effusions associated with vascular erosion from improper catheter position most commonly occur on the right and are associated with left-sided venous cannulations when the catheter comes in contact with the lateral border of the SVC with an angle of greater than 40°.[2,27,28] In these cases the accumulated fluid is often mixed and may be a combination of blood and infused fluids, though predominately appears to be non-bloody effusion.[22,27,28,29] Injury to the thoracic duct or other lymphatics may also present as a pleural effusion, in a delayed fashion with fluid characteristic of chylothorax.

Diagnosis

History and physical examination

Over 90% of patients who are neurologically intact and develop hemothorax or pleural effusion will display symptoms.[27] The most common symptoms include chest pain, dyspnea, and tachypnea.

The physical examination findings that should alert the practitioner to the possibility of hemothorax include: unilateral decrease in breath sounds, dullness to percussion, tachycardia, hypotension, hypoxemia, cyanosis, and pallor.

Most patients who develop delayed perforation/erosion will present with a new or rapidly increasing unilateral pleural effusion within the first seven days after catheter placement, with the majority becoming evident within the first three days.[27] Physical examination findings will be similar to the acute setting, though their development may be more insidious.

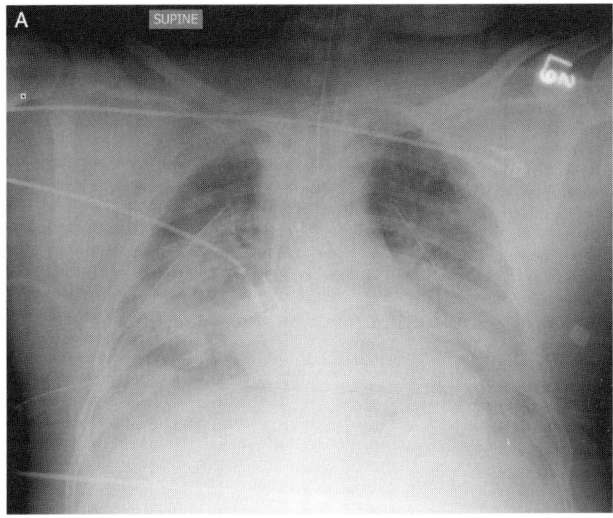
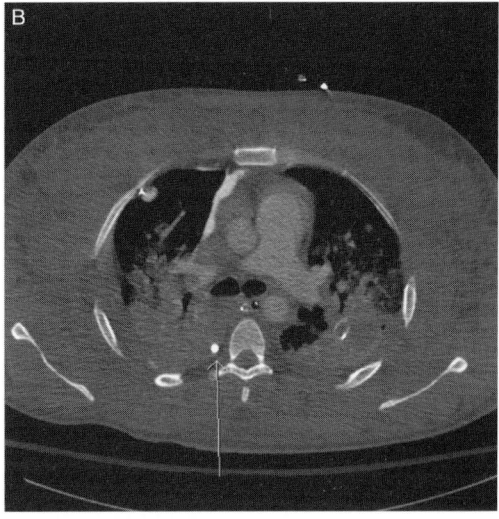

Figure 27.3 (A) After insertion, right subclavian CVC appears appropriately placed on AP chest X-ray. (B) Due to inability to draw blood from catheter and development of pleural effusion, a CT of the chest was obtained and showed an extravascular course of the catheter. The catheter took a transvenous course, and was removed under fluoroscopic guidance with placement of a subclavian venous stent.

Laboratory examination

New onset of anemia after placement of CVCs should prompt evaluation for hemothorax. When delayed pleural effusion develops, in the setting of a poorly positioned line as described above, fluid should be sent for routine analysis including: pH, glucose, protein, albumin, LDH, amylase, lipids, cell count/differential, and gram stain. Unfortunately, there is no definitive pattern of pleural analysis that is diagnostic of delayed venous perforation, as the content will be dependent on the type of infused fluid and degree of hemothorax. Generally the pleural fluid glucose is more elevated than serum, and protein content is more consistent with transudative effusion (< 2 g/dL).[27]

Imaging

CXR. Significant hemothorax should be readily demonstrated on routine AP chest X-ray. Catheters that contact the medial or lateral border of the SVC at an angle of greater than 40° should alert the physician to the potential for development of vascular erosion. Catheters that appear well positioned on CXR may still lie outside the vasculature (Figure 27.3A,B), and a high index of suspicion is warranted.

Ultrasound. Compared to CXR, ultrasound is more specific and as sensitive for diagnosing pleural fluid.[30] In the post-CVC-insertion patient with tachycardia or hypotension, it can be used for early diagnosis and decision for treatment.

Computed tomography. CT is both sensitive and specific for diagnosing pleural fluid and catheter malposition.

Emergency department management

Hemothorax

- **Leave catheter in place** as it may be partially occluding an injury.[22]
- Place a large-bore (32 French or greater) chest tube thoracostomy on the affected side.
- Treat hypovolemia and hypotension with intravenous fluid resuscitation, auto-transfusion of collected hemothorax, and transfusion with packed red blood cells.
- If there is concern for ongoing hemorrhage, hypotensive resuscitation (SBP 80–90 mmHg) should be used to minimize ongoing blood loss until definitive control can be obtained.
- Aggressively correct coagulopathy.
- Obtain emergent vascular/thoracic surgery consultation.
- In stable patients:
  - transduce the catheter and obtain blood gas analysis to evaluate for arterial cannulation;
  - assess with contrast CT to define the anatomic location of the catheter and define the injury.

Delayed hemothorax/pleural effusion

For the patient who presents with delayed or rapid accumulation of unilateral pleural effusion within seven days of CVC insertion:

- **Leave the catheter in place.**
- If asymptomatic, perform thoracentesis with fluid analysis.
- If symptomatic, place a chest tube thoracostomy or a percutaneously placed pleural drain and send fluid for analysis.
- Obtain a contrast CT scan or venogram to evaluate for catheter tip position/vascular injury.
- Obtain vascular/cardiothoracic surgery consultation for catheters that have migrated through the vessel wall, chylothorax, or if there is concern for venous erosion at the insertion site.

Definitive treatment and inpatient care

All patients who develop hemothorax after CVC placement should be monitored in an ICU level of care until the hemothorax is adequately drained, the patient is resuscitated, and the underlying cause is diagnosed and definitively treated.

Treatment will be dictated by the underlying cause of the hemothorax or pleural effusion. In cases of arterial injury where the patient is hemodynamically stable or stabilizable, most will be amenable to angiographic evaluation and treatment with balloon tamponade, stenting, or percutaneous closure devices.[20,21,26,31] Patients who are hemodynamically unstable may require thoracostomy and direct vascular repair.

Most patients who present with delayed venous perforation/erosion and pleural effusion will be treatable with only pleural drainage and CVC removal.[27] It is prudent to obtain venography at the time of catheter removal to ensure no ongoing vascular leak.

Retroperitoneal hematoma

The most common significant mechanical complication of femoral CVC placement is retroperitoneal hematoma, which occurs in up to 1.3% of cases.[4] This may occur when dilators or catheters are placed through the iliac veins (Figure 27.4), or related to arterial puncture above the inguinal ligament. Rarely, intraperitoneal hemorrhage may occur when catheters or dilators are placed through the iliac veins into the abdominal cavity.

Diagnosis

History and physical examination

The presentation of retroperitoneal hematoma after CVC insertion can be insidious due to the lack of clinical signs that may be present. The neurologically intact patient may complain of abdominal pain or pressure. The development of hypotension, tachycardia, or hematoma at the insertion site, known arterial puncture, or difficult-to-advance catheters or guidewires during placement should alert the practitioner to the possibility of injury or risk for retroperitoneal hematoma. Grey–Turner's and Cullen's signs (flank and peri-umbilical ecchymosis) may occur 24–48 hours after the development of retroperitoneal hematoma. Additionally, poorly functioning catheters should be evaluated for proper placement.

Imaging

Abdominal X-ray may reveal a catheter that takes an abnormal course (Figure 27.5). Ultrasound may be used to diagnose free intra-abdominal fluid, and, in advanced hands, retroperitoneal fluid may be observable. CT will definitively diagnose retroperitoneal hematoma and catheter misplacement. Angiography will definitively diagnose vascular injury and catheter malposition.

Laboratory examination

Coagulopathy, anemia, and metabolic acidosis may be present in patients who develop retroperitoneal hematoma.

Emergency department management

In the patient that develops hypotension, tachycardia, or instability after femoral CVC placement:

- **Leave the catheter in place**.
- Treat hypovolemia and hypotension with intravenous fluid resuscitation and transfusion with packed red blood cells.
- If there is concern for ongoing hemorrhage, hypotensive resuscitation (SBP 80–90 mmHg) should be used to minimize ongoing blood loss until definitive control can be obtained.
- Aggressively correct coagulopathy.
- Obtain vascular surgery consultation.

For the stable patient who develops unexplained anemia after femoral CVC placement, or for lines that are non- or poorly functioning after placement:

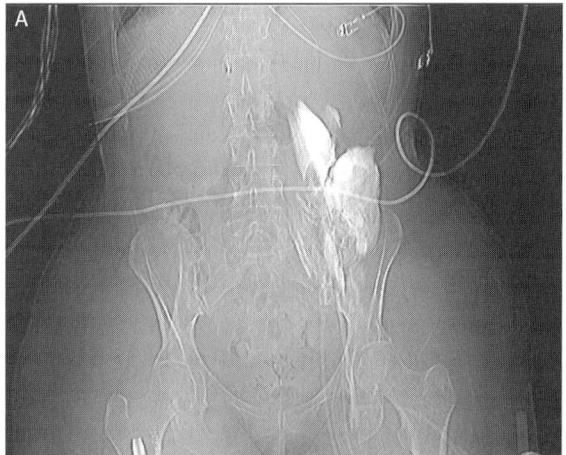

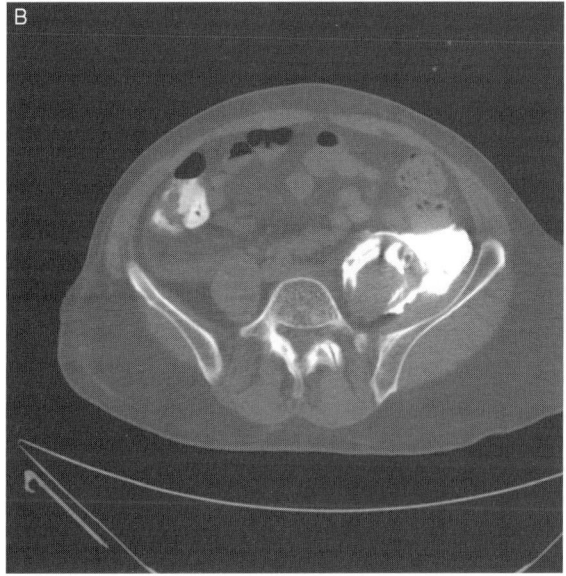

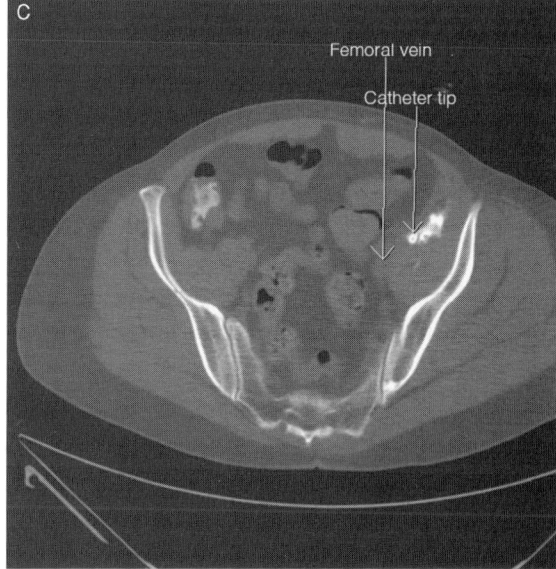

Figure 27.4 (A) A scout film from a CT obtained as part of the trauma workup after an "uneventful" placement of a left femoral CVC shows extravasation of contrast into the peritoneal cavity. (B) Computed tomography image showing same. (C) Computed tomography image showing relationship of the catheter to the femoral vein.

- **Leave the catheter in place**.
- Transfuse to correct anemia, if indicated.
- Attempt to withdraw blood from the catheter, send for blood gas analysis, and transduce the line to assure venous placement.
- Obtain abdominal X-ray to follow the course of the catheter.
- Perform bedside ultrasound to demonstrate that the catheter enters the venous system.
- Obtain duplex ultrasound to evaluate for arterial injury.

- If clinical suspicion is high, obtain a CT scan with contrast through a separate IV site to evaluate for the presence of retroperitoneal hematoma and check catheter tip position.
- Obtain vascular surgery consultation.

Definitive treatment and inpatient care

In the absence of major venous laceration or arterial injury/catheterization, most cases of retroperitoneal hematoma are self-limited by surrounding structures

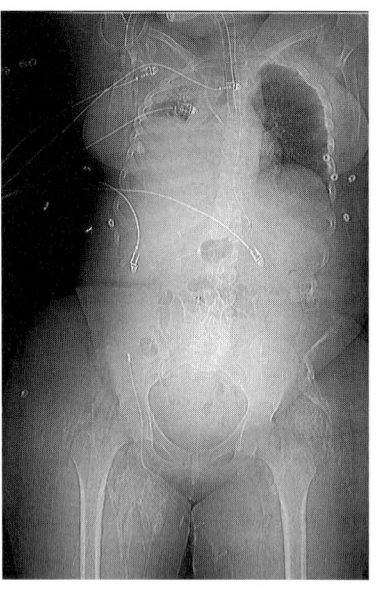

Figure 27.5
Abdominal X-ray demonstrating an abnormal course laterally, after placement of a right femoral CVC. Subsequent CT demonstrated a total extravascular retroperitoneal course.

and do not require intervention. Catheters should be left in place until angiographic assessment can be performed to evaluate for injury, and in many cases provide definitive treatment. Occasionally, operative treatment will be required for retroperitoneal hematoma associated with major arterial vascular injury or when placement of the catheter into the peritoneal space has occurred. Patients who develop retroperitoneal hematoma as a result of major vascular injury or are unstable should be monitored in an ICU level of care until the injury is definitively managed. Stable patients with retroperitoneal hematoma without major vascular injury should be monitored in a step-down setting until their hematocrit is stable for more than 24 hours. Further imaging in the stable patient is not mandatory.

Pericardial tamponade

Pericardial tamponade is a devastating injury that may occur at the time of CVC insertion due to venous laceration or arterial injury below the pericardial reflection. Most of these injuries are related to mishandling of the dilator due to insertion beyond the subcutaneous tissue into the vasculature, and poor attention to careful Seldinger technique.[2] They may also occur as a result of delayed perforation/erosion through the SVC when a malpositioned catheter tip lies below the pericardial reflection. In the acute setting, as little as 50–100 mL of fluid can cause tamponade, and cases

associated with CVC placement have a mortality rate of up to 90%.[2]

Diagnosis

History and physical examination

Neurologically intact patients will generally complain of chest pain or pressure and associated dyspnea. Orthopnea is frequent, and tamponade should be suspected in any patient who is unable to lie flat due to anxiety or agitation after the insertion of a CVC. Common signs include tachycardia, jugular venous distension, diminished heart sounds, hypotension, and pulsus paradoxus. Electrocardiogram findings that may be seen include ST wave changes, decreased QRS amplitude, and electrical alternans. Cardiac tamponade should be immediately ruled out in any patient who develops cardiac arrest after CVC insertion.

Imaging

CXR. Concerning findings on chest X-ray after CVC insertion include a widened mediastinum, enlarged or globular cardiac silhouette, and an apical cap.

Ultrasound/echocardiography. The diagnosis of cardiac tamponade can be made with high sensitivity and specificity utilizing echocardiography. Focused ultrasound can diagnose pericardial fluid with high accuracy.

Emergency department management

In any patient with hypotension, tachycardia, dyspnea, orthopnea, cardiac arrest, or who is suspected of having pericardial tamponade after CVC insertion:

- **Leave the catheter in place** as it may be partially occluding vascular injury.
- Immediately perform focused ultrasonography of the heart and pleural spaces.
- Obtain a CXR if stable/stabilizable.
- Treat arrest as per ACLS protocols.
- Treat hypotension with fluid resuscitation (not through the previously placed CVC as this may worsen tamponade).

If pericardial fluid is noted in the unstable or arresting patient:

- Perform ultrasound-guided pericardiocentesis and place a drainage catheter.

- Proceed with resuscitative thoracostomy in the arresting patient not responsive to pericardiocentesis, if no other cause is identified.
- Obtain emergent vascular/cardiothoracic surgery consultation.

If pericardial fluid is noted in the stable patient, obtain emergent vascular/cardiothoracic surgery consultation.

Definitive treatment and inpatient care

Patients with pericardial tamponade from CVC insertion will almost always require open surgical drainage and repair of the injury.[22] Stabilizable patients should be monitored in an ICU setting until definitive management.

Pericardial effusion is not uncommon in the elderly, critically ill patient undergoing CVC placement. The stable patient who is found to have pericardial fluid after placement of a CVC should have formal echocardiography and fluid aspiration. In the absence of hemo-pericardium or tamponade physiology, further radiographic workup with CT and angiography is warranted. In these cases the fluid may be physiologic and not related to injury. Triage judgment is needed, but these patients should be admitted to at least a step-down level of monitored care until injury can be ruled out.

Cardiac arrhythmias

Arrhythmias are common during CVC insertion and are most frequently related to direct myocardial stimulation by a guidewire that is placed too deeply. The incidences of atrial and ventricular arrhythmias are 40% and 25%, respectively, and there is a greater than 75% incidence when the guidewire is placed more than 25 cm from a left internal jugular vein insertion site.[2,22] Arrhythmias occur in up to 0.9% of indwelling lines, but appear to be more common with peripherally inserted central catheters (PICCs) due to their tendency to move significant distances (up to 9 cm) with changes in arm position.[2,3,22]

Though the placement of pulmonary arterial catheters has become uncommon, it is important to remember that approximately 50% of patients will develop self-limited arrhythmias during their insertion. Pulmonary arterial catheters may cause right bundle branch block (RBBB), and in the patient with pre-existing left bundle branch block (LBBB), complete heart block may result. The practitioner should be prepared to immediately pace patients with LBBB who are undergoing placement of a pulmonary arterial catheter.[3]

Fortunately, most arrhythmias associated with CVC insertion are transient and treated by partially withdrawing the wire or catheter.

Diagnosis

History and physical examination

When feasible, electrocardiograms should be obtained prior to CVC insertion to evaluate for underlying conduction abnormalities, arrhythmias, and evidence of injury, ischemia, or previous myocardial infarction. Cardiac monitoring should be performed during CVC insertion and will immediately reveal any arrhythmias.

Patients who develop arrhythmias after insertion should have their CXRs carefully reviewed for catheter tip position. In these patients, a careful history related to timing of arrhythmia and patient position should be obtained, as catheter tip position on static CXR may not be reflective of the position at the time of arrhythmia. For example, abduction of the arm may cause a significant increase in insertion depth of peripherally inserted central catheter (PICC), and the mediastinal contents move upward in relation to a centrally placed catheter during exhalation and supine positioning. These changes may allow the tip of a catheter at the atrio-caval junction or distal SVC to move into the atrium, despite a normal appearance on static CXR.

Imaging

CXR. A chest X-ray should reveal most cases of catheter tip malposition, but changes in tip position with movement as discussed above should be considered.

Emergency department management

For the patient who develops arrhythmias during catheter insertion:

- **Partially or completely withdraw the guidewire or catheter.**
- Manage continued arrhythmia as per ACLS guidelines.
- Manage the development of complete heart block with catheter withdrawal, and immediate external

pacing. Follow with internal pacing if external is insufficient or pacing is required for a prolonged period.

- Consider other causes of arrhythmia: cardiac tamponade, air embolization, mediastinal hematoma, direct cardiac injury, catheter/guidewire fracture and embolization, etc.

For patients who develop arrhythmias with an indwelling catheter:

- Obtain an ECG.
- Treat as per ACLS guidelines.
- Obtain and carefully review a CXR for catheter tip position, fracture, or embolization.
- Partially withdraw or remove catheters that lie at the atrio-caval junction or distal SVC, if arrhythmias are intermittent and positional.
- Consider other causes.

Air embolism

Small volumes of air are commonly introduced during central venous catheterization and generally cause no harm to the patient. However, major air embolus can occur during catheter insertion, at the time of removal, in a delayed fashion due to catheter tracks after catheter removal, or as a result of disruption of indwelling lines.[2,22,32] Deep inspiration, coughing, or a snore can allow sudden decreases in intrathoracic pressure that can allow 90 mL of air to pass through a 4-cm, 18-gauge needle in 1 second.[3] The risk of air embolism is increased with significant hypovolemia. Some case reports suggest the lethal dose of air embolism to be 3–5 mL/kg, though fatal events have been reported with as little as 50 to 100 mL of air.[3,32] Patients may present with complete outflow obstruction of the right heart and cardiovascular collapse when high-volume air embolus occurs. Far smaller amounts of air may cause myocardial infarction or CVA in patients who have intrapulmonary shunts or cardiac septal defects.

The most effective treatment for air embolism is prevention. Attention to detail in technique, positioning of the vein intended for cannulation below the heart, and assuring adequate hydration of the patient minimizes risk of air embolism. In patients who are uncooperative, have an uncontrollable cough, or are unable to tolerate the Trendelenburg position,

alternative access to an upper venous central catheter should be considered.

Diagnosis

History and physical examination

A whoosh of air heard during insertion should alert the practitioner to the possibility of air embolism. It should be considered in any patient who is undergoing CVC insertion, removal, or with an indwelling central line when any of the following occur *during or within several minutes of the procedure*: the acute development of shortness of breath with anxiety, tachycardia, arrhythmia, hypotension, chest pain, loss of consciousness, CVA, cardiopulmonary arrest, and death. A "mill wheel" murmur, jugular venous distension, ST-T wave changes, ECG evidence of right heart strain, elevated right cardiac pressures, a decrease in cardiac output, an acute decrease in end tidal carbon dioxide, and hypoxemia may be observed.

Symptoms can occur at any time in a patient who develops an air embolism as a result of a fractured catheter or a catheter track after removal of a chronically indwelling line. This makes the diagnosis significantly more difficult due to the non-specific signs and symptoms, and clinicians should always be aware of this potential complication.

Laboratory and diagnostic examination

There are no specific laboratory tests that are diagnostic of air embolism. Cardiac enzymes may be positive in cases of myocardial ischemia due to air embolism, but are not diagnostic of cause. Electrocardiogram may show evidence of sinus tachycardia, right heart strain (peaked P-wave), non-specific ST-segment and T-wave changes, and acute myocardial ischemia or infarction.

Imaging

Ultrasound/echocardiography. While TEE is the most sensitive diagnostic test, transthoracic ultrasound can readily diagnose air within the cardiac chambers.

Computed tomography. CT of the head and neck may assist in ruling out other causes for neurologic changes after CVC placement, but is not diagnostic of air embolism; CT of the chest will readily demonstrate air in the cardiac chambers but is of little utility in the unstable patient.

Emergency department management

For the patient with suspected air embolism:

- Prevent further embolization.
- Provide hemodynamic support with dobutamine or epinephrine.
- Treat arrhythmia and arrest as per ACLS protocols.
- Place the patient in left-side-down Trendelenburg position (or Trendelenburg position alone if in arrest), to allow air to move out of the pulmonary outflow tract.
- Begin 100% oxygen therapy to eliminate nitrogen and decrease the size of the embolus.
- Attempt to aspirate intracardiac air if there is an existing CVC in place. Due to the poor success with this technique, placing a catheter for this purpose is generally not recommended, though in the patient who is deteriorating despite supportive care it should be considered.[32]

In the stable patient with cerebral or myocardial ischemia related to air embolism, hyperbaric oxygen should be considered to improve the acute and delayed associated injury.[32]

Unstable patients, and stable patients who develop cerebral or myocardial ischemia as a result of air embolism, should be monitored in an ICU level of care.

Guidewire/catheter retention and embolus

Guidewire retention and embolization is uncommon and most often described when there is failure to adequately control it during insertion. Other causes are internal kinking/looping/knotting, entanglement with other devices (internal pacers and IVC catheters), and entrapment within the inserted catheter with subsequent shear and fracture. Indwelling catheter fracture and embolization may occur in a delayed fashion related to "pinch off," when the catheter becomes compressed between the clavicle and the first rib.[1,22] Characteristic appearance of kinking or compression on CXR (Figure 27.6) should prompt catheter removal with the arm in the abducted position, which opens the angle between the first rib and clavicle.[3] Direct needle damage, fracture, and embolization of catheters already in place may rarely occur during subsequent line attempts.[22]

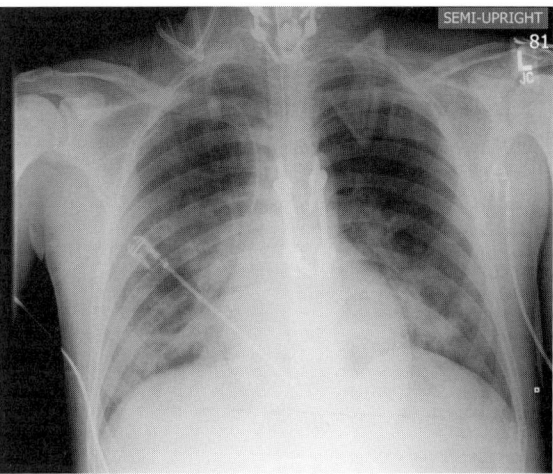

Figure 27.6 Typical appearance of a subclavian catheter being pinched between the clavicle and first rib. To avoid subsequent fracture and embolization, the catheter should be removed with the arm in the abducted position.

Diagnosis

History and physical examination

Practitioners should investigate for the presence of an implantable cardioverter defibrillator/pacer, IVC filter, or other implantable device prior to inserting CVCs. Undue resistance while inserting or withdrawing the guidewire should raise the possibility of guidewire kinking or entrapment. The entire needle guidewire complex should be withdrawn and carefully inspected to ensure no shearing or fracture. Even in the seamless procedure, the guidewire should always be carefully inspected after removal to ensure that it is intact. Intermittent catheter functionality with changes in arm position should make the clinician suspicious for "pinch off" syndrome. Patients who develop pain, erythema, or subcutaneous swelling near catheter insertion sites during fluid administration should be suspected of having internal fracture of the catheter. Pulmonary embolus, myocardial infarction, cardiac/vessel rupture, and pulmonary infarction may all result from catheter or guidewire embolization, and patients who develop these conditions should be critically evaluated for this as a cause.

Imaging

Guidewire retention is readily apparent on CXR (Figure 27.7), though sometimes overlooked, especially when it remains within a CVC catheter. Catheter narrowing or kinking where it passes over the first

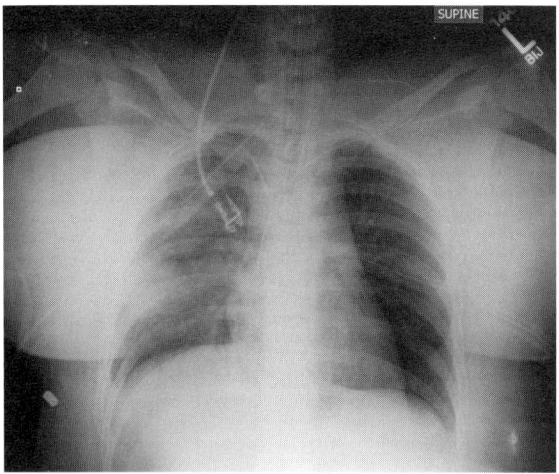

Figure 27.7 An anteroposterior CXR, after an initial failed attempt at left subclavian CVC and subsequent right CVC placement, demonstrated a retained guidewire on the left. The wire was able to be extracted at bedside after a small cutaneous cut-down.

rib is indicative of compression. Embolized fragments may be difficult to see on CXR and may require CT imaging for diagnosis. Embolization may also occur into the IVC and may not be apparent on chest imaging.

Emergency department management

Guidewire/catheter entrapment

- If the wire is caught within the needle or catheter, gently remove the entire complex, and inspect for signs of shear/fracture.
- If the wire is entrapped in a vessel or implanted device, remove the needle. If through a catheter, leave the catheter in place.
- Secure the wire to ensure no embolization.
- Cover with an occlusive dressing to prevent air embolism.
- Obtain CXR and/or abdominal X-ray.
- Obtain emergent vascular/cardiothoracic surgery consultation.

Guidewire/catheter embolization

- Carefully inspect all removed guidewires and catheters to ensure that they are intact.
- Treat acute complication of embolization.
- Obtain CXR and abdominal X-ray. Consider CT if a fragment is not seen and suspicion is high.
- Maintain patient on telemetry until embolization is ruled out or definitive treatment occurs.

- Obtain emergent vascular/cardiothoracic surgery consultation.

Definitive treatment and inpatient care

Fortunately, most retained and embolized guidewires, catheters, and fragments can be retrieved with percutaneous endovascular techniques. Patients should be monitored with telemetry while awaiting extraction. Occasionally, open surgical extraction will be necessary. For select instances in asymptomatic patients where small fragments have embolized distally into the lung or extraction would be dangerous, it may be advisable to leave them *in situ*.

Thrombosis and infection

Due to the increased frequency of indwelling lines in outpatient care, emergency medicine providers will encounter catheter-related thrombosis and infection. Catheter-related thrombotic complications occur more commonly with femoral sites of access (21.5%) when compared to subclavian (1.9%).[4] In the case of thrombosis, the patient may present with unilateral limb swelling or catheter malfunction. This should prompt duplex ultrasonography, and in selected cases venography.

Catheter-related infections occur in 3 to 8% of inserted catheters, with an associated mortality of 10 to 20%.[2,3,4,33] Their incidence is decreased by: adherence to hand hygiene, use of maximal barrier precautions during insertion, avoidance of mechanical complications during insertion, and use of protocols for catheter insertion maintenance and removal.[33] Catheter-related sepsis should be suspected in any patient with an indwelling line and SIRS (systemic inflammatory response syndrome) criteria. In these cases, blood cultures should be drawn from the catheter and peripherally.

Acute thrombosis and suspected catheter-related sepsis should generally lead to catheter removal. Catheters may be left in place in select cases where there is ongoing need for access and other options are limited.

Antimicrobial treatment should be instituted immediately when infection is suspected. Patients should be treated with vancomycin (or alternative MRSA coverage in areas of high endemic resistance to vancomycin), as coagulase-negative staphylococcus and *Staphylococcus aureus* are the most common cause of CVC-related infection. Gram-negative coverage

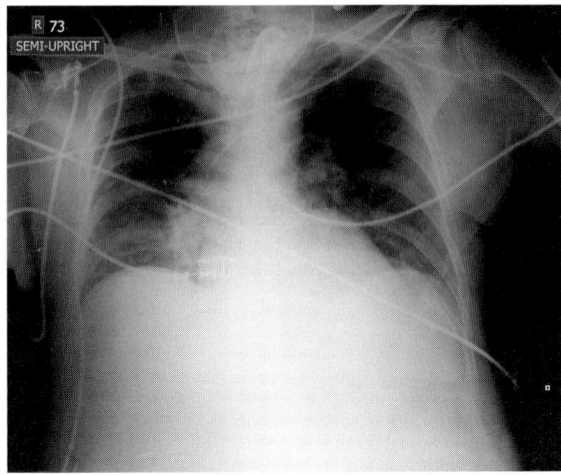

Figure 27.8 AP chest X-ray shows a left subclavian catheter in contact with the lateral border of the SVC at greater than a 40° angle. The catheter should be removed or repositioned due to the risk of subsequent vascular erosion.

should be considered in patients with severe sepsis, a known or suspected focus of Gram-negative infection, or femoral catheterization, in internal jugular vein catheterization in patients with tracheostomy, and in patients with an immunocompromised state such as malignancy or neutropenia. Double coverage should be considered in severe sepsis, or in areas where multi-drug resistant *Pseudomonas* or *Acinetobacter* are endemic. *Candida* coverage should be instituted for patients with severe sepsis and femoral catheterization, or who have been on total parenteral nutrition, receiving prolonged broad-spectrum antibiotics, have hematologic malignancy, or have received transplantation.[34]

In the absence of contraindications, anticoagulation should be started for acute thrombosis, though there is some evidence to suggest that it does not affect the rate of embolization, resolution, or outcomes in upper extremity catheter-related thrombosis.[35]

Catheter malposition

The emergency medicine practitioner should be aware of CXR markers for appropriate catheter position and the role malposition plays in the development of delayed mechanical complications. Clinicians should be alerted to the increased risk of erosion and perforation when catheters abut the wall of the SVC with an angle > 40° (Figure 27.8).[2,27] Perforation of the SVC above the pericardial reflection can lead to pleural

effusion or hemothorax, and below can lead to cardiac tamponade with a high associated mortality. Catheter tips above the SVC can lead to thrombosis, and compressed catheters can lead to fracture and embolization. The carina appears to be a reliable marker for the SVC above the pericardial reflection.[28,29]

Injury to other anatomic structures

Any anatomic structure that lies in close proximity to the major central veins commonly accessed for CVCs may be injured. There are reports of injury to the bladder, intestine, trachea, and esophagus after attempts at CVC placement. Injuries to the nervous system and brachial plexus are regularly reported, and most are related to infiltration of local anesthetic for CVC insertion and are self-limited. There are reports of permanent peripheral neurologic injury from needle laceration and due to external compression from hematoma development. All mechanical complications are reported with decreasing frequency when ultrasound guidance is used for CVC placement.

What to do with limited resources

Most complications from CVC insertion are clinically diagnosable without advanced imaging. In areas where routine radiographic imaging is unavailable, practitioner ultrasound can be an invaluable tool in both preventing and diagnosing most significant complications. Fortunately, the most common complications are treatable with percutaneous bedside techniques like tube thoracostomy and pleural drainage. The use of routine bedside manometry will help prevent most arterial catheterizations, and the majority of arterial punctures and small-gauge catheterizations are treatable by simply removing the needle or catheter and holding pressure. When large-gauge arterial catheterization occurs in areas where advanced radiographic interventions, surgical intervention, or transfer to higher level of care are not available; removal of the catheter with directed pressure is the only option but has a significant rate of morbidity and attributable mortality.

Summary

Central venous catheterization is a common procedure that is utilized in many patients who are critically ill and injured. Though complications related to their placement are uncommon, the frequent use of

CVCs means that they will be seen regularly. Most of these are preventable by careful attention to technique and correction or optimization of modifiable patient factors.

While not eliminating all complications, the use of ultrasound guidance minimizes most mechanical complications and, if available, should be utilized for all central venous catheterization attempts. Though ultrasound is easiest and most commonly described with internal jugular and femoral access, there are increasing reports of its successful use in axillary vein access just lateral to the clavicle.[8]

Clinicians must have a high incidence of suspicion for the complications related to central venous access, and aggressively investigate any concerning signs or symptoms with focused physical examination, the liberal use of X-ray, bedside ultrasound, and laboratory investigation. Computed tomography and angiography should be used in select cases but generally should be obtained in conjunction with consultation from general, vascular, or cardiothoracic surgery services. Most complications will be manageable with minimally invasive percutaneous or angiographic techniques; however, some patients will require open surgical management.

Critical actions and pearls

- Routine use of ultrasound nearly eliminates mechanical complications related to CVC insertion.
- Correct modifiable patient factors prior to attempts at CVC insertion.
- Monitor patients with continuous ECG and pulse oximetry to help diagnose complications during insertion.
- Pneumothorax may be rapidly diagnosed with bedside ultrasound.
- Do not redirect introducer/finder needles midcourse, as this may lead to tissue laceration.
- Do not advance dilators beyond the subcutaneous position into the vasculature.
- The internal jugular and subclavian veins are generally preferred due to the reduction in thrombotic and infectious complications.
- Routine use of manometry will eliminate almost all inadvertent arterial cannulations.
- Re-adjust CVCs that come in contact with the SVC at an angle greater than 40°, and those that are positioned below the pericardial reflection.

- Suspect tamponade in any patient who develops the inability to lie flat due to anxiety or agitation after the insertion of a CVC.
- Cardiac arrest after CVC insertion should prompt emergent evaluation for pericardial tamponade, massive hemothorax, tension pneumothorax, and massive air embolus. In trained hands, bedside ultrasound will allow rapid diagnosis, differentiation, and treatment.

References

1. McGee DC, Gould MK. Preventing complications of central venous catheterization. *N Engl J Med* 2003; 348: 1123–33.

2. Kusminsky RE. Complications of central venous catheterization. *J Am Coll Surg* 2007; 204: 681–96.

3. Polderman KH, Girbes AR. Central venous catheter use Part 1: mechanical complications. *Intensive Care Med* 2002; 28: 1–17.

4. Merrer J, De Jonghe B, Golliot F, *et al.* Complications of femoral and subclavian venous catheterization in critically ill patients. *JAMA* 2001; 286: 700–7.

5. Timsit JF, Farkas JC, Boyer JM, *et al.* Central vein catheter-related thrombosis in intensive care patients: incidence, risk factors and relationship with catheter-related sepsis. *Chest* 1998; 114: 207–13.

6. Leung J, Duffy M, Finckh A. Real-time ultrasonographically-guided internal jugular vein catheterization in the emergency department increases success rates and reduces complications: a randomized, prospective study. *Ann Emerg Med* 2006; 48: 540–7.

7. Miller AH, Roth BA, Mills TJ, *et al.* Ultrasound guidance versus the landmark technique for the placement of central catheters in the emergency department. *Acad Emerg Med* 2002; 9: 800–5.

8. Fragou M, Gravvanis A, Dimitriou V, *et al.* Real-time ultrasound-guided subclavian vein cannulation versus the landmark method in critical care patients: a prospective randomized study. *Crit Care Med* 2011; 39: 1607–12.

9. Eisen LA, Narasimhan M, Berger JS, *et al.* Mechanical complications of central venous catheters. *J Intensive Care Med* 2006; 21: 40–6.

10. Sange M, Langrish CJ. Pneumothorax in the critially ill. In McLuckie A, ed. *Respiratory Disease and its Management*. London: Springer London; 2009: 73–8.

11. Carr JJ, Reed JC, Choplin RH, *et al.* Plain and computed radiography for detecting experimentally induced pneumothorax in cadavers: implications for detection in patients. *Radiology* 1992; 183: 193–9.

12. Wilkerson RG, Stone MB. Sensitivity of bedside ultrasound and supine anteroposterior chest radiographs for the identification of pneumothorax after blunt trauma. *Acad Emerg Med* 2010; 17: 11–17.

13. Xirouchaki N, Magkanas E, Vaporidi K, *et al*. Lung ultrasound in critically ill patients: comparison with bedside chest radiography. *Intensive Care Med* 2011; 37: 1488–93.

14. Ballarino GJ, Khosla R. Chest ultrasonography for the detection of post procedural iatrogenic pneumothorax. *Am J Respir Crit Care Med* 2010; 181: A4575.

15. Lin Y, Tu C, Liang S, *et al*. Pigtail catheter for the management of pneumothorax in mechanically ventilated patients. *Am J Emerg Med* 2010; 28: 466–71.

16. Cho S, Lee EB. Management of primary and secondary pneumothorax using a small bore thoracic catheter. *Interact Cardiovasc Thorac Surg* 2010; 11: 146–9.

17. Noppen M, De Keukeleire T. Pneumothorax. *Respiration* 2008; 76: 121–7.

18. Zehtabchi S, Rios CL. Management of emergency department patients with primary spontaneous pneumothorax: needle aspiration or tube thoracostomy? *Ann Emerg Med* 2008; 51: 91–100.

19. Moore FO, Goslar PW, Coimbra R, *et al*. Blunt traumatic occult pneumothorax: is observation safe? – results of a prospective, AAST multicenter study. *J Trauma* 2011; 70: 1019–25.

20. Guilbert M, Elkouri S, Bracco D, *et al*. Arterial trauma during central venous catheter insertion: case series, review, and proposed algorithm. *J Vasc Surg* 2008; 48: 918–25.

21. Nicholson T, Ettles D, Robinson G. Managing inadvertent arterial catheterization during central venous access procedures. *Cardiovasc Intervent Radiol* 2004; 27: 21–5.

22. Bodenham AR, Simcock L. Complications of central venous access. In Hamilton H, Bodenham AR, eds. *Central Venous Catheters*. Chichester: Wiley-Blackwell; 2009: 175–205.

23. Heath KJ, Woulfe J, Lownie S, *et al*. A devastating complication of inadvertent carotid artery puncture. *Anesthesiology* 1998; 89: 1273–5.

24. Zaida NA, Khan M, Naqvi HI, *et al*. Cerebral infarct following central venous cannulation. *Anaesthesia* 1990; 45: 458–9.

25. Ezaru CS, Mangione MP, Oravitz TM, *et al*. Eliminating arterial injury during central venous catheterization using manometry. *Anesth Analg* 2009; 109: 130–4.

26. Wicky S, Meuwly JY, Doenz F, *et al*. Life-threatening vascular complications after central venous catheter placement. *Eur Radiol* 2002; 12: 901–7.

27. Duntey P, Siever J, Korwes ML, *et al*. Vascular erosion by central venous catheters. Clinical features and outcome. *Chest* 1992; 101: 1633–8.

28. Vesely TM. Central venous catheter tip position: a continuing controversy. *J Vasc Interv Radiol* 2003; 14: 527–34.

29. Schuster M, Nave H, Piepenbrock S, *et al*. The carina as a landmark in central venous catheter placement. *Brit J Anaesth* 2000; 85: 192–4.

30. McEwen K, Thompson P. Ultrasound to detect haemothorax after chest injury. *Emerg Med J* 2007; 24: 581–2.

31. Yu H, Stavas JM, Dixon RG, *et al*. Temporary balloon tamponade for managing subclavian arterial injury by inadvertent central venous catheter placement. *J Vasc Interv Radiol* 2011; 22: 654–9.

32. Mirski MA, Lele AV, Fitzsimmons L, *et al*. Diagnosis and management of vascular air embolism. *Anesthesiology* 2007; 106: 164–77.

33. Frasca D, Dahyot-Fizelier C, Mimoz O. Prevention of central venous catheter-related infection in the intensive care unit. *Crit Care* 2010; 14: 212.

34. Han Z, Liang SY, Marschall J. Current strategies for the prevention and management of central line-associated bloodstream infections. *Infect Drug Resist* 2010; 3: 147–63.

35. Malinowski DJ, Ewing T, Patel MS, *et al*. The natural history of upper extremity deep venous thrombosis in critically ill surgical and trauma patients: what is the role of anticoagulation? *J Trauma* 2011; 71: 316–21.

Chapter

28

Complications of cardiac catheterization

James T. DeVries

Background

More than 1.3 million percutaneous coronary intervention (PCI) procedures were performed in the United States in 2010, with that number approximately doubling when worldwide PCIs are totaled.[1] Moreover, with minimally invasive vascular procedures rapidly replacing open surgical procedures, a growing number of non-coronary catheter-based procedures are being performed via endovascular means, including peripheral vascular interventions (non-cardiac angioplasty and stenting, embolizations, atherectomy), diagnostic angiograms, and electrophysiology-based procedures. As a result, a familiarity with complications related to endovascular procedures is important for emergency physicians and other acute care providers.

For the purposes of this chapter, endovascular complications will be considered as a group, with a particular focus on complications in the time period days to weeks post-cardiac catheterization. Complications related to catheterization can be divided into several broad categories, including access-site complications (pseudoaneurysm, vessel occlusion, arteriovenous fistula, hematoma, infection, chronic pain), dermatologic complications (delayed contrast reaction, clopidogrel hypersensitivity reactions, radiation skin burns), and "other" procedural complications (cholesterol embolization syndrome, acute stroke, acute stent thrombosis, cardiac tamponade, contrast-induced nephropathy).

Access-site complications

Diagnosis

Vascular access is a necessary requirement for endovascular procedures. As a result, many of the complications which may be seen in the emergency department following these procedures are related to vascular access. It is estimated that major bleeding occurs in about 5% of all cardiac catheterizations, with the majority of that bleeding occurring at the access site.[2] In the United States, the majority of cardiac catheterizations are performed via the femoral approach, utilizing the common femoral artery; whereas in other countries alternative access sites such as the radial artery are more commonly utilized. Radial artery catheterization has been shown to lower the risk of vascular access complications,[3] and as a result is growing in popularity in the United States. Access complications can be divided further into those involving bleeding, such as hematoma, pseudoaneurysm formation, and arteriovenous fistula (AVF). Other access-site complications include infections, thrombosis of the access site, or chronic pain syndromes which develop at the site of vascular access.

Vascular closure devices have been widely adopted for use following endovascular procedures, and allow for more rapid ambulation following femoral arterial access[4] when compared with manual hemostasis. All vascular closure devices leave foreign material either within the artery or in the skin dermotomy tract and as such have the potential to act as a nidus for infection. They can also cause pain at the access site which persists for days or even months post-procedure. Finally, if not deployed correctly, they can result in partial or total occlusion of the femoral artery and therefore cause claudication or acute limb ischemia (Figure 28.1).

History and physical examination

Patients who present with an access-site complication generally complain of pain, tenderness, or a palpable

Vascular Emergencies, ed. Robert L. Rogers, Thomas Scalea, Lee Wallis, and Heike Geduld. Published by Cambridge University Press. © Cambridge University Press 2013.

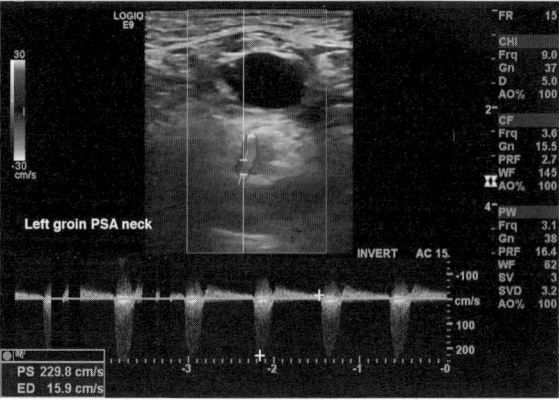

Figure 28.1 Duplex showing pseudoaneurysm (PSA) neck with "to and fro" Doppler flow pattern. (Image courtesy of Sarah Rust, RVT.) See plate section for color version.

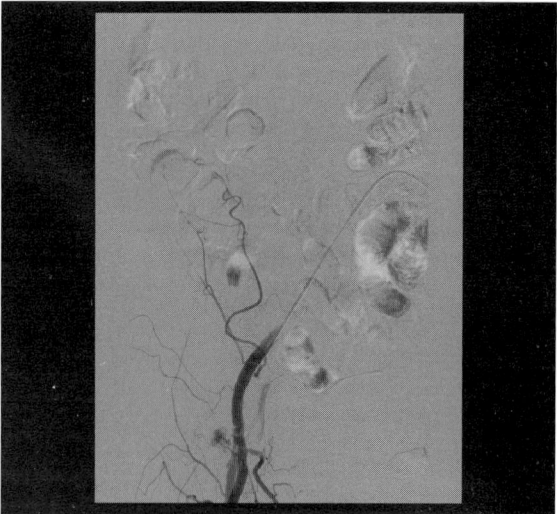

Figure 28.2 Angiogram demonstrating right common femoral pseudoaneurysm (PSA).

lump at the access site. Other associated symptoms to elicit include recent fever, erythema, frank bleeding, sudden pain in the groin (may represent late closure-device failure), or new claudication symptoms in the ipsilateral leg. Often there is extensive ecchymosis which can extend into the soft tissues of the affected leg. Important questions regarding the procedure include the timing relative to presentation and if a vascular closure device was used. Bleeding risks are higher for patients who underwent an intervention (stent insertion or angioplasty) versus a diagnostic procedure, because interventions require full systemic anticoagulation to prevent catheter thrombosis during coronary vessel manipulation, and also typically require dual antiplatelet therapy post-procedure. If the procedure was performed locally, it is very helpful to obtain a copy of the procedure report, which can contain details the patient may not recall regarding access-site manipulation, including sheath size (larger sheath sizes result in a higher risk of bleeding complications), anticoagulation used, and mechanism of vessel closure. The differential diagnosis for access-site complication includes the following: hematoma, active bleeding (including retroperitoneal), pseudoaneurysm, AVF, arterial thrombosis, infection, and femoral nerve injury.

Physical examination findings should include a full set of vital signs. A fever should raise suspicion of access-site infection. Tachycardia with or without hypotension may be associated with active bleeding and is cause for immediate stabilization with volume resuscitation, large-bore venous access, and blood product matching. Pulses should be documented in

all four extremities and any differences in the affected limb noted. Examination of the access site should include inspection, palpation, and auscultation. If a hematoma is present, it should be traced on the surface of the skin and the diameter measured. Anything larger than 5 cm diameter needs very close monitoring for signs of expansion and hemodynamic instability. Erythema surrounding the access site, particularly when streaking or associated regional lymphadenopathy is present, can indicate infection. On palpation, the area should feel soft to touch with no surrounding firmness which indicates hematoma formation. A firm, pea-sized lump at the access site can be normal for several weeks following the procedure, but anything larger than a walnut-sized lump over the access site is a cause for concern and may indicate the presence of a pseudoaneurysm. Significant tenderness to light pressure is indicative of pseudoaneurysm, as is a bruit heard over the access site. AVF may be asymptomatic or associated with a thrill and bruit, depending on size. Lack of a pulse at the access site or distal to the access site is highly suggestive of vessel thrombosis (Figure 28.2). In patients with a radial access site, the radial artery and ulnar artery provide parallel blood flow to the hand, and roughly 5 to 10% of patients will occlude the radial artery post-procedure.[5] Normally this is asymptomatic, provided the patient has adequate collateral flow via the ulnar artery. Infection and pseudoaneurysm are very uncommon following radial artery access.[6]

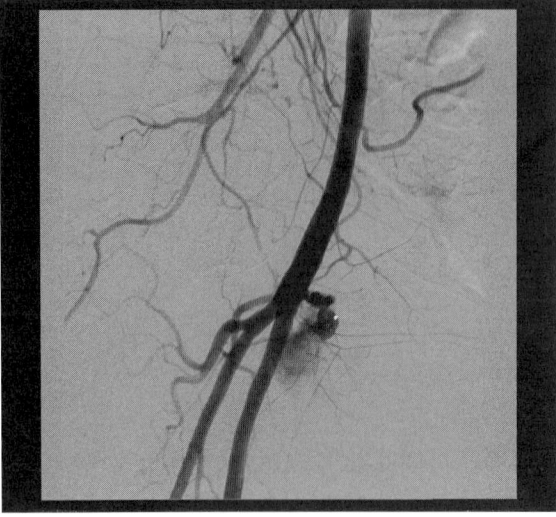

Figure 28.3 Ruptured pseudoaneurysm (PSA) with active bleeding.

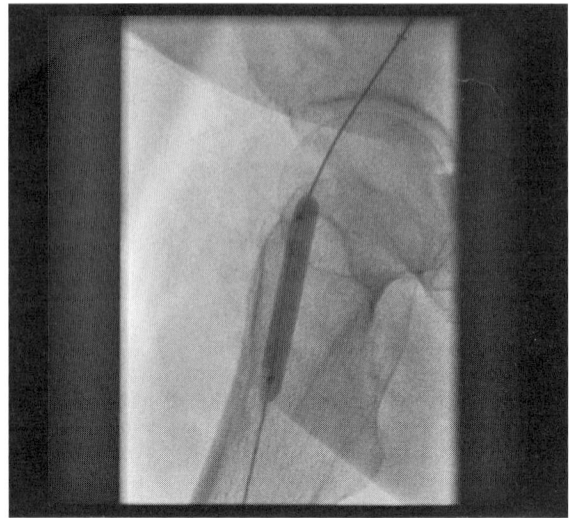

Figure 28.4 Balloon occlusion of common femoral artery to control access-site bleeding.

Laboratory and imaging

Basic blood work should include a complete blood count, basic metabolic panel, and PT/INR for all patients. For those with suspicion of infection, blood cultures should be ordered as well. Patients who are hypotensive with suspected active bleeding should be typed and screened for blood products.

The imaging of choice to assess an access-site complication is vascular duplex. This allows rapid and safe (radiation-free) interrogation of the vascular bundle for diagnosis of pseudoaneurysm, AVF, and arterial or venous thrombosis (Figure 28.3). Because ultrasound imaging above the inguinal ligament and in the retroperitoneal space is difficult, if bleeding into the retroperitoneal space is suspected, a CT scan without contrast can allow for rapid visualization (Figure 28.4). A Doppler probe can be used to assess for distal pulses in a patient who has non-palpable pedal pulses, and can be used to calculate an ankle-brachial index (ABI) at the bedside, which allows quantification of the degree of blood-flow obstruction to the foot.

Emergency department management

Emergency department management should focus on stabilization of an actively bleeding patient. Any hematoma with active bleeding (externally or internally) should have manual pressure applied to the site

to control the bleeding. Frequent vital signs, large-bore IV access, and hemodynamic support with crystalloid and blood products should be given. Coagulopathies should be corrected with blood products as needed. If a diagnosis of pseudoaneurysm is made, options in management include serial observation if small (< 1 cm diameter), or ultrasound-guided manual compression in the emergency department. Arteriovenous fistulas rarely require intervention and can safely be conservatively managed in most cases, with only extremely high-flow AVFs requiring surgical repair. Clues to presence of high-flow fistulas include a palpable thrill and significantly diminished arterial pulse in the distal vasculature due to shunting. If femoral artery occlusion is suspected or diagnosed, consultation with the local endovascular care provider (vascular surgery, interventional radiology, interventional cardiology) should be obtained, and the patient should be started on intravenous heparin (bolus 50–70 units/kg IV then infuse to target PTT of 60–90 seconds) in the interim, in preparation for revascularization (Figure 28.5). Importantly, bedside Doppler probes are inadequate to make the diagnosis of AVF or pseudoaneurysm, as color flow imaging is crucial for detection.

Infection of an access site, particularly one where a closure device was used, mandates immediate IV antibiotic administration and admission for observation and possible surgical debridement. Skin flora in

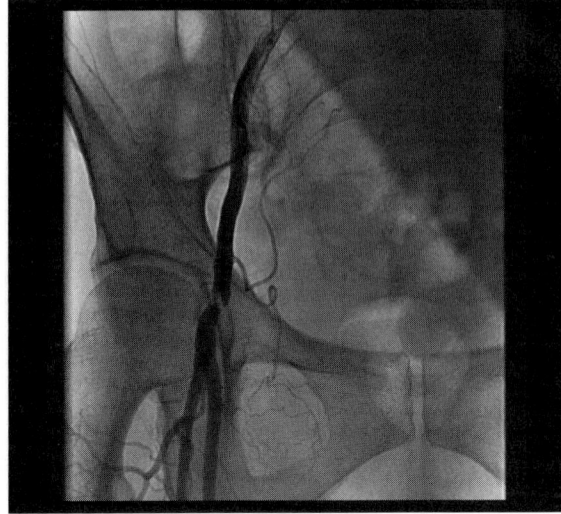

Figure 28.5 Angiogram demonstrating subtotal occlusion of common femoral artery after failed closure device.

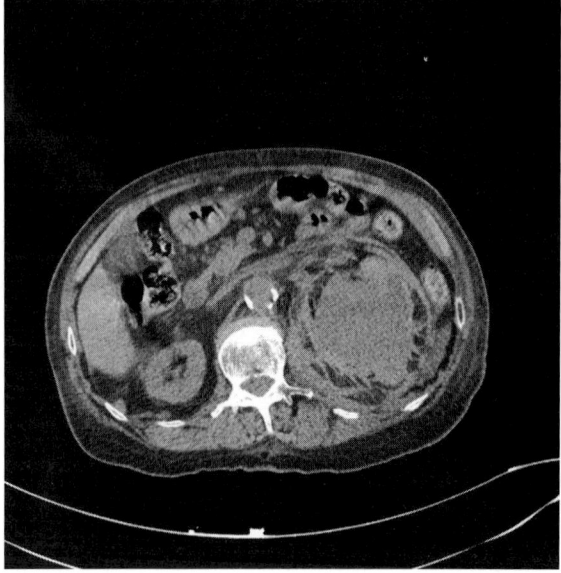

Figure 28.6 CT scan demonstrating retroperitoneal hemorrhage in the area of the left kidney.

addition to Gram-negative bacteria are the usual culprits, so antibiotics should be adequately broad to treat these organisms, keeping in mind local resistance patterns. Because of the serious nature of vascular infection, these patients must be triaged and treated rapidly to prevent irreversible complications including limb loss.

Because manipulation of the groin vasculature is inherently painful, it is important to be mindful of adequate analgesia during diagnosis and treatment of groin complications. Intravenous narcotics such as fentanyl often provide adequate pain control in appropriate patients.

Definitive therapy

Definitive therapy for a pseudoaneurysm involves a careful and slow thrombin injection directly into the pseudoaneurysm. Direct pressure can also be attempted in situations where thrombin injection is not readily available or the pseudoaneurysm is small in size (< 1 cm). To accomplish successful compression, occlusive pressure is held over the pseudoaneurysm for at least 20 minutes to attempt to induce thrombosis, after providing adequate sedation and pain control for the patient. This effectively seals the cavity and prevents further expansion and possible rupture. Very large pseudoaneurysms (> 3 cm) often do not respond to direct pressure or thrombin injection and may require open surgical repair. AVFs rarely require

surgical repair unless there is very high flow documented by duplex ultrasound, which can cause distal limb ischemia or high-output heart failure from shunting. If other groin bleeding (expanding hematoma) or retroperitoneal bleeding cannot be controlled via direct pressure, either surgical exploration for vascular control or endovascular balloon occlusion may be required (Figure 28.6). If no surgical or endovascular back up is immediately available, the patient should be immediately triaged to a tertiary care facility.

Femoral artery occlusion is typically approached via the contralateral femoral artery, which permits cross-over angiography to confirm the diagnosis and allow for endovascular or surgical approaches to management.[7] Following stabilization, these patients are admitted for observation and documentation of normal flow in the femoral artery.

Pearls and pitfalls

- Pseudoaneurysm formation is more commonly seen in patients taking systemic anticoagulants, such as warfarin, dabigatran, enoxaparin, or dual antiplatelet therapy.
- Infection with a known closure device mandates an aggressive approach with IV antibiotics and admission for infected foreign body.
- Vascular duplex is the modality of choice for diagnosing most access-site complications.

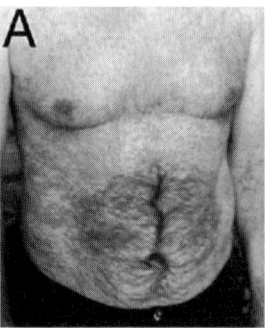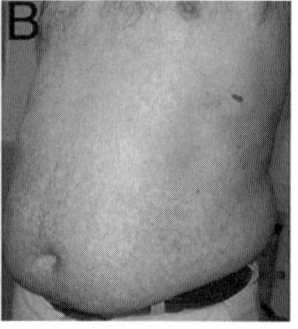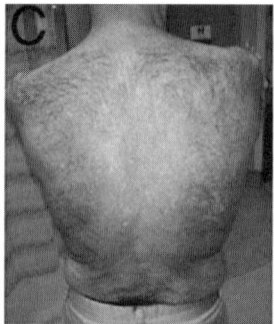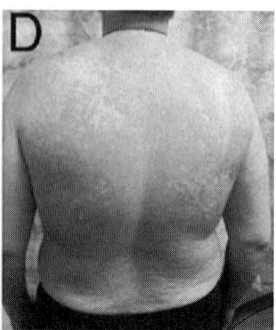

Figure 28.7 (A–D) Clopidogrel hypersensitivity rash in four patients.

Dermatologic complications

Diagnosis

Patients who undergo catheterization are by default exposed to ionizing radiation and iodinated contrast, both of which are necessary for visualization of the arterial anatomy. In addition, patients with myocardial infarction are often discharged on multiple new medications, including a thienopyridine such as clopidogrel, which is important in the medical management of heart attack.[8] Both intravenous contrast and thienopyridines are well known for causing rash several days after exposure. As a result, it is not uncommon for patients to present to the emergency department with a new rash a few days after catheterization. Because the skin manifestations and timing of each reaction are very similar, the etiology of the rash can often be difficult to diagnose. Radiation-induced skin burns are now a recognized late complication of radiographic procedures, particularly ones which involve lengthy amounts of fluoroscopic imaging.

Late adverse reactions to contrast media are defined as reactions occurring one hour to one week following exposure to the agent,[9] with most occurring within three days of exposure.[10] While these reactions can manifest in multiple ways, such as nausea, headache, fever, and muscular pain, the most common presentation is skin rash. It is estimated that the incidence of late reactions following contrast exposure is between 2% and 4%.[11] The typical findings on examination include maculopapular rash, erythema, and pruritus. The rash can present in a variety of locations, but tends to be located on the trunk and arms preferentially. Most late reactions to contrast are mild and self-limiting, and resolve with conservative therapy within seven days.[12]

Hypersensitivity reactions to clopidogrel are well described in the literature. Recent data have suggested that clopidogrel hypersensitivity occurs in less than 2% of patients who are exposed to the drug.[13] Three distinct clinical patterns of presentation occur, with the vast majority (80%) of patients presenting with a generalized pruritic rash on the trunk and extremities (Figure 28.7). These patients present an average of five days post-exposure, while patients who present with angioedema (5%) tend to present within one day of exposure. There is also a subset of patients (15%) who present with localized rash in discreet areas of the body. The histological process is a lymphocyte-mediated delayed hypersensitivity reaction.[13] It is crucially important to avoid stopping clopidogrel in the setting of a recent coronary stent, because early discontinuation of clopidogrel post-stenting is highly correlated with stent thrombosis, which carries a high risk of morbidity and mortality.[14] Switching to an alternative thienopyridine such as ticlopidine or prasugrel is not always feasible because of a high likelihood of cross-reactivity.[15]

Radiation-induced skin burns are a rare but important complication of fluoroscopic procedures (Figure 28.8). As coronary and other vascular procedures have become more complex, the amount of radiation which is delivered to patients has increased. Case reports have highlighted the potential for radiation-induced skin necrosis, which can be difficult to diagnose, difficult to treat, and ripe for litigation.[16] Factors which contribute to the development of radiation burns include the amount of radiation delivered, the size of the patient, and the amount the radiation beam was varied in projection. Typically, the first sign of radiation burn occurs one week following the procedure, with local erythema in the shape of the X-ray

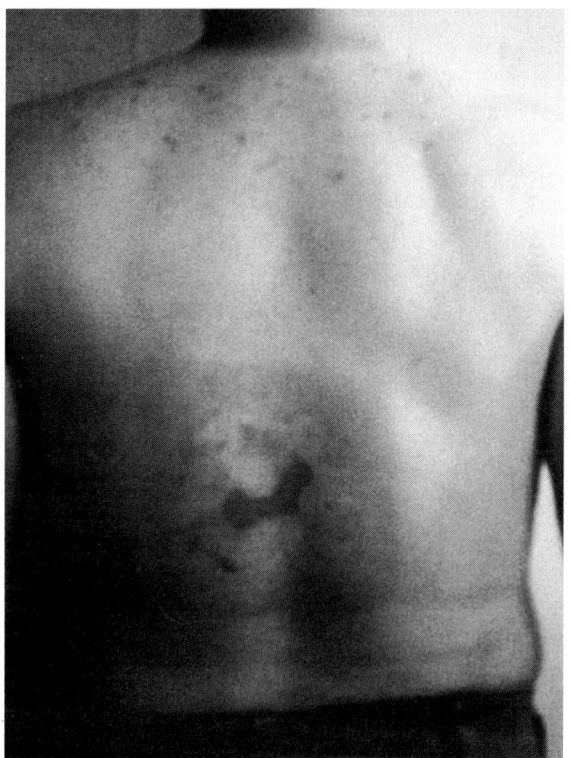

Figure 28.8 Radiation-induced skin burn. (Downloaded from: http://www.fda.gov/Radiation-EmittingProducts/ RadiationEmittingProductsandProcedures/MedicalImaging/ MedicalX-Rays/ucm116682.htm.) See plate section for color version.

generator at the location of beam entry to the patient (frequently the back).[17] The peak effects usually develop around three to six weeks post-procedure, and can result in pain, erythema, and skin necrosis. Patients with diabetes mellitus and known connective tissue disorders may be at particularly high risk. Key factors which can help make the diagnosis are the location and shape (typically the upper back and the same shape as the X-ray generator), the timing (one to six weeks post-procedure), and a history of a lengthy fluoroscopic time during a single procedure (will be noted in the procedure report). Multiple fluoroscopic procedures in a short timeframe can have the same effect.

History and physical

When taking a history from a patient with a new skin finding, there are several important questions. First, the timing of the procedure relative to presentation is crucial. Delayed contrast reactions tend to occur the earliest, at an average of one to three days post-procedure. Clopidogrel hypersensitivity reactions occur around five days post-procedure, and can manifest very similarly to contrast reactions in appearance. A careful medication history is important to verify that no other new medications were started at the time of the procedure. A high suspicion is necessary for correctly diagnosing skin burns, as there may not be an obvious connection to the procedure due to their delayed presentation (one to six weeks post-procedure). Any airway compromise suggests a more severe reaction, and is not likely to be related to a delayed contrast reaction or clopidogrel hypersensitivity.

Physical examination findings for both delayed contrast reaction and clopidogrel hypersensitivity reaction are similar: a diffuse maculopapular rash on the trunk and extremities. It is pruritic and blanches to direct pressure. There is no associated fever, tachycardia, or tachypnea. Radiation skin burns present as very focal areas of erythema and tenderness. They have discrete edges which have the shape of the beam from the X-ray generator. They are usually located on the mid to upper back region, or whichever area was closest to the X-ray generator.

Laboratory and imaging

A complete blood count can be helpful to rule out other processes, but is not necessary to make the diagnosis. There is no imaging which is required. Biopsy of an equivocal rash in the emergency department is rarely helpful and is not recommended.

Emergency department management

Supportive care for delayed contrast reactions, using oral antihistamines and topical steroids as required to treat the pruritus, which can be particularly bothersome at night when patients are trying to sleep. Clopidogrel hypersensitivity should be treated with a three-week course of steroids, starting at a dose of 30 mg of prednisone twice daily for five days. Clopidogrel should not be discontinued in patients with a recent cardiac stent, because discontinuation of dual antiplatelet therapy can result in stent thrombosis. Antihistamines can also be prescribed depending on the severity of pruritus. Diphenhydramine at a dose of 25–50 mg orally every 4–6 hours is usually sufficient for the first 24–48 hours, at which time the dosing frequency can be decreased. Patients who present with either of these conditions can be safely discharged to home, with outpatient follow-up in three to five days to assess for recovery.

For patients with suspected radiation-induced skin burns, topical agents should not be used. They can be treated with oral analgesics for pain control and referred to a dermatology or burn care physician for further follow-up. Biopsy should not be performed, to avoid inadequate healing at the site. These patients can also be discharged from the emergency department, provided adequate outpatient follow-up can be arranged.

Definitive therapy

Patients with severe radiation-induced skin burns may require skin grafting for adequate healing and should be referred to local skin-care experts for close follow-up. Because of the late presentation, these rashes do not require acute admission to burn units.

Pearls and pitfalls

- Do not stop clopidogrel or aspirin in patients with a recent cardiac stent, as this can lead to subacute stent thrombosis.
- Most patients with clopidogrel rash can be managed with oral steroids and continuation of clopidogrel.
- Delayed contrast reactions are self-limited and occur one hour to one week post-exposure.
- Radiation-induced skin burns are difficult to diagnose because of late presentation and require a high index of suspicion.

Cholesterol embolization syndrome

Diagnosis and management

Cholesterol embolization syndrome, or systemic atheroembolization syndrome, is caused by release of 100–200 μm cholesterol emboli from the arterial vessel walls due to endovascular instrumentation. It is a well-described complication of catheterization which can result from guide catheter trauma to the plaque-lined vessel wall, cardiac surgery, or spontaneously after fibrinolytic therapy in patients with severely atheromatous aortas.[18,19] The timeframe for presentation is immediately after or within one to two days of instrumentation, although it can also occur spontaneously with no instrumentation.

Overall incidence is estimated to be less than 1% of all patients undergoing catheterization; although incidence can vary dramatically depending on patient subset. Patients with known severe vascular disease, "shaggy" thoracic aortas, and abdominal aneurysm with thrombus are presumed to be at higher risk.

History and physical

The clinical sequelae vary widely, from no symptoms to multiorgan failure. The most commonly affected organs are the abdominal viscera, the kidneys, and the skin of the lower extremities. The classic presentation is livedo reticularis with acrocyanosis of the legs and feet.[20] The syndrome is often referred to as "blue toe syndrome" because of the blue discoloration which can develop in the distal digits, typically the toes. Distal pulses are usually maintained, as the emboli tend to be in small vessels of the skin. There is not typically pain in the affected toes.

Laboratory and imaging

Laboratory measurement can demonstrate elevated serum creatinine indicative of renal failure, leukocytosis, and eosinophilia. There is no specific imaging test which is helpful in making the diagnosis. Eosinophilia is one of the hallmarks of this disease and is usually present to varying degrees. More severe cases which involve the gut or other visceral organs can present in shock with severe acidosis.

Emergency department management

Management in the ED is largely supportive. Because the presentation can range from asymptomatic blue toes to multiorgan failure, there is no overall guidance algorithm. Mild cases with little systemic involvement can be discharged to home; while more severe cases require inpatient admission for monitoring and support. Critical care admission is required for patients with diffuse showering of emboli and multiorgan failure.

Definitive therapy

Skin biopsy can confirm the diagnosis by demonstrating cholesterol crystals in the small vessels of the dermis. There is no definitive treatment for cholesterol embolization syndrome, and treatment is supportive. Multiple therapies have shown promise in small case series, such as low-density lipoprotein apheresis,[21] iloprost vasodilator therapy,[22] or steroids with high-dose statin therapy.[23] The need for admission and inpatient management is determined by the degree of systemic compromise, with some patients requiring renal replacement therapy or hemodynamic support due to multiorgan failure. In general, additional arterial endovascular procedures should be avoided in this patient population.

Pearls and pitfalls

- Cholesterol embolization syndrome often presents with blue toes, livedo reticularis, and eosinophilia.

Acute stroke and acute myocardial infarction

Acute stroke and acute myocardial infarction from stent thrombosis can both occur following catheterization. Both of these conditions are commonly seen in the ED setting, and treatment does not vary significantly from the "standard" therapy just because of recent catheterization. The etiology of acute stroke when temporally close to catheterization is very likely to be embolic, typically from a plaque-liberated embolus which was disrupted by catheter manipulation in the ascending aorta or aortic arch. Depending on the degree of impairment, activation of the stroke team may be appropriate for consideration of advanced therapies including thrombolysis or catheter-facilitated reperfusion.[24,25] Timing of symptom onset is crucial in stroke evaluation, and patients who present within three hours of symptom onset have the highest chances of receiving benefit from acute reperfusion therapies.

Patients with recent coronary stent placement are at risk for subacute stent thrombosis, defined as stent thrombosis within 24 hours to 30 days post-implantation. Risks factors for subacute thrombosis include low ejection fraction, renal failure, cardiogenic shock, and lack of dual antiplatelet therapy.[26,27] These patients typically present with chest pain and ST elevation on the electrocardiogram. Mortality for this patient subset can be as high as 25%, so expedited care is crucial.[28] Management should follow local practices for coronary reperfusion, including rapid triage to a PCI-capable catheterization laboratory or administration of intravenous thrombolysis.

History and physical

History for stroke or acute stent thrombosis should focus on the timing of symptom onset. Patients benefit the most from advanced therapies if they present within three hours of symptom onset for stroke and six hours of symptom onset with acute MI. Any relative or absolute contraindications to thrombolysis should be quickly assessed, such as recent major surgeries, history of intracranial bleeding, intracranial neoplasm, or active bleeding. For stroke patients, a quantitative stroke scale should be used to assess the degree of impairment, such as the National Institutes of Health Stroke Scale (NIHSS).[29]

Laboratory and imaging

Lab work should include a complete blood count and metabolic panel including renal function. Coagulation panel should also be obtained in preparation for possible thrombolytic therapy. An ECG is diagnostic for ST-elevation myocardial infarction, and should be obtained in all patients with chest pain. For patients with suspected stroke, an emergent non-contrast head CT should be obtained to evaluate for intracranial hemorrhage or other mass effect which would disqualify the patient from consideration of reperfusion therapies.

Emergency department management

Rapid assessment and triage is crucial for patients with acute stroke or acute MI. In both cases, time delays can directly impact patient outcomes. Once the diagnosis is suspected, calls should be made to the appropriate consultant, such as the neurology stroke team or cardiology interventional team. If these resources do not exist locally, either telephone consultation or transfer to a medical center with capability for acute management of ischemic stroke or acute MI should be made. For most ischemic stroke patients, systolic blood pressure should be maintained between 150 and 160 mmHg systolic to facilitate cerebral perfusion.

Patients with acute MI should be monitored on telemetry and have standard cardiac therapies, including oxygen therapy, nitrates as needed, and antiplatelet therapy with aspirin, administered. Antithrombin therapy with IV unfractionated heparin or low-molecular-weight heparin should be administered while awaiting definitive therapy, depending on local practice. Triage to the cardiac catheterization lab should be expedited. If not available, reperfusion therapy with IV thrombolytics should be delivered according to local practice.

Definitive therapy

Definitive therapy for acute stroke in appropriate patients includes IV thrombolysis in conjunction with monitoring on a stroke care unit.[30,31] Certain patient subsets may benefit from catheter-directed reperfusion techniques, depending on local availability.[32,33] For patients with acute MI, catheterization is the standard of care, with rapid reperfusion of the culprit artery. These patients are typically admitted to a critical-care-level bed for the initial phase of their hospitalization following successful catheter-based reperfusion.

Cardiac tamponade

Cardiac tamponade is a clinical diagnosis which presents with hypotension, elevated jugular venous pressure, and muffled heart sounds (Beck's triad). It is a potential complication of cardiac interventional procedures, including coronary intervention and permanent pacemaker or ICD (implantable cardioverter defibrillator) placement. It can be seen days or even weeks following pacer implantation, and may present gradually or abruptly. Typically the mechanism is slow leak into the pericardial space from an active fixation lead which perforates the thin-walled myocardium of the right ventricular free wall or right atrial wall. The physiologic process involves compression of the cardiac chambers by fluid in the surrounding pericardial space, which leads to compromise of cardiac inflow and equalization of diastolic pressures in the heart.[34] The clinical spectrum of presentation can vary widely, from cough, to anorexia, to tachypnea and air hunger, to syncope.[35]

History and physical

Physical examination findings generally include tachycardia, hypotension, distal heart sounds, and marked distension of the neck veins; interestingly, a friction rub is generally not heard.[36] Pulsus paradoxus is a key finding, and is defined as an inspiratory fall in systolic blood pressure by 10 to 15 mmHg during normal breathing.[37] This can be difficult to assess in patients who are profoundly tachypneic or hypotensive. Tamponade is a continuum, and presentation can vary between mild hypotension to overt cardiogenic shock, depending on where a patient is along the spectrum.

Laboratory and imaging

Findings on imaging studies include an enlarged cardiac silhouette with clear lung fields on chest X-ray, and low voltage, tachycardia, and electric alternans on ECG. The diagnostic test of choice is transthoracic echocardiogram, which will allow visualization of the pericardial effusion and can reveal echocardiographic signs of tamponade such as sustained right atrial collapse and widely varied mitral inflow velocities.[38] Labs should be collected, including coagulation parameters, in preparation for pericardial drainage.

Emergency department management

Treatment for symptomatic tamponade is immediate pericardiocentesis, which relieves the pericardial pressure to allow for normalization of the cardiac function and recovery of hypotension. While preparing for pericardiocentesis, IV fluids (normal saline) should be given to help stabilize blood pressure, and coagulopathies can be reversed if time permits.

Definitive therapy

Definitive therapy for pericardial tamponade is drainage of the pericardial space, which relieves the constriction and allows for normalization of cardiac function. This is typically achieved via a standard subxyphoid approach, using an 18- or 20-gauge needle directed toward the left mid-axillary line just below the costal margin. Once the pericardial space is entered, a wire is placed through the needle into the pericardial space and a small fenestrated drain is tracked over the wire and used to drain the pericardial space. Hemodynamic function is usually restored quickly as pericardial pressure is relieved. Depending on the etiology of the effusion, the drain can be left in place for several days to ensure adequate resolution of the effusion.

Contrast nephropathy

Contrast-induced nephropathy (CIN), which is now also referred to as contrast-induced acute kidney injury, is the third leading cause of acute kidney injury in hospitalized patients and affects patient morbidity and overall mortality. It is defined as an increase in serum creatinine $> 25\%$ above baseline or $> 0.5 \, mg/dL$ within 48 hours after contrast administration.[39] For ED physicians, it is important to recognize that patients are often discharged to home the same day or one day following coronary procedures, and as such are not in the hospital at the 48–72 hour timeframe when the peak incidence of CIN occurs. Risk calculators have demonstrated that the risk of contrast nephropathy increases with diabetes, contrast volume, baseline renal function, and hypotension at the time of contrast administration.[40] Patients typically have no symptoms with CIN, but it remains an important predictor of long-term survival and is important to document, as further contrast exposure should be avoided in this patient population. The majority of patients with CIN will recover renal function with supportive care and avoidance of nephrotoxic agents.

History and physical

History in contrast nephropathy should focus on the timing of recent contrast exposure from catheterization, keeping in mind that the peak incidence occurs 48–72 hours post-exposure. Risk factors for CIN should be assessed, including presence of diabetes, history of renal dysfunction, and contrast volume used for procedure, which should be available in the procedure report. Patients should be questioned about urine output, as falling urine output may herald anuric renal failure which prompts a more aggressive approach.

Laboratory and imaging

A basic metabolic panel including renal function is necessary to diagnose acute kidney injury. Urinalysis typically shows epithelial cell casts and non-specific debris, but can show eosinophiluria.[41] No specific imaging is diagnostic, although retained contrast in the renal system (persistent nephrogram) can be suggestive of contrast nephropathy.

Emergency department management

Management in the ED is largely supportive, and admission may be required in certain cases for monitoring of electrolytes and recovery of renal function. Importantly, contrast exposure from other diagnostic testing should be avoided in this patient population.

Definitive therapy

Most cases of contrast-induced nephropathy resolve spontaneously in 5 to 10 days, but patients can progress to permanent renal dysfunction and need for dialysis. Functionally, these patients should be managed in the same manner as other patients with acute renal failure.

Pearls and pitfalls

- Contrast-induced nephropathy is a marker for increased mortality, and its incidence peaks 48–72 hours post-contrast exposure.

References

1. Levine GN, Bates ER, Blankenship JC, *et al*. 2011 ACCF/AHA/SCAI Guideline for Percutaneous Coronary Intervention: Executive Summary: a report of the American College of Cardiology Foundation/American Heart Association Task Force on Practice Guidelines and the Society for Cardiovascular Angiography and Interventions. *J Am Coll Cardiol* 2011; 58(24): 2550–83.

2. Budaj A, Eikelboom JW, Mehta SR, *et al*. Improving clinical outcomes by reducing bleeding in patients with non-ST-elevation acute coronary syndromes. *Eur Heart J* 2009; 30(6): 655–61.

3. Jolly SS, Yusuf S, Cairns J, *et al*. Radial versus femoral access for coronary angiography and intervention in patients with acute coronary syndromes (RIVAL): a randomised, parallel group, multicentre trial. *Lancet* 2011; 377(9775): 1409–20.

4. Shroff A. Vascular access closure devices: in search of "perfect" closure. *J Invasive Cardiol* 2011; 23(4): 156.

5. Agostoni P, Biondi-Zoccai GG, de Benedictis ML, *et al*. Radial versus femoral approach for percutaneous coronary diagnostic and interventional procedure: systematic overview and meta-analysis of randomized trials. *J Am Coll Cardiol* 2004; 44(2): 349–56.

6. Rao SV, Ou FS, Wang TY, *et al*. Trends in the prevalence and outcomes of radial and femoral approaches to percutaneous coronary intervention: a report from the National Cardiovascular Data Registry. *JACC Cardiovasc Interv* 2008; 1(4): 379–86.

7. Kiernan TJ, Ajani AE, Yan BP. Management of access site and systemic complications of percutaneous coronary and peripheral interventions. *J Invasive Cardiol* 2008; 20(9): 463–9.

8. Yusuf S, Zhao F, Mehta SR, *et al*. Effects of clopidogrel in addition to aspirin in patients with acute coronary syndromes without ST-segment elevation. *N Engl J Med* 2001; 345(7): 494–502.

9. Bellin MF, Stacul F, Webb JA, *et al*. Late adverse reactions to intravascular iodine based contrast media: an update. *Eur Radiol* 2011; 21(11): 2305–10.

10. Hosoya T, Yamaguchi K, Akutsu T, *et al*. Delayed adverse reactions to iodinated contrast media and their risk factors. *Radiat Med* 2000; 18(1): 39–45.

11. Namasivayam S, Kalra MK, Torres WE, Small WC. Adverse reactions to intravenous iodinated contrast media: a primer for radiologists. *Emerg Radiol* 2006; 12(5): 210–5.

12. Idée JM, Pinès E, Prigent P, Corot C. Allergy-like reactions to iodinated contrast agents. A critical analysis. *Fundam Clin Pharmacol* 2005; 19(3): 263–81.

13. Cheema AN, Mohammad A, Hong T, *et al*. Characterization of clopidogrel hypersensitivity reactions and management with oral steroids without clopidogrel discontinuation. *J Am Coll Cardiol* 2011; 58(14): 1445–54.

14. Iakovou I, Schmidt T, Bonizzoni E, *et al*. Incidence, predictors, and outcome of thrombosis after successful implantation of drug-eluting stents. *JAMA* 2005; 293(17): 2126–30.

15. Lokhandwala JO, Best PJ, Butterfield JH, *et al*. Frequency of allergic or hematologic adverse reactions to ticlopidine among patients with allergic or hematologic adverse reactions to clopidogrel. *Circ Cardiovasc Interv* 2009; 2(4): 348–51.

16. Berlin L. Radiation-induced skin injuries and fluoroscopy. *AJR Am J Roentgenol* 2001; 177(1): 21–5.

17. Wagner LK, Eifel PJ, Geise RA. Potential biological effects following high X-ray dose interventional procedures. *J Vasc Interv Radiol* 1994; 5(1): 71–84.

18. Enomae M, Takeda S, Yoshimoto K, Takagawa K. Chronic cholesterol crystal embolism with a spontaneous onset. *Intern Med* 2007; 46(14): 1123–6.

19. Fukumoto Y, Tsutsui H, Tsuchihashi M, *et al*. The incidence and risk factors of cholesterol embolization syndrome, a complication of cardiac catheterization: a prospective study. *J Am Coll Cardiol* 2003; 42(2): 211–16.

20. Fukumoto Y, Tsutsui H, Tsuchihashi M, Masumoto A, Takeshita A. 3P-0867 The incidence and risk factors of cholesterol embolization syndrome, a complication of cardiac catheterization: a prospective study. *Atheroscler Suppl* 2003; 4(2): 252.

21. Tsunoda S, Daimon S, Miyazaki R, *et al*. LDL apheresis as intensive lipid-lowering therapy for cholesterol embolism. *Nephrol Dial Transplant* 1999; 14(4): 1041–2.

22. Elinav E, Chajek-Shaul T, Stern M. Improvement in cholesterol emboli syndrome after iloprost therapy. *BMJ* 2002; 324(7332): 268–9.

23. Matsumura T, Matsumoto A, Ohno M, *et al*. A case of cholesterol embolism confirmed by skin biopsy and successfully treated with statins and steroids. *Am J Med Sci* 2006; 331(5): 280–3.

24. Mathews MS, Sharma J, Snyder KV, *et al*. Safety, effectiveness, and practicality of endovascular therapy within the first 3 hours of acute ischemic stroke onset. *Neurosurgery* 2009; 65(5): 860–5; discussion 865.

25. Khatri P, Taylor RA, Palumbo V, *et al*. The safety and efficacy of thrombolysis for strokes after cardiac catheterization. *J Am Coll Cardiol* 2008; 51(9): 906–11.

26. Dangas GD, Caixeta A, Mehran R, *et al*. Frequency and predictors of stent thrombosis after percutaneous coronary intervention in acute myocardial infarction. *Circulation* 2011; 123(16): 1745–56.

27. Zhu ZB, Zhang RY, Zhang Q, *et al*. Moderate-severe renal insufficiency is a risk factor for sirolimus-eluting stent thrombosis. The RIFT study. *Cardiology* 2009; 112(3): 191–9.

28. Biondi-Zoccai GG, Sangiorgi GM, Chieffo A, *et al*. Validation of predictors of intraprocedural stent thrombosis in the drug-eluting stent era. *Am J Cardiol* 2005; 95(12): 1466–8.

29. The Internet Stroke Center. Stroke assessment scales: NIH stroke scale (NIHSS). Available at www.strokecenter.org/trials/scales/nihss.html. Accessed on September 30, 2012.

30. Hacke W, Kaste M, Bluhmki E, *et al*. Thrombolysis with alteplase 3 to 4.5 hours after acute ischemic stroke. *N Engl J Med* 2008; 359(13): 1317–29.

31. Furlan AJ, Katzan IL, Caplan LR. Thrombolytic therapy in acute ischemic stroke. *Curr Treat Options Cardiovasc Med* 2003; 5(3): 171–80.

32. Edgell R, Yavagal DR. Acute endovascular stroke therapy. *Curr Neurol Neurosci Rep* 2006; 6(6): 531–8.

33. DeVries JT, White CJ, Cunningham MC, Ramee SR. Catheter-based therapy for acute ischemic stroke: a national unmet need. *Catheter Cardiovasc Interv* 2008; 72(5): 705–9.

34. Spodick DH. Acute cardiac tamponade. *N Engl J Med* 2003; 349(7): 684–90.

35. Cooper JP, Oliver RM, Currie P, Walker JM, Swanton RH. How do the clinical findings in patients with pericardial effusions influence the success of aspiration? *Br Heart J* 1995; 73(4): 351–4.

36. Spodick DH. Pericardial rub. Prospective, multiple observer investigation of pericardial friction in 100 patients. *Am J Cardiol* 1975; 35(3): 357–62.

37. Shabetai R. Pericardial and cardiac pressure. *Circulation* 1988; 77(1): 1–5.

38. Pepi M, Muratori M. Echocardiography in the diagnosis and management of pericardial disease.

J Cardiovasc Med (Hagerstown) 2006; 7(7): 533–44.

39. Rundback JH, Nahl D, Yoo V. Contrast-induced nephropathy. *J Vasc Surg* 2011; 54(2): 575–9.

40. Mehran R, Aymong ED, Nikolsky E, *et al.* A simple risk score for prediction of contrast-induced nephropathy after percutaneous coronary intervention: development and initial validation. *J Am Coll Cardiol* 2004; 44(7): 1393–9.

41. Tublin ME, Murphy ME, Tessler FN. Current concepts in contrast media-induced nephropathy. *AJR Am J Roentgenol* 1998; 171(4): 933–9.

Chapter

29

Vascular manifestations of systemic autoimmune diseases

Raymond Flores and Sharon Dowell

Introduction

The systemic autoimmune diseases are a group of disorders of unknown cause that are characterized by a dysregulation within the immune system. A wide array of immunological mechanisms have been implicated, and genetic and environmental factors have also been shown to play a role in the pathogenesis of disease. In addition, some of these conditions are characterized by the presence of autoantibodies that are directed at various cellular constituents (i.e., anti-dsDNA [anti-double-stranded DNA]) and may be related to the underlying pathogenesis of the disease. The clinical picture often reflects the principal immunopathologic lesion, and can be varied.

Many autoimmune diseases have predominant vascular manifestations and, on occasion, the first point of contact is the emergency physician. It is important that the emergency medicine professional be aware of these disorders, and give them due consideration when compiling a list of differential diagnoses. In some cases, late diagnosis can lead to exacerbation of symptoms with irreversible loss of function and/or significant morbidity and mortality. There are protean manifestations of these disorders and significant overlap in clinical presentations. We have attempted to present a comprehensive overview of these disorders with predominant vascular manifestations via unique case presentations. It is our hope, that on completion of this chapter, the reader will have a greater understanding of autoimmune disorders and feel confident when confronted with these patients in the emergency department (see Table 29.1).

Case presentation 1

A 66-year-old Caucasian gentleman with a history of hypertension and diabetes presents to the emergency department with a two-week history of a throbbing frontal headache, and a one-day history of sudden painless right vision loss. He gives an additional history of fatigue for one month, and stiffness and pain in his shoulders and hips for two months. He also complains of neck and jaw pain when eating, which he believes is due to poorly fitting dentures that he has been unable to change. On examination, his blood pressure is elevated and he has a low-grade fever. He is unable to see with his right eye, and has a notable right afferent pupillary defect. There is tenderness to palpation over the right temple, and his right temporal artery appears tortuous. His physical examination is otherwise unremarkable except for decreased range of motion at the shoulders secondary to pain.

In patients presenting with acute non-traumatic visual loss, there should be a high clinical suspicion for underlying retinal and/or optic nerve ischemia. The conduits to vascular ischemia are diverse and may include large artery occlusion (atherosclerosis, dissection, and embolus), small artery occlusion (vasculitis), venous disease, and hypercoagulable states. Consideration should also be given to optic neuritis, papilledema, and retinal detachment. In the case described, the presence of constitutional symptoms suggests a chronic systemic process, and makes an acute atherothrombotic event or carotid artery dissection less likely. The described history of pain with mastication (jaw claudication) and proximal limb girdle pain and stiffness (suggestive of polymyalgia rheumatica) is very characteristic of giant cell arteritis (GCA), a vasculitis of large and medium-sized vessels. This disease should always be suspected in patients over 50 years of age presenting with new headache and acute visual loss or change in vision.

Vascular Emergencies, ed. Robert L. Rogers, Thomas Scalea, Lee Wallis, and Heike Geduld. Published by Cambridge University Press. © Cambridge University Press 2013.

Table 29.1 Vascular manifestations of systemic autoimmune diseases

Disease	Vascular manifestations
Systemic lupus erythematosus (SLE)	Vasculitis involving any organ Arterial and venous thrombosis
Antiphospholipid antibody syndrome (APS)	Venous and arterial thrombosis Can have a catastrophic presentation with multiorgan involvement and high mortality rate (48%) Recurrent pregnancy losses
Large vessel vasculitis	
Giant cell arteritis (GCA)	Predominantly extracranial artery involvement Temporal pain and tenderness Acute mono-ocular vision loss
Takayasu's arteritis	Peripheral ischemia with pulselessness Aortic aneurysm and/or aortic dissection Severe aortic incompetence with heart failure
Polyarteritis nodosa (PAN)	Usually involves splanchnic circulation, with mesenteric ischemia Aortic aneurysms and dissection Renal artery involvement with renal failure and hypertension
ANCA-associated vasculitis (AAV)	Upper airway involvement is common Respiratory distress due to pulmonary alveolar hemorrhage Renal failure due to glomerulonephritis Disease may be limited to one organ
Other vasculitides	
Behçet's disease	Arterial and venous thromboses Pulmonary artery aneurysms with severe pulmonary hemorrhage
Rheumatoid arthritis Sjogren's syndrome	Rare associated vasculitis of the small vessels with predominant cutaneous and nerve involvement
Drug-induced	May induce P-ANCA antibodies Full spectrum of disease may be seen in the presence of positive anti-myeloperoxidase antibodies Commonly implicated drugs include propylthiouracil, methimazole, and hydralazine
Kawasaki disease	Most common in children Strawberry tongue Erythema and desquamation of the palms and soles Coronary artery aneurysms; arrhythmias; heart failure; sudden death
Goodpasture's syndrome	Pulmonary alveolar hemorrhage due to damage to alveolar basement membrane Glomerulonephritis
Systemic sclerosis	Severe Raynaud's disease Digital ischemia with ischemic ulcers and gangrene Hypertension and acute renal failure herald scleroderma renal crisis, a medical emergency

ANCA, antineutrophil cytoplasmic antibody; P-ANCA, perinuclear antineutrophil cytoplasmic antibody.

GCA predominantly involves the cranial arteries, and may result in permanent vision loss due to involvement of the posterior ciliary artery or central retinal artery. Visual disturbances may vary, and patients may present with temporary vision loss or blurred vision. The incidence increases with age, and it is rarely seen before 50 years of age. There is a female-to-male preponderance of 2 : 1. Patients often have constitutional symptoms and may have an overlapping syndrome of polymyalgia rheumatica, which manifests as pain and stiffness of the muscles of the neck, shoulders, and the hips. More than 60% of patients will describe a new headache, which may be temporal, frontal, or global. The subclavian and axillary arteries may occasionally be involved, and these patients will present with signs of arm claudication. Aortitis and aortic aneurysms have also been reported as a late complication of GCA. Clinical examination may reveal tenderness or induration of the temporal arteries with decreased pulsation, carotid bruits, and decreased pulses in the upper

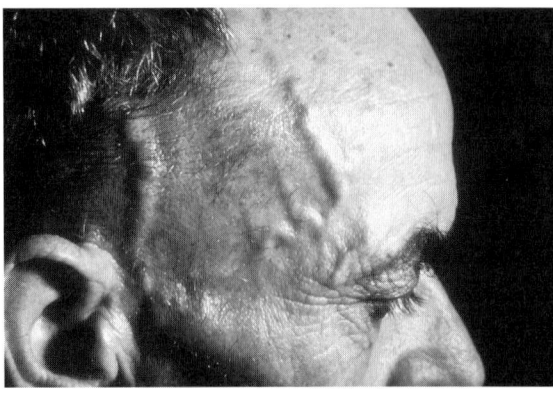

Figure 29.1 Giant cell arteritis: forehead. Dilated branches of this temporal artery are seen. On palpation they were tender and indurate, but pulsations were still felt. These characteristic signs of swelling, tenderness, and inflammation may not always be present, even when biopsy results of the temporal artery are abnormal. In many patients, pulsations are absent in the affected arteries. Giant cell arteritis is frequently associated with headaches, jaw claudication, visual changes, and polymyalgia rheumatica. (Rheumatology Image Bank Reference number: 99–12–0035.)[1,2]

extremities. A relative afferent pupillary defect may be noted in patients with vision loss (Smetana and Shmerling, 2002).[3] The physical examination signs with the highest positive predictive value for disease involve the temporal artery and include beading, enlargement, and lack of pulsation (Figure 29.1).

The presence of three out of five criteria shown in Table 29.2 is associated with a high sensitivity and specificity for diagnosis.

Investigations

Initial diagnostic tests should include an erythrocyte sedimentation rate (ESR), usually elevated to > 100 mm/h, and a complete blood count (CBC), which may reveal a normocytic anemia, thrombosis, and mild leukocytosis. These are all indicators of systemic inflammation. It is important to note that patients with temporal arteritis may have a normal ESR (Ciccarelli *et al.*, 2009).[4,5] In the literature, an ESR < 50 mm/h has been reported in 4.8 to 10.4% of patients with temporal arteritis.[6,7] The entire clinical picture should be considered when making a diagnosis, rather than an ESR alone. The ESR may be falsely low in the setting of polycythemia, congestive cardiac failure, and NSAID use.[4]

Diagnostic confirmation requires a temporal artery biopsy which may be done after initiating treatment. A temporal artery ultrasound can be obtained

Table 29.2 The American College of Rheumatology (ACR) criteria for diagnosis of giant cell arteritis [8]

1. Age greater than or equal to 50 years.
2. Localized headache of new onset.
3. Tenderness or decreased pulse of the temporal artery.
4. Erythrocyte sedimentation rate greater than 50 mm/h.
5. A biopsy revealing necrotizing granulomatous arteritis.

in the emergency department, but is not diagnostic. This tool may detect changes in blood flow and areas of vascular insufficiency, and may help direct the site of temporal artery biopsy. The role of color duplex ultrasonography of the temporal artery in the diagnosis of GCA is currently being investigated.

Management

In the emergency department, the prednisone equivalent of 60 mg should be started immediately by the oral route, or intravenously if the patient is unable to tolerate oral medications. This patient will require timely follow-up with rheumatology and vascular surgery, and may be discharged from the emergency department in the setting of a well-orchestrated plan for continued care (temporal artery biopsy and medication review). Treatment should not be delayed in order to obtain a definitive diagnosis by temporal artery biopsy. In cases of clinically active disease, biopsy results may remain abnormal two to four weeks after initiation of corticosteroid therapy.[9,10]

The presence of vision disturbances mandates an urgent ophthalmology consult in the emergency department. Patients should receive more aggressive therapy with pulse intravenous methylprednisolone 1 g IV for three days followed by prednisone 60 mg by mouth once daily. This is done to prevent progression of the disease, with an aim to preserve vision in the contralateral eye. Patients presenting with partial vision loss or blurred vision can progress to permanent vision loss in a mean of 8.5 days if left untreated,[11] and these patients require hospital admission for a higher level of immediate care.

Critical points

- Consider giant cell arteritis in patients presenting with mono-ocular vision changes and headache.
- Inquire about scalp tenderness, pain with chewing, proximal muscle pain, and stiffness. The

presence of jaw claudication is very suggestive of the diagnosis.

- Assess the character of the temporal arteries on physical examination. Listen for carotid bruits, and check for diminished upper extremity pulses.
- Request blood work for CBC and ESR.
- Obtain urgent referral to ophthalmology if the patient has symptoms/signs of visual disturbances.
- Organize referral to vascular surgery or neuro-ophthalmology for temporal artery biopsy (may be done as an outpatient, ideally within one week).
- Refer to rheumatology for urgent evaluation.
- Start oral prednisone 60 mg once daily; do not delay starting treatment until after the temporal artery biopsy is done.
- Start pulse methylprednisolone 1 g IV for three days if there is vision change or loss, then continue prednisone 60 mg once daily.
- The presence of vision loss mandates admission to hospital for IV methylprednisolone and urgent ophthalmological evaluation.

Case presentation 2

A 24-year-old African American female is brought to the emergency department by the emergency medical service. She is an avid tennis player, but has been having increasing pain in her right arm whenever she plays. The pain usually resolves with rest. She complained of chest pain and mild shortness of breath while at work, and was sent to the emergency department. She has an antecedent history of fever, malaise, and night sweats for six months, and has lost more than 20 pounds (9 kg) over the same timeframe. She denies recent travel, or sick contacts. On examination, her temperature is elevated to 38.2 °C, and her blood pressure (taken in the left arm) is 160 / 72 mmHg. It is difficult to palpate a right radial or brachial pulse, but she has normal capillary refill. She has a diastolic murmur heard best at the fourth right intercostal space, and bibasilar pulmonary crepitations are heard on auscultation.

This clinical scenario describes upper limb claudication, indicative of underlying arterial compromise of the innominate or subclavian arteries. Atherosclerosis is the most common cause of arterial disease in the older population. In the absence of trauma, it is worthwhile to consider a thrombotic event and evaluate for an underlying prothrombotic condition. Consideration should also be given to vasculitis, including Takayasu's arteritis, giant cell arteritis, and congenital malformations. Signs of a systemic process with fever, malaise, and weight loss once again raise the specter of a chronic inflammatory syndrome. In the scenario described, the patient's young age makes Takayasu's arteritis a top consideration in the list of differential diagnoses.

Takayasu's arteritis is a granulomatous vasculitis of the large vessels and typically involves the aorta and its branches, although the coronary and pulmonary arteries can also be affected. It is most commonly seen in young women (between ages 10 and 40), and has an 8 : 1 female-to-male predominance. The highest incidence rates have been reported in Asia, but it can occur in all races and in all geographic regions.

The most common pathologic lesion is that of arterial stenosis, but injury to the vessel wall can also lead to vessel dilation and aneurysmal formation. There are two phases of the disease: an initial "inflammatory" phase characterized by constitutional symptoms with fever, weight loss, and malaise (weeks to months), and a "pulseless" phase characterized by symptoms and/or signs of vascular insufficiency.

Clinical symptoms may be initially vague, and include fever, malaise, fatigue, weight loss, anorexia, and night sweats. These symptoms often prompt an infectious workup, and patients are often misdiagnosed unless the clinician has a high index of suspicion for vasculitis. Most patients are diagnosed months to years later, during the sclerotic ("pulseless") phase of their disease when they present with signs of arterial ischemia. Clinical examination may reveal retinopathy, hypertension, pulselessness, unequal blood pressures, and arterial bruits.

One of the main complications of the disease is the development of aortic aneurysms, and severe aortic incompetence may be noted when there is concomitant involvement of the root of the aorta. There are case reports of patients presenting with clinical features of aortic dissection as the first indicator of disease.[12]

Investigations

Diagnosis is made in the absence of tissue pathology and is based on the clinical symptoms and characteristic findings on imaging studies (see Table 29.3). Conventional angiography is the gold

Table 29.3 American College of Rheumatology (ACR) criteria for Takayasu's arteritis[13]

- Age at disease onset ≤ 40 years.
- Claudication of the extremities.
- Decreased pulsation of one or both brachial arteries.
- Difference of at least 10 mmHg in systolic blood pressure between the arms.
- Bruit over one or both subclavian arteries or the abdominal aorta.
- Arteriographic narrowing or occlusion of the entire aorta, its primary branches, or large arteries in the proximal upper or lower extremities, not due to arteriosclerosis, fibromuscular dysplasia, or other causes.

Patients should have at least three of the six criteria.

standard for evaluation of the arterial lesions, and provides a clear outline of the lumen of involved arteries (See Figure 29.2). It is, however, an invasive procedure with concomitant risks associated with arterial puncture and receiving a contrast dye load. Magnetic resonance imaging/angiography (MRI/MRA), Doppler ultrasound, computed tomography angiography (CTA), and positron emission tomography (PET) are all useful imaging modalities in the evaluation of these patients. MRI/MRA and CTA have the advantage of identifying arterial wall thickening at a pre-stenotic stage, and tend to be most often used in the initial diagnostic assessment of these patients.[14]

Management

High-dose prednisone, 40–60 mg per day, is the mainstay of treatment in the initial "inflammatory" phase.

Patients should also receive low-dose aspirin or other antiplatelet therapy.

Stenotic lesions are irreversible, and surgical intervention (angioplasty or stent placement) may be necessary in some patients. This is often not necessary due to the extensive collateral vessel formation characteristic of this disease. Patients presenting to the emergency department with acute vascular symptoms should be admitted for the initial diagnostic workup and determination of need for surgery. The presence of critical limb ischemia, arterial dissection, organ failure due to arterial compromise, or severe symptomatic aortic incompetence will clearly mandate hospital admission for urgent medical or surgical intervention.

Once initiated, steroid therapy is gradually tapered over time and maintenance doses are tailored to the individual patient. Steroid sparing agents such as azathioprine, methotrexate, and tumor necrosis factor alpha inhibitors have been used with varying degrees of success.

Critical points

- Suspect Takayasu's arteritis in young women presenting with constitutional symptoms and signs of peripheral ischemia.
- One may note absent pulses on clinical examination.
- Check blood pressures in all extremities, but at least in both arms, and auscultate over major arteries (carotid, subclavian, renal) for bruits.

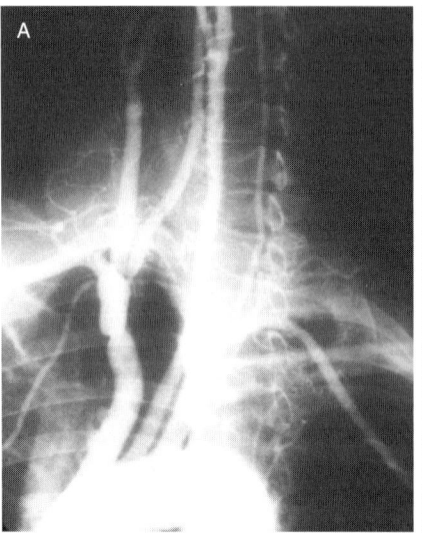
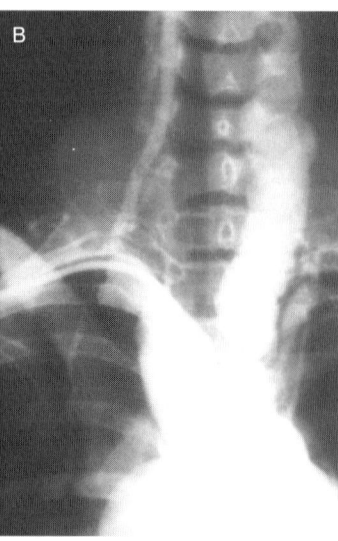

Figure 29.2 Takayasu's disease: arteritis. Aortograms of two patients with Takayasu's disease demonstrate disease progression. (A) Moderate ectasia and stenosis of the innominate artery have developed, and the aortic arch is intact. (B) In a later stage, disease progression is marked by large aneurysms of the aortic arch, left common carotid artery, and innominate artery. A long segment of the left subclavian artery is narrowed. (Rheumatology Image Bank Reference number: 99–12–0088.)

- Aortic incompetence may be a sign of an aortic aneurysm with involvement of the aortic root.
- There is no diagnostic laboratory investigation, but signs of inflammation may be noted on routine blood work (anemia, thrombocytosis, leukocytosis, high ferritin, increased ESR and C-reactive protein).
- CTA or MRI may reveal aneurysmal dilation and stenotic lesions.
- Surgery should be avoided in the inflammatory stages (unless there is a life-threatening event), as surgical outcomes during this stage are generally poor.[15]
- Initial therapy should include prednisone at 40–60 mg once daily and admission to hospital in the presence of new vascular events.

Case presentation 3

A 42-year-old Hispanic lady presents to the emergency department with a complaint of sudden onset of difficulty in breathing and chest pain. She has been coughing up blood-tinged sputum for one day. Her primary care physician saw her four weeks prior to presentation, and noted new renal insufficiency, thought to be secondary to dehydration. She was also noted to have mild hematuria. She admits to weight loss, fever, night sweats, and malaise for the last few months. On clinical examination she is hypotensive, and in visible respiratory distress. Her mucous membranes are pale, and she is tachycardic. Lung auscultation is significant for coarse, widespread crepitations.

The possible causes of non-traumatic hemoptysis are diverse, and bleeding can arise from the airways (bronchitis, bronchiectasis, foreign body, tumor), the pulmonary parenchyma (pneumonia, abscess, pneumonitis, capillaritis), and the pulmonary vasculature (pulmonary embolism, pulmonary hypertension, arteriovenous malformation). Drug-induced lung injury can also occur, and cocaine use has been associated with diffuse alveolar hemorrhage. Behçet's disease can present with severe, life-threatening hemoptysis secondary to rupture of a pulmonary artery aneurysm. The presence of longstanding constitutional symptoms raises the possibility of infection, malignancy, and autoimmune disorders to the top of the list of differential diagnoses. The presence of concurrent renal dysfunction further highlights the possibility of one of the pulmonary–renal syndromes.

The pulmonary–renal syndromes comprise a group of disorders which are typically associated with both pulmonary (diffuse alveolar hemorrhage, lung cavitations) and renal (glomerulonephritis) involvement. The term is classically used in reference to Goodpasture's syndrome and the antineutrophil cytoplasmic antibody (ANCA)-associated vasculitides. Other diseases, including systemic lupus erythematosus (SLE), essential mixed cryoglobulinemia, and antiphospholipid antibody syndrome (APS) can present similarly.

The ANCA-associated vasculitides (AAV) are a group of vasculitides of small-to-medium-sized vessels, with overlapping clinical features and anticytoplasmic antibodies directed against neutrophils. Granulomatosis with polyangiitis (GPA; formerly Wegener's granulomatosis), microscopic polyangiitis (MPA), and Churg–Strauss syndrome (CSS) predominantly affect older individuals (mean age of diagnosis is 55 years), and are more frequently seen in whites.

As with all vasculitides, patients may present with vague constitutional symptoms of anorexia, weight loss, arthralgias, and fever. All three vasculitides may have substantial ear, nose, and throat manifestations (so-called upper-airway involvement), but this is particularly characteristic of patients with GPA. Inflammation of the nose can result in nasal perforations and nasal bridge collapse, with the characteristic saddle-nose deformity (see Figure 29.3). In CSS, allergic rhinitis is seen early in the disease course. Pulmonary capillaritis often results in diffuse alveolar hemorrhage and respiratory distress, and is more often associated with MPA and GPA.[16] Churg–Strauss syndrome typically manifests with obstructive airway disease and fleeting infiltrates on a background of new-onset or worsening asthma. Renal involvement is common, and patients may have renal failure with hematuria and proteinuria on presentation. The underlying lesion on renal biopsy is a pauci-immune crescentic glomerulonephritis. In the absence of early recognition and treatment, patients may develop advanced glomerulosclerosis and fibrosis with end-stage renal disease, requiring hemodialysis.

Investigations

Laboratory studies will reveal signs of systemic inflammation, with anemia, leukocytosis, thrombocytosis, and elevated inflammatory markers. Anemia may be

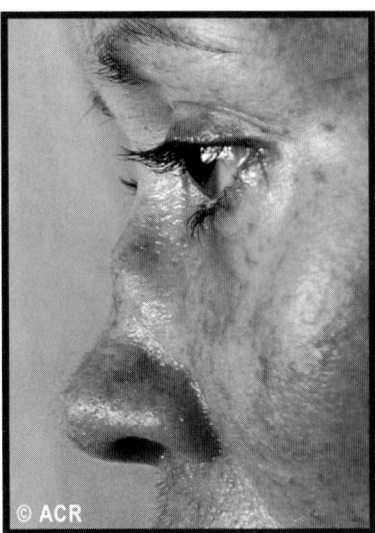

Figure 29.3 Wegener's granulomatosis: saddle-nose deformity, face. This patient developed a saddle-nose deformity with destruction of the dorsal nasal cartilage. Other nasal complications include perforated nasal septum, mucosal ulceration, epistaxis, and boggy nasal turbinates with purulent nasal discharge. (Rheumatology Image Bank Reference Number: 01–12–0033.)

In addition to clinical features and positive serology, biopsy of the involved organ (usually lung or kidney) will show the characteristic lesion of the disease and confirm the diagnosis. Bronchoscopy is often undertaken in the setting of pulmonary hemorrhage, and as part of the workup to rule out an infectious etiology. Fibrinoid necrosis accounts for damage to the vessel walls, and necrotizing granulomatous vasculitis seen on open lung biopsy is diagnostic.

Management

In this case scenario, emergent intervention to stabilize the patient's blood pressure and support her respiratory status is appropriate. A chest X-ray (CXR) may reveal diffuse interstitial infiltrates (pulmonary hemorrhage) or pulmonary nodules with cavitations (GPA). These lesions may be better delineated on a CT scan of the chest.

Pulse methylprednisolone at 1 g IV per day for three days is warranted in the setting of pulmonary hemorrhage, or renal failure. This can be initiated in the emergency department if there is a high index of suspicion for disease.

Cyclophosphamide has long been the therapy of choice in patients with major organ involvement, and is usually started after biopsy confirmation of disease. More recently, rituximab has been approved as a first-line agent in patients with AAV with renal disease. It is not currently indicted as a first-line therapy in patients who have concomitant pulmonary alveolar hemorrhage. Plasmapheresis may also have a role in the treatment of patients with pulmonary hemorrhage. The rheumatology, pulmonary, and nephrology services should be urgently consulted with respect to further diagnostic workup and management of these patients.

Goodpasture's syndrome may also present with alveolar hemorrhage and renal failure. The underlying mechanism is the presence of antibodies that attack the alveolar and renal glomerular basement membranes. The initial treatment of these patients is the same as for the patient with suspected ANCA-associated vasculitis, including plasmapheresis. In the emergency department it is often difficult to distinguish between these disorders if other specific characteristic symptoms or signs are absent. Anti-glomerular basement membrane (anti-GBM) antibodies should be requested in patients with features of both pulmonary and renal involvement.

marked in the presence of ongoing pulmonary alveolar hemorrhage. The presence of ANCA antibodies will assist in making the diagnosis when there is a high clinical suspicion. These tests may be sent off in the emergency department, but the results are usually not readily available to assist the emergency medicine physician. There are three patterns of fluorescence recognized with the immunofluorescence assay: the cytoplasmic (C-ANCA), perinuclear (P-ANCA), and atypical patterns. The C-ANCA pattern tends to correspond with the detection of antibodies to proteinase-3 (PR3), and is the pattern that is most often seen in GPA. The P-ANCA pattern is seen in the presence of antibodies to myeloperoxidase (MPO), and is most commonly associated with microscopic polyangiitis. ANCA antibodies are seen in 80 to 90% of patients with GPA or MPA, but may only be seen in 50% of patients with CSS.

It is worthwhile to note that certain drugs (pharmacologic and illicit) can induce antineutrophil cytoplasmic antibodies, and may also induce vasculitis. There have been multiple reports in the literature of a cocaine-induced vasculitis characterized by hemorrhagic skin lesions and positive atypical P-ANCA antibodies.

Critical points

- Suspect AAV in patients presenting with a pulmonary–renal syndrome. Most patients will have an antecedent history of chronic constitutional symptoms.
- ANCA antibodies can be induced by certain drugs, and if specific antibodies to MPO or (more rarely) PR3 are found in these patients, they may have the full spectrum of disease. Elicit a history of cocaine use, or exposure to propylthiouracil or hydralazine.
- Check labs for P-ANCA, C-ANCA, and more specifically for anti-MPO and anti-PR3 antibodies.
- One should also request antinuclear antibodies (ANA), anti-GBM antibodies, complement levels, antiphospholipid antibodies, and cryoglobulins, as SLE, Goodpasture's disease, APS and mixed essential cryoglobulinemia may present with alveolar hemorrhage with or without renal involvement.
- Provide supportive treatment for patients in respiratory distress; some patients may require intubation and ventilatory support.
- Obtain referral to the pulmonary service for bronchoscopy and diagnostic bronchoalveolar lavage.
- Refer to nephrology for evaluation of renal failure, initiation of hemodialysis if warranted, and renal biopsy.
- Refer to rheumatology for further evaluation and workup.
- Start pulse methylprednisolone 1 g IV for three days, followed by prednisone equivalent of 1 mg/kg.

Case presentation 4

A 31-year-old Spanish-speaking female is brought to the hospital by the emergency medical service. She had sudden onset of right-sided weakness with slurred speech, and change in consciousness that morning. Her distraught husband reports that she has no significant past medical history. She is recovering from a recent miscarriage at 11-weeks gestation. This is the second miscarriage in three years. Her review of systems is otherwise only positive for an erythematosus facial rash thought to be rosacea, as this runs in her family. She also has a history of daily joint pain, and

self-medicates with acetaminophen. On clinical examination, she has an elevated blood pressure and a dense right hemiparesis, with slurred speech and expressive aphasia. Her clinical examination is otherwise unremarkable except for mottling of the skin of her lower extremities.

The occurrence of a cerebrovascular accident (CVA) at a young age is unusual, and raises the suspicion of an underlying hypercoagulable state or hematologic disorder, cardiac defects, vasculopathy, hypertension, drug use, or migrainous attacks. Premature atherosclerosis is also possible, but other causes should be ruled out first. In the case scenario, the associated history of late first-trimester pregnancy losses makes APS a possibility. This is an autoimmune syndrome characterized by the presence of antibodies to phospholipids, with resultant arterial and venous thrombotic events and fetal losses or pregnancy morbidity. It may be primary, or it may be secondary to an underlying connective tissue disorder, most often SLE. There is a female predilection for both forms of the disease. The case scenario raises the possibility of underlying SLE with reference to a concomitant facial rash and arthralgias.

Antiphospholipid antibody syndrome (Table 29.4) may present in multiple ways, but should always be suspected in young women with thrombotic events. In older patients, vascular ischemia or thrombosis is more likely secondary to atherosclerosis or malignancy.

The clinical spectrum is wide. The most common cutaneous manifestation is that of livedo reticularis, a reddish, lace-like discoloration of the skin, which is more readily apparent on the limbs and torso.

Venous thromboses occur more frequently than arterial thromboses, and may affect the deep veins of the lower extremities, as well as the renal and hepatic veins (Budd–Chiari syndrome).[17] The brain is the most common site of arterial thromboses, and this may be primary or secondary to embolization from an affected cardiac valve.

More than 50% of thrombotic events occurring in women happen during pregnancy, the postpartum period, or while on oral contraceptive pills. Patients may have unexplained recurrent fetal loss (usually after the 10th week of gestation), intrauterine fetal death, fetal growth retardation, or premature delivery.

This syndrome may also present with renal insufficiency secondary to thrombotic microangiopathy, and

Table 29.4 Revised classification criteria for antiphospholipid antibody syndrome (2006)[18]

Antiphospholipid antibody syndrome (APS) is present if at least one of the clinical criteria and one of the laboratory criteria that follow are met

Clinical criteria

1. Vascular thrombosis : one or more clinical episodes of arterial, venous, or small-vessel thrombosis confirmed by objective validated criteria
2. Pregnancy morbidity
    a. One or more unexplained deaths of a morphologically normal fetus at or beyond the 10th week of gestation, or
    b. One or more premature births of a morphologically normal neonate before the 34th week of gestation because of eclampsia, severe pre-eclampsia, or placental insufficiency, or
    c. Three or more unexplained consecutive spontaneous abortions before the 10th week of gestation

Laboratory criteria

1. Lupus anticoagulant present in plasma, on two or more occasions at least 12 weeks apart
2. Anticardiolipin (aCL) antibody of IgG and/or IgM isotype in serum or plasma, present in medium or high titer on two or more occasions, at least 12 weeks apart
3. Anti-beta-2-glycoprotein 1 antibody of IgG and/or IgM isotype in serum or plasma present on two or more occasions, at least 12 weeks apart

Classification criteria for definite APS proposed by international consensus conferences and intended primarily for research purposes.

is associated with malignant hypertension and thrombotic thrombocytopenic purpura.

Catastrophic APS is a rare presentation with thrombosis within multiple organs, and is a medical emergency requiring urgent intervention. There is an associated mortality of approximately 48%.[19]

Investigations

Thrombocytopenia is a very common manifestation in the antiphospholipid antibody syndrome, with platelet counts ranging from 50,000 to 140,000 / μL.[20] Interestingly, thrombosis still occurs in the presence of thrombocytopenia and may represent consumption by clot.

The complete blood count may reveal thrombocytopenia and anemia (which may be hemolytic). Specific diagnostic tests would include demonstration of the presence of lupus anticoagulant, or medium-to-high titers of IgG or IgM antibodies to cardiolipin or beta-2-glycoprotein 1. The lupus anticoagulant can be screened for in the emergency department with either a prolonged activated partial thromboplastin time (aPTT) or dilute Russell viper venom time (dRVVT). A prolonged time in the absence of other pathology will add weight to the suspected diagnosis. Confirmation of this result must be shown by failure to correct with a mixing study, and normalization with a platelet neutralization test. These confirmatory tests will not be available in the acute setting.

Initial imaging studies should include Doppler studies of the lower extremities, as well as targeted imaging of the organ involved. In this case scenario, an MRI/MRA of the brain would be obtained.

In cases of renal involvement, renal biopsy may reveal evidence of thrombotic microangiopathy. The renal biopsy is important in patients who have underlying SLE, as renal injury may be secondary to underlying glomerulonephritis, which requires a different treatment strategy.

Management

Anticoagulation should be initiated immediately and, in the emergency setting, IV heparin tends to be the agent of choice. In the setting of an acute stroke, the timing of initiation of anticoagulation is unclear, and a neurologist should be consulted prior to initiating therapy. It has been the accepted strategy to hold anticoagulation therapy for up to two weeks after a large infarct due to the increased risk of hemorrhagic conversion. Some case series and observational data suggest that this strategy is not necessary, and anticoagulation should not be withheld in cases where there are no contraindications and there is a high risk of recurrent stroke or ongoing thrombosis.[21,22] Most patients will require lifelong anticoagulation.

Catastrophic APS (CAPS) is a medical emergency and requires urgent intervention. In addition to anticoagulation with heparin, and identifying and treating precipitating causes, patients should be started on high-dose methylprednisolone 1 g IV for three days followed by oral prednisone of 1–2 mg/kg per day.

Plasmapheresis is recommended as first-line therapy for patients with CAPS, and is used with or without IV immunoglobulin in cases of microthrombotic angiopathy.[21] There are reports of patients with refractory APS and CAPS who responded favorably to therapy with rituximab.[22]

Immunosuppressive therapy is also indicated in APS secondary to another autoimmune disorder (SLE).

Critical points

- Suspect APS in patients (especially young women) presenting with recurrent thrombotic events.
- Elicit a history of recurrent fetal loss (at around 10 weeks gestation), or increased pregnancy morbidity for unknown reasons.
- Evaluate all organ systems for potential involvement.
- Look for signs of an underlying connective tissue disease (malar rash or other skin lesions, arthritis).
- Check CBC; thrombocytopenia may be noticed.
- Screen for lupus anticoagulant with a dRVVT or aPTT.
- Request tests to detect anticardiolipin antibodies and anti-beta-2-glycoprotein 1 antibodies. Also request ANA to screen for underlying SLE.
- Perform imaging studies to confirm thrombosis or embolism based on clinical symptoms.
- Start anticoagulation with IV heparin.
- Recognize catastrophic APS when there is involvement of three or more organ systems.
- Obtain urgent referral to hematology for plasmapheresis in the event of catastrophic APS.
- May start pulse methylprednisolone 1 g IV for three days in the event of catastrophic APS.
- Refer to rheumatology for further workup and evaluation.

Case presentation 5

A 48-year-old lady presents to the emergency department complaining of painful dusky fingers of the right hand for three days. She initially noted a sharp and throbbing pain in her right second finger, then right third finger with numbness and tingling at the fingertips. This sensation persisted and was followed by a bluish discoloration of her fingertips two days later. Over the past five years, she has frequently experienced a bluish and sometimes white discoloration of her fingertips in the cold, which usually resolves with warming of her hands. She has a history of gastro-esophageal reflux disease and self-medicates with over-the-counter antacid therapy. She has some small ulcers at her fingertips, which she attributes to trauma from her work as a typist. Clinical examination is significant for a dusky discoloration of the second and third right fingers, which are also cool to touch. The skin of her distal phalanges is taut and

slightly thickened. Her peripheral pulses are palpable but diminished in volume. There are old stellate scars involving the fingertips of both hands.

Digital ischemia occurs when there is compromise to the distal arterial tree, most often secondary to stenosis or thrombotic occlusion. It occurs more commonly in the lower extremity than in the upper extremity, where its occurrence poses a diagnostic and therapeutic challenge. About 70% of the symptomatic peripheral arterial occlusion in the upper extremities affects the small arteries distal to the wrist.[23] The differential diagnosis of digital ischemia is broad and includes embolic phenomenon (including cholesterol emboli), local thrombosis, thrombophilic disorders, and systemic diseases like systemic sclerosis, cryoglobulinemia, and chronic renal failure.

In the clinical scenario above, Raynaud's phenomenon, characterized by digital color changes induced by cold temperature or emotional stress, is described. It is thought to be secondary to abnormal vasoconstriction of digital arteries due to a local defect in normal vascular responses.

Raynaud's phenomenon may be primary or idiopathic, most likely due to an exaggerated normal vasoconstrictive response to cold exposure. Primary Raynaud's phenomenon is generally not associated with digital ischemia or other injurious clinical sequelae.

Secondary Raynaud's disease may occur in the setting of connective tissue diseases, hematologic conditions, vascular disease, medications or illicit drugs, and environmental factors (frostbite, use of vibrating tools).

Secondary Raynaud's phenomenon may be complicated by digital ischemia and ischemic digital tip ulcers. The connective tissue disorders of primary concern in this clinical scenario are systemic sclerosis and SLE. Antiphospholipid antibody syndrome with thrombus formation and distal microemboli, Buerger's disease (thromboangiitis obliterans), and Takayasu's arteritis should also be considered.

Buerger's disease is a non-atherosclerotic, segmental, inflammatory disease that most often affects middle-aged men with a history of tobacco use, and hence it is less likely in the clinical scenario outlined.

Systemic sclerosis is an autoimmune disorder characterized by the presence of thickened sclerotic skin (scleroderma) and varying degrees of associated internal organ involvement. Systemic sclerosis may have either diffuse or limited skin involvement, and may be

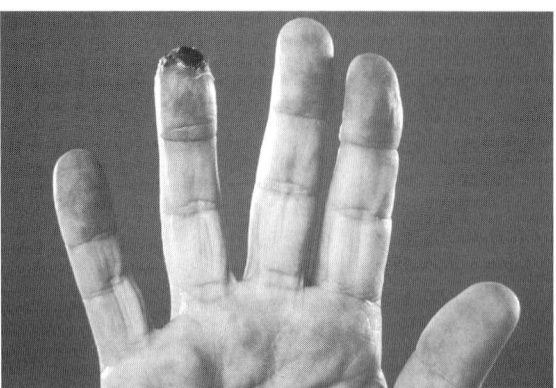

Figure 29.4 Juvenile scleroderma: digital gangrene, hand. Digital gangrene of the right fourth finger is seen in this 20-year-old male who developed scleroderma at the age of 12 years. Note also the dusky erythema of the pulps of each of the finger pads and thumb and the palmar surfaces of the metacarpophalangeal joints. (Rheumatology Image Bank Reference no: 99–06–0075.)[24]

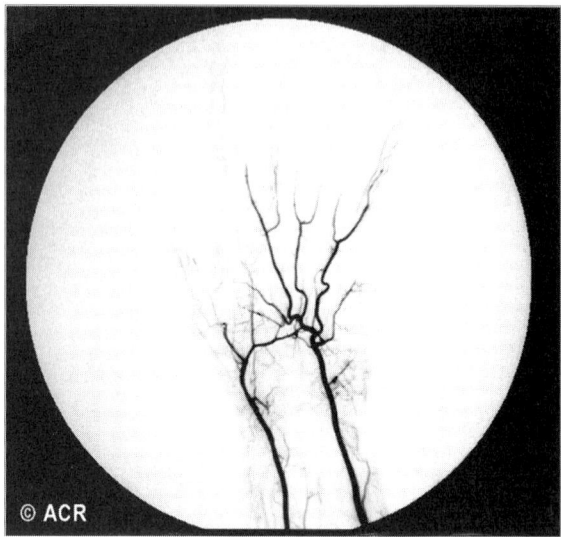

Figure 29.5 Raynaud's phenomenon: hand. Digital angiogram in a patient with Raynaud's phenomenon shows cutoff of digital blood flow. These angiographic changes resolved with the use of intra-arterial vasodilators. (Rheumatology Image Bank Reference number: 01–10–0045.)

associated with pulmonary hypertension, interstitial lung disease, gastrointestinal dysmotility, and renal failure. Secondary Raynaud's phenomenon is seen in most patients with systemic sclerosis and is mediated by the underlying obliterative vasculopathy seen in this disease. Chronic ischemia may lead to reduction of the finger pad. Patients may have evidence of frank digital ischemia with pitting scars, recurrent ischemic and traumatic ulcers, and digital gangrene (see Figure 29.4).

In the patient with systemic sclerosis, taut skin and abnormal nail-fold capillaries may be seen on physical examination. Old digital scars may also be seen.

Investigations

Initial blood work should include a complete blood count, basic metabolic panel, and urinalysis. The diagnosis of systemic sclerosis would be suggested primarily by the presence of scleroderma, although systemic manifestations and a characteristic positive serologic assay may be present. Blood should be drawn for ANA, and specific tests for anti-topoisomerase 1 (antiScl-70) and anti-centromere antibodies should be requested.

Doppler US should be obtained to evaluate the arterial supply, and the patient should undergo angiography of the affected limb to determine the level of occlusion (see Figure 29.5).

Management

In the setting of severe Raynaud's with digital ischemia, it is important to keep the digits warm, minimize anxiety, and avoid sympathomimetic drugs that may exacerbate the patient's symptoms.

In the emergency department, antithrombotic therapy with aspirin and vasodilator therapy is indicated. The non-dihydropyridine calcium channel blockers remain the drugs of first choice in patients with Raynaud's phenomenon.[25,26] Adjunct therapies include the phosphodiesterase inhibitors, topical nitrates, and pentoxifylline. Endothelin antagonists and prostaglandin analogues have also been incorporated into the treatment paradigm, but are reserved for patients with severe disease and digital ischemic ulcers. Prostaglandins are potent vasodilators, and acute digital ischemia can be managed with intermittent intravenous iloprost or epoprostenol.

Anticoagulant therapy with IV heparin for 24–72 hours may be instituted in the acute setting for cases of advancing ischemia; although there are no formal studies in the literature to support this.[26]

In refractory cases, surgical interventions such as proximal or distal sympathectomy and arterial reconstruction can be considered. Recent literature suggests a role for local botulinum toxin A injections in the treatment of digital ischemia associated with Raynaud's phenomenon. Three case series have reported decreased frequency of vasospastic effects and healing of digital ulcers in patients treated with botulinum toxin A.[27–29] This is an area of ongoing investigation. There is no role for prednisone therapy or chronic anticoagulation in these patients.

Critical points

- Secondary Raynaud's phenomenon may be associated with digital ischemia and ischemic ulcers.
- Systemic sclerosis may lead to severe digital ischemia secondary to an underlying vasculopathy, as well as exaggerated vasoconstriction on exposure to cold ambient temperatures.
- Patients should be kept in a calm environment, and sympathomimetic drugs (e.g., β-blockers) should be avoided.
- In the setting of acute ischemia which is limb threatening, hospital admission is required, and it is reasonable to start anticoagulation with heparin.
- Calcium channel blockers are the drugs of first choice (amlodipine 5 mg or nifedipine XR 30 mg), and dose is titrated for symptom effect.
- Intravenous vasodilator therapy can also be used in the emergency setting as the patient's blood pressure tolerates.
- The prostaglandin analogue epoprostenol can be given intravenously in the setting of an acute ischemic digital ulcer but this should only be done after consultation with a specialist (rheumatology or pulmonary).
- Referrals should be made to the vascular service for further evaluation of the ischemic digit.

Case presentation 6

A 58-year-old gentleman presents to the emergency department with cramping lower abdominal pain for several months. He describes it as waxing and waning initially, but he noted increasing severity in the past two weeks, prompting his visit to the emergency department. The pain appears to be exacerbated by eating meals. He has tried Tums and over-the-counter antacid treatment with no relief. He denies fever, vomiting, or melena. He has lost 15 pounds (6.8 kg) in the

last two months. He admits to a vague sense of malaise and easy fatigability, but this has been a very busy time for his business, and he has been working long hours. His review of systems is positive for left leg numbness with paresthesias for two months, and intermittently severe muscle cramps. Clinical examination is unremarkable except for mild diffuse abdominal tenderness and diminished peripheral pulses in the left lower extremity.

Intestinal ischemia most commonly occurs in the setting of atherosclerosis or mesenteric artery thrombosis. In the case presentation given, the constitutional symptoms of weight loss and malaise raise the suspicion of an underlying systemic inflammatory process. As noted in the prior case scenarios, these constitutional symptoms make a systemic vasculitic process a main contender on the list of differential diagnoses. Mesenteric artery involvement suggests at least a medium-vessel vasculitis, and is most likely indicative of polyarteritis nodosa (PAN), although Takayasu's arteritis and giant cell arteritis may rarely involve these vessels. The age and sex of this patient makes Takayasu's arteritis unlikely, and the distribution is highly atypical of giant cell arteritis. Thrombotic occlusion secondary to an underlying connective tissue disease or thrombophilic state is also possible.

Polyarteritis nodosa is a systemic necrotizing vasculitis of medium-to-small muscular vessels. It can affect all age groups, although it is predominantly seen in older men. The spectrum of PAN can range from cutaneous-only disease, to systemic disease with multiorgan involvement. It is most often idiopathic, although it can occur secondary to hepatitis B or hepatitis C infection. The pathologic lesion of PAN is fibrinoid necrosis of the arterial wall with segmental transmural occlusion of muscular arteries. Disruption of the internal and external elastic lamina contributes to the development of aneurysms.

The symptoms are non-specific (fever, malaise, weight loss) or related to the organ system involved. Some of the more common clinical features include myalgias or leg muscle tenderness, mononeuropathy, hypertension, testicular pain, and skin lesions or ulcers.

The criteria given in Table 29.5 are not meant to be used for diagnostic purposes but have been shown to have a sensitivity of 82% and specificity of 87% for the diagnosis of polyarteritis when applied to patients

Table 29.5 The American College of Rheumatology (ACR) criteria for the classification of polyarteritis nodosa in a patient with vasculitis (at least three of the following)[30]

Otherwise unexplained weight loss greater than 4 kg

Livedo reticularis

Testicular pain or tenderness

Myalgias (excluding that of the shoulder and hip girdle), weakness of muscles, tenderness of leg muscles, or polyneuropathy

Mononeuropathy or polyneuropathy

New-onset diastolic blood pressure greater than 90 mmHg

Elevated levels of serum blood urea nitrogen (> 40 mg/dL or 14.3 mmol/L) or creatinine (> 1.5 mg/dL or 132 μmol/L)

Evidence of hepatitis B virus infection via serum antibody or antigen serology

Characteristic arteriographic abnormalities not resulting from non-inflammatory disease processes

A biopsy of small or medium-sized artery containing polymorphonuclear cells

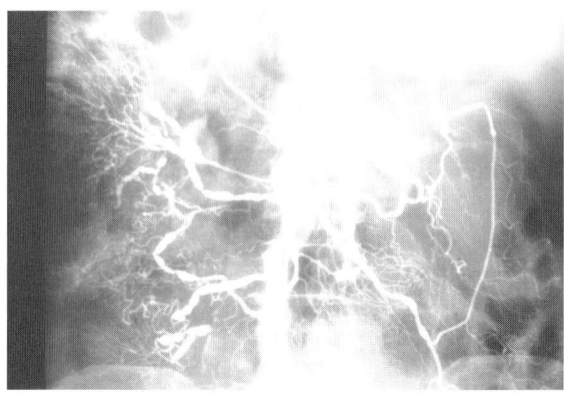

Figure 29.6 Polyarteritis nodosa. A selective angiogram of the superior mesenteric artery shows multiple saccular aneurysms that vary in size and shape. Note the irregularity of the vascular lumens with areas of stenosis and dilation. (Rheumatology Image Bank Reference number: 99–12–0081.)

with documented vasculitis in whom at least three of the criteria are present.

Investigations

Initial blood work should include a complete blood count, erythrocyte sedimentation rate, and C-reactive protein. Hepatitis B surface antigen and hepatitis C antibodies should also be requested. There is no diagnostic laboratory test for PAN.

Diagnosis maybe confirmed by biopsy of the involved organ, but this is rarely done. Imaging should be guided by the site of involvement, and in most cases the diagnosis is confirmed by typical changes on angiography (see Figure 29.6). CT and MRA can also be utilized in the diagnostic workup of these patients.[31]

One major differential for PAN, which can present with signs of ischemia and have similar imaging features (multiple aneurysms of the involved vasculature), is segmental arterial mediolysis (SAM). The incidence of this rare disease is unknown. It affects middle-aged and elderly patients with no male or female predilection, and commonly involves the splanchnic vessels. This is a non-inflammatory disease with vacuolar degeneration of the smooth muscle in the outer media that results in gaps in the arterial wall. Some authors have suggested that SAM represents a variant or precursor to fibromuscular dysplasia (FMD).[32]

Management

High-dose steroids followed by oral cyclophosphamide therapy is the mainstay of treatment. Oral prednisone at 1 mg/kg can be initiated in patients with mild to moderate disease, and this can be done in an outpatient setting. Pulse methylprednisolone 1 g IV for three consecutive doses followed by oral prednisone at 1 mg/kg is reserved for those patients with severe, life-threatening manifestations or evolving neuropathic complications. These patients will require hospital admission. Patients with underlying active hepatitis B and hepatitis C should receive targeted antiviral therapy.

Critical points

- Suspect PAN in middle-aged men presenting with signs of mesenteric ischemia and a history of chronic constitutional symptoms.
- Classical history may include testicular pain, neuropathy (sensory and/or motor), skin rash, and hypertension.
- One should evaluate for differential blood pressures in the extremities and bruits over the large vessels.
- There is no diagnostic blood work, but hepatitis B and C should be ruled out as the precipitant of this disease in some patients. Inflammatory markers are likely to be elevated.
- Imaging studies will reveal the characteristic saccular aneurysms of the affected vessels.
- Tissue is rarely available for pathology.

- Patients with severe disease or arterial compromise should be admitted to hospital and started on methylprednisolone 1 g IV once daily for three consecutive days, then oral prednisone at 60 mg per day.
- Therapy with cyclophosphamide is indicated, and can be started once the diagnosis is confirmed.
- Referrals to vascular surgery and rheumatology for further evaluation and management are in order.

Miscellaneous

Behçet's disease

Behçet's disease is a rare disease of unknown etiology. It is characterized by recurrent oral ulcers and protean systemic manifestations. Most of the clinical features of Behçet's disease are believed to be due to vasculitis, which may involve any caliber vessel (small, medium, large), and both arteries and veins. Venous involvement is more common than arterial involvement, and disease can occur both in the form of endovascular inflammation as well as thrombus formation. The carotid, pulmonary, aortic, and femoral arteries are commonly involved. Pulmonary artery involvement is of special concern as these patients may have aneurysms involving the large branches of the pulmonary trunk. Patients may present with hemoptysis and may have both thrombosis and aneurysms of the pulmonary artery on presentation. A misdiagnosis of pulmonary embolism and subsequent anticoagulation can have catastrophic consequences. If suspected, pulmonary arteriography is diagnostic.[33]

In the case of acute venous thrombosis in this disease, immunosuppressive agents such as corticosteroids and azathioprine are recommended. There is currently little support for the use of anticoagulation in these patients. Emergency surgery for ruptured pulmonary aneurysms has a very high mortality rate and should be avoided unless hemorrhage is life threatening.[34]

Kawasaki disease

Kawasaki disease is an acute, self-limited vasculitis of childhood, which may be occasionally seen in adults. It is characterized by systemic inflammation, and patients may present with prolonged fever, cervical lymphadenopathy, erythema of the hands and feet, involvement of the lips or tongue (strawberry tongue), non-purulent conjunctivitis, and a diffuse polymorphous skin rash. The inflammatory process has a predilection for the coronary arteries, with development of coronary artery aneurysms, arrhythmias, heart failure, and sudden death. Early intervention and therapy with aspirin and IV immunoglobulin decreases the incidence of coronary artery damage.[35,36]

Levamisole-contaminated cocaine-induced vasculitis

There are a few drugs which can induce a vasculitic syndrome. Cocaine has long been associated with various rheumatic conditions, but recently there has been a significant increase in cases of cutaneous vasculitis associated with cocaine use. The culprit appears to be the contaminant levamisole, which was first documented as an adulterant to cocaine in 2002. Many of these patients have a positive perinuclear ANCA assay (P-ANCA), with reactivity to human neutrophil elastase.[37] The cutaneous vasculitis is characterized by purpuric bullous lesions with areas of skin necrosis, and may be associated with neutropenia. It is important to recognize this syndrome, as the skin lesions can occasionally be widespread with superimposed infection and sepsis. Withdrawal of the offending agent is paramount.

Limited resources

In places with limited resources and poor access to imaging facilities and confirmatory blood work, the diagnosis will be based predominantly on clinical grounds. It would be important to rule out infection in patients presenting with chronic constitutional symptoms. If the index of suspicion for an underlying autoimmune disease is high, then the application of the appropriate classification criteria should be helpful in arriving at a most likely diagnosis. Patients may be treated with prednisone therapy at the appropriate doses while awaiting confirmatory tests, once infection has been excluded.

Pearls and pitfalls

1. Suspect GCA in patients greater than 50 years of age presenting with mono-ocular vision loss.
2. The most common complaint in patients with GCA (> 60%) is a new headache, which may be

temporal, frontal, or global. Jaw claudication is very suggestive.

3. Aortitis and aortic aneurysms have also been reported as a late complication of GCA.

4. The physical examination sign with the highest positive predictive value for GCA is an abnormal examination of the temporal artery (beading, prominence, enlargement).

5. A small fraction of patients with GCA temporal arteritis may have a normal ESR and, in the literature, 4.8 to 10% of patients may have an ESR < 50 mm/h.

6. The erythrocyte sedimentation rate may be falsely low in the setting of polycythemia, congestive cardiac failure, and NSAID use.

7. Takayasu's arteritis occurs in young women (age < 40), but the age at first presentation may be older.

8. Takayasu's arteritis may mimic aortic dissection. Patients may develop aortic aneurysms, and severe aortic incompetence may be noted when there is concomitant involvement of the root of the aorta.

9. The top differential diagnoses for patients presenting with respiratory symptoms (hemoptysis) and renal insufficiency (pulmonary–renal syndromes) include the ANCA-associated vasculitides (AAVs) and Goodpasture's disease.

10. Thrombocytopenia is a very common manifestation of the antiphospholipid antibody syndrome (APS), with platelet counts ranging from 50,000 to 140,000 / μL. Thrombosis continues to occur in the presence of thrombocytopenia.

11. In patients with secondary Raynaud's with digital ischemia, it is important to keep the digits warm, minimize anxiety, and avoid sympathomimetic drugs.

12. The non-dihydropyridine calcium channel blockers are the drugs of first choice in patients with Raynaud's phenomenon.

13. There is no role for prednisone therapy or chronic anticoagulation in patients with digital ischemia due to systemic sclerosis and secondary Raynaud's disease.

14. One major differential for polyarteritis nodosa (PAN), which can present with signs of ischemia and have similar imaging features, is the non-inflammatory syndrome of segmental arterial mediolysis (SAM).

15. Behçet's disease may present with arterial and venous thrombosis; the mainstay of treatment in this situation is immunosuppressive medications and not anticoagulation.

16. Patients with suspected Behçet's disease presenting with hemoptysis should be evaluated for pulmonary artery aneurysms. A misdiagnosis of pulmonary emboli and subsequent anticoagulation can have catastrophic consequences.

Summary

Patients with vascular disease presenting with signs of systemic inflammation with no clear precipitating cause should be evaluated for an underlying autoimmune disease/vasculitis. Emergency procedures and interventions are initially supportive and directed to the organ system involved. If surgery is warranted, it should be postponed until the inflammatory process is addressed unless there is a significant life-threatening or limb-threatening event. High-dose corticosteroid therapy is indicated emergently in patients presenting with acute vision loss secondary to giant cell arteritis. Anticoagulation with heparin should be started in the emergency department in patients presenting with an acute thrombotic event. Otherwise, in most cases, targeted medical therapy can be delayed until the emergency workup and evaluation is complete.

References

1. Wilske KR. Clinical spectrum of giant cell arteritis. *Intern Med Spec* 1982; 3(10): 82–97.

2. Healey LA. *The Systemic Manifestations of Giant Cell Arteritis*. New York, NY: Grune and Stratton; 1978.

3. Smetana GW, Shmerling RH. Does this patient have temporal arteritis? *JAMA* 2002; 287(1): 92–101.

4. Ciccarelli M, Jeanmonod D, Jeanmonod R. Giant cell temporal arteritis with a normal erythrocyte sedimentation rate: report of a case. *Am J Emerg Med* 2009; 27(2): 255.e1–3.

5. Zweegman S, Makkink B, Stehouwer CD. Giant-cell arteritis with normal erythrocyte sedimentation rate: case report and review of the literature. *Neth J Med* 1993; 42(3-4): 128–31.

6. Martínez-Taboada VM, Blanco R, Armona J, *et al.* Giant cell arteritis with an erythrocyte sedimentation rate lower than 50. *Clin Rheumatol* 2000; 19(1): 73–5.

7. Salvarani C, Hunder GG. Giant cell arteritis with low erythrocyte sedimentation rate: frequency of occurence in a population-based study. *Arthritis Rheum* 2001; 45: 140–5.

8. Hunder G, Bloch D, Michel B, *et al.* The American College of Rheumatology 1990 criteria for the classification of giant cell arteritis. *Arthritis Rheum* 1990; 33: 1122–8.

9. Achkar AA, Lie JT, Hunder GG, O'Fallon WM, Gabriel SE. How does previous corticosteroid treatment affect the biopsy findings in giant cell (temporal) arteritis? *Ann Intern Med* 1994; 120(12): 987–92.

10. Narváez J, Bernad B, Roig-Vilaseca D, *et al.* Influence of previous corticosteroid therapy on temporal artery biopsy yield in giant cell arteritis. *Semin Arthritis Rheum* 2007; 37(1): 13–19.

11. Harder N. Temporal arteritis: an approach to suspected vasculitides. *Prim Care* 2010; 37(4): 757–66.

12. Reichman EF, Weber JM. Undiagnosed Takayasu's arteritis mimicking an acute aortic dissection. *J Emerg Med* 2004; 27(2): 139–42.

13. Arend WP, Michel BA, Bloch D, *et al.* The American College of Rheumatology 1990 criteria for the classification of Takayasu arteritis. *Arthritis Rheum* 1990; 33(8): 1129.

14. Kissin EY, Merkel PA. Diagnostic imaging in Takayasu arteritis. *Curr Opin Rheumatol* 2004; 16(1): 31–7.

15. Safi AM, Kwan T, Afflu E, Feit A, Clark LT. Takayasu's arteritis: an unusual manifestation – a case report. *Angiology* 1999; 50: 341–4.

16. Seo P, Stone JH. The antineutrophil cytoplasmic antibody-associated vasculitides. *Am J Med* 2004; 117(1): 39–50.

17. Gromnica-Ihle E, Schössler W. Antiphospholipid syndrome. *Int Arch Allergy Immunol* 2000; 123(1): 67–76.

18. Miyakis S, Lockshin MD, Atsumi T, *et al.* International consensus statement on an update of the classification criteria for definite antiphospholipid syndrome (APS). *J Thromb Haemost* 2006; 4(2): 295–306.

19. Erkan D, Cervera R, Asherson RA. Catastrophic antiphospholipid syndrome: where do we stand? *Arthritis Rheum* 2003; 48(12): 3320–7.

20. Cervera R, Piette JC, Font J, *et al.* Antiphospholipid syndrome: clinical and immunologic manifestations and patterns of disease expression in a cohort of 1,000 patients. *Arthritis Rheum* 2002; 46(4): 1019–27.

21. Chamorro A, Vila N, Saiz A, Alday M, Tolosa E. Early anticoagulation after large cerebral embolic infarction: a safety study. *Neurology* 1995; 45(5): 861–5.

22. Arboix A, Alió J. Cardioembolic stroke: clinical features, specific cardiac disorders and prognosis. *Curr Cardiol Rev* 2010; 6(3): 150–61.

21. Bucciarelli S, Espinosa G, Cervera R, *et al.* European Forum on Antiphospholipid Antibodies. Mortality in the catastrophic antiphospholipid syndrome: causes of death and prognostic factors in a series of 250 patients. *Arthritis Rheum* 2006; 54(8): 2568–76.

22. Rubenstein E, Arkfeld DG, Metyas S, *et al.* Rituximab treatment for resistant antiphospholipid syndrome. *J Rheumatol* 2006; 33(2): 355–7.

23. Keo HH, Umer M, Baumgartner I, Willenberg T, Gretener SB. Long-term clinical outcomes in patients diagnosed with severe digital ischemia. *Swiss Med Wkly* 2011; 141: w13159. DOI: 10.4414/smw.2011.13159.

24. Cassidy JT, Petty RE. *Textbook of Pediatric Rheumatology,* 3rd edition. Philadelphia, PA: WB Saunders Co; 1995.

25. Hummers LK, Wigley FM. Management of Raynaud's phenomenon and digital ischemic lesions in scleroderma. *Rheum Dis Clin North Am* 2003; 29(2): 293–313.

26. Thompson AE, Shea B, Welch V, *et al.* Calcium-channel blockers for Raynaud's phenomenon in systemic sclerosis. *Arthritis Rheum* 2001; 44: 1841–7.

27. Iorio ML, Masden DL, Higgins JP. Botulinum toxin A treatment of Raynaud's phenomenon: a review. *Semin Arthritis Rheum* 2012; 41(4): 599–603.

28. Fregene A, Ditmars D, Siddiqui A. Botulinum toxin type A: a treatment option for digital ischemia in patients with Raynaud's phenomenon. *J Hand Surg Am* 2009; 34(3): 446–52.

29. Neumeister MW, Chambers CB, Herron MS, *et al.* Botox therapy for ischemic digits. *Plast Reconstr Surg* 2009; 124(1): 191–201.

30. Lightfoot RW Jr, Michel BA, Bloch DA *et al.* The American College of Rheumatology 1990 criteria for the classification of polyarteritis nodosa. *Arthritis Rheum* 1990; 33(8): 1088.

31. Schmidt WA. Use of imaging studies in the diagnosis of vasculitis. *Curr Rheumatol Rep* 2004; 6(3): 203.

32. Kalva SP, Somarouthu B, Jaff MR, Wicky S. Segmental arterial mediolysis: clinical and imaging features at presentation and during follow-up. *J Vasc Interv Radiol* 2011; 22(10): 1380–7.

33. Koç Y, Güllü I, Akpek G, *et al.* Vascular involvement in Behçet's disease. *J Rheumatol* 1992; 19(3): 402–10.

34. Calamia KT, Schirmer M, Melikoglu M. Major vessel involvement in Behçet disease. *Curr Opin Rheumatol* 2005; 17(1): 1–8.

35. Yeung RS. Kawasaki disease: update on pathogenesis. *Curr Opin Rheumatol* 2010; 22(5): 551–60.

36. Gomard-Mennesson E, Landron C, Dauphin C, *et al.* Kawasaki disease in adults: report of 10 cases. *Medicine (Baltimore)* 2010; 89(3): 149–58.

37. Ullrich K, Koval R, Koval E, Bapoje S, Hirsh JM. Five consecutive cases of a cutaneous vasculopathy in users of levamisole-adulterated cocaine. *J Clin Rheumatol* 2011; 17(4): 193–6.

Index

343
IV